PSYCHIATRY - THEORY, APPLICATIONS AND TREATMENTS

PERSPECTIVES IN PSYCHIATRY RESEARCH

Psychiatry - Theory, Applications and Treatments

Additional books in this series can be found on Nova's website
under the Series tab.

Additional E-books in this series can be found on Nova's website
under the E-books tab.

PSYCHIATRY - THEORY, APPLICATIONS AND TREATMENTS

PERSPECTIVES IN PSYCHIATRY RESEARCH

NICOLE M. LEVINE
AND
DONNA J. CAMPBELL
EDITORS

Nova Science Publishers, Inc.
New York

For permission to use material from this book please contact us:
Telephone 631-231-7269; Fax 631-231-8175
Web Site: http://www.novapublishers.com

LIBRARY OF CONGRESS CATALOGING-IN-PUBLICATION DATA

Perspectives in psychiatry research / editors, Nicole M. Levine and Donna J. Campbell.
p. ; cm.
"PSYCHIATRY RESEARCH JOURNAL VOLUME 1, ISSUE 1 / 2 "
Includes bibliographical references and index.
ISBN 978-1-61209-236-2 (hardcover)
1. Psychiatry. I. Levine, Nicole M. II. Campbell, Donna J.
[DNLM: 1. Psychiatry. 2. Research. 3. Mental Disorders--psychology. WM 100]
RC454.P433 2011
616.89--DC22

2010048380

Published by Nova Science Publishers, Inc. † New York

CONTENTS

Preface		**vii**
Chapter 1	Lessons Learned After Ten Years of Telepsychiatry Practice *Carlos De las Cuevas*	**1**
Chapter 2	Fear Emotional Expression in Psychopathy and Antisocial Personality Disorder *Laurent Servais, Edith Stillemans, Stephan De Smet, Bruno Piccinin, Pierre Fossion, Jérôme Laville, Pierre Titeca, Jacques Titeca and Elsa Hoffmann*	**15**
Chapter 3	Fear and Anxiety in Psychiatric Disorders, Cognitive-Behavioral Concepts and Treatments *A. Velardi, R. Willis and V. Pomini*	**37**
Chapter 4	On the Possibility of Direct Memory *Stephen E. Robbins*	**77**
Chapter 5	The Montreal Adolescent Depression Development Project (MADDP): School Life and Depression Following High School Transition *Alexandre J.S. Morin, Michel Janosz and Serge Larivée*	**141**
Chapter 6	The Relationship Between Societal Crime and Socio-Economic Status, Income Inequality and Education: A Cross-National Study *Ajit Shah*	**189**
Chapter 7	Development of an Epidemiological Transition Model to Explain Cross-National Variations in Elderly Suicide Rates, Time Trends in Elderly Suicide Rates and Age-Associated Trends in Suicide Rates *Ajit Shah and Ravi Bhat*	**197**
Chapter 8	Psychotropic Analgesic Nitrous Oxide [PAN] for Substance Abuse Withdrawal: Current Status *Mark A Gillman*	**213**
Index		**249**

PREFACE

This book presents and discusses current research in the field of psychiatry. Topics discussed include fear and anxiety in psychiatric disorders; developments in telepsychiatry; emotional expression of psychopathy and antisocial personality disorder and the relationship between societal crime and socio-economic status, income inequality and education.

Chapter 1 - It has long been accepted that improvements in medical care cannot be made merely by adding professionals to healthcare systems but also require restructuring the patterns of healthcare delivery. The incorporation of relevant technological innovations into medical practice is an essential part of this reorganization.

Telepsychiatry is the branch of telemedicine that focuses on mental health applications and can be considered to be the use of electronic communication and information technologies to provide or support clinical psychiatric care at a distance. Videoconferencing, i.e. the real-time transmission of voice, data, and video images between two or more users at some distance from one another, constitutes the principal, although not the only, communication method in telepsychiatry. Other communication modalities include: phone, fax, email, and the Internet.

Chapter 2 - The brain's structure, function and development are the result of the interactions of several factors, including genetic, physiological and experiential variables. At the neurobiological level it has been well demonstrated that the quality of early interaction will determine the structure and wiring of the brain and, therefore, the cerebral functions as well.

As regards the cerebral functions involved in the emotions, the developmental neurosciences have demonstrated the importance of cooperative communication of infant-caregiver attachments for emotional and cognitive development. This gradual emotional and cognitive development is due in no small measure to social interactions in which attachment to the caregivers predominates in the early years of life, subsequently diversifying during infancy and adolescence.

Chapter 3 - Who has never been afraid? No one without a doubt; fear being such an integral part of existence. Fear is essential to the survival of the species because it helps to identify and avoid dangers that can compromise existence. Everyone recognizes the necessity of fear; even if it is an unpleasant experience we prefer avoiding. And when fear no longer has an object, when it is prolonged without any apparent reason and progressively invades an individual's daily life until he can't work, go out or meet other people, it ends up loosing its functional aspect and usefulness: fear then becomes a disease.

Chapter 4 - Is experience stored in the brain? The answer to this question is critical, for it strongly constrains possible theories of the nature and origin of consciousness. If the answer is "yes," conscious experience *must* be generated from stored "elements" within the neural structure. If the answer is "no," Searle's principle of neurobiological sufficiency, as one example, carries no force. On the other hand, a theory of direct perception can be construed to actually require a "no" answer, but then would require a theory of memory not reliant on brain storage. Perception research is reviewed which describes the invariance laws defining the elementary, time-extended, perceived events that must be "stored" and which speaks simultaneously to the nature of the qualia of these events. To support this description of perceived, external events, a model of "direct memory" is described, wherein the brain is viewed as supporting a modulated reconstructive wave passing through a holographic matter-field. The modulation pattern is determined or driven by the invariance laws defining external events. The model is applied to several areas of memory theory in cued-recall, to include verbal paired-associate learning, concreteness and imagery, subject performed tasks and priming. Some implications are reviewed for cognition in general, mental imagery, eye-witness phenomena and the question of whether everything experienced is "stored." The model is predictive and at the very least holds its own relative to current theory without appealing to storage of experience within the brain.

Chapter 5 - The present study was designed to evaluate the relationship between school life and depression development in adolescents. More precisely, this study sought to determine which specific aspects of school life (in-school psychological characteristics, school-related socialization experiences, perceived school environment) could be considered as risk factors for depression development once students' background characteristics are taken into account. The possibility that these relationships could be moderated by gender and by students' previous levels of depression was also evaluated. These exploratory questions were evaluated with data from the transitional component of the Montreal Adolescent Depression Development Project (MADDP), a one-year follow-up study of 1167 seventh grade students having just experienced high school transition. The results clearly suggested that various aspects of students' school life represent significant predictors of depression development, particularly among girls. One of the main conclusions from this study is that school-based prevention programs, would be likely to diminish students' risk of developing depression following high school transition.

Chapter 6 - Low socio-economic status, socio-economic inequality and poor educational attainment may be associated with crime. The main findings were: (i) the percentage of the population victimised by most categories of crimes was significantly correlated with the Education Index (negative), male and female life expectancy (negative), male and female child mortality rates (positive), GDP (negative) and Gini coefficient (positive); and, (ii) the percentage of the population victimised by the crime of assault was not significantly correlated with any of the measured variables. The impact of socio-economic factors, socio-economic inequality and educational attainment on crime may occur through interaction with other factors, mediation of the effects of other factors, or by their effects being mediated by other factors, and requires further study. If a causal link can be substantiated then these associations potentially offer strategies for improvement.

Chapter 7 - There are cross-national variations in elderly suicide rates, trends over time in elderly suicide rates and age-associated trends in suicide rates. A developmental model of epidemiological transition for elderly suicide rates with four sequential stages was formulated: (i) low elderly suicide rate-low socio-economic society; (ii) high elderly suicide rate-low socio-economic society; (iii) high elderly suicide rate-high socio-economic society; and (iv) low elderly suicide rate-high socio-economic society. It is likely that different countries will be at different stages of development within this model. It is envisaged that each country would progress through each of these four developmental stages over time. This model is complimentary to, and does not preclude, other proximal and distil aetiological risk factors for elderly suicides.

Chapter 8 - PAN is high concentrations of oxygen (O_2) plus low concentrations of nitrous oxide (N_2O) individually titrated to an endpoint where the subject is relaxed and at which they are fully conscious and co-operative throughout inhalation of the gases. PAN is not merely administering nitrous oxide/oxygen. It also specifically excludes using nitrous oxide at a fixed preconceived dose. Instead, PAN uses titration to provide the nitrous oxide using the individual clinical response of each patient as the guide to the optimal concentration required. Thus, optimal concentrations of nitrous oxide vary widely from individual to individual. Titrating to the correct endpoint usually requires hands-on training or very careful attention to the instructions given in previous papers or in a textbook dealing with dental conscious sedation with nitrous oxide, because the inhaled concentrations of N_2O required to achieve the correct endpoint varies between 10-70%. Although this technique has been used safely and effectively in South Africa (S.A.) for more than 25 years and in Finland for over a decade, there has been strong published criticisms of the technique, from armchair academic critics in S. A., Finland and Sweden. Despite their widely published opposition on theoretical grounds alone, it took almost 10 years before the Finnish group attempted to replicate the use of PAN for treating alcoholic withdrawal states. However, although they used nitrous oxide, they failed to use the PAN technique correctly. This review will cover the published criticisms and work on PAN for alcohol withdrawal, as well as detailing the latest research supporting its efficacy. Evidence will be presented that the PAN therapy is safe and rapidly effective and can be applied by a trained registered nurse, without direct physician supervision, making PAN an ideal cost-effective method for First and Third World countries, saving unnecessary in-patient admissions. Although more controlled trials using the correct method are needed, evidence will be presented that PAN is an effective treatment of the acute withdrawal state from most substances of abuse including alcohol, opioids, cannabis, cocaine, methaqualone/cannabis combinations, nicotine and polydrug abuse. PAN is recognised by the Health Professions Council of South Africa (official tariff code: 0203/0204) and is therefore accepted by medical insurance organisations in S.A. Because it has been used safely (with no more than trivial adverse effects) and effectively on thousands of outpatients in S.A. and Finland the review will highlight how potentially large cost-savings can be made because many more patients can be treated safely as outpatients than with the currently favoured sedative therapies because the:

1) Patient improves within minutes of administration and is often well enough to have the next meal;
2) Use of addictive sedative medications such as the benzodiazepines (e.g. diazepam) are reduced by 90% plus. This obviates the danger of secondary addiction in this highly susceptible group;
3) Extreme rapidity of recovery enables nurses/physicians to distinguish those patients requiring intensive inpatient therapy from those that do not; since 90%

plus patients respond positively to one administration of the gases, usually on admission;

4) Rapidity of response enables the patient to abandon the sick role speedily (often within an hour of gas treatment) and enter the essential next phase of rehabilitation; usually requiring social, psychological and/or psychiatric therapy;
5) Placebo (oxygen) alone ameliorates withdrawal in approximately 30-50% of patients who require no further pharmacological therapy.

PAN is usually given on one occasion only for inpatients. Depending on the drug of abuse, out-patients may require more than one application of the gases, but usually no more than 2 applications during the first week of withdrawal. PAN has been used successfully on more than 50,000 patients in South Africa, Finland and the USA. The rationale for using PAN, as a gaseous partial opioid agonist will be discussed. The review concludes by placing the PAN method in the wider perspective of substance withdrawal states and craving, dealing with its current status and ending with an appeal for more studies to be done on this promising therapy.

Versions of these chapters were also published in *Psychiatry Research Journal*, Volume 1, Numbers 1-3, edited by Frank Columbus, published by Nova Science Publishers, Inc. They were submitted for appropriate modifications in an effort to encourage wider dissemination of research.

In: Perspectives in Psychiatry Research
Editors: Nicole M. Levine and Donna J. Campbell
ISBN: 978-1-61209-236-2

Chapter 1

LESSONS LEARNED AFTER TEN YEARS OF TELEPSYCHIATRY PRACTICE

Carlos De las Cuevas
Department of Psychiatry, University of La Laguna
Telepsychiatry Service
Canary Islands Health Service
Canary Islands, Spain

As Arthur Schopenhauer said (1788-1860) "There are three steps in the revelation of any truth: first, it is ridiculed; in the second, resisted; in the third, it is considered self-evident"

It has long been accepted that improvements in medical care cannot be made merely by adding professionals to healthcare systems but also require restructuring the patterns of healthcare delivery [Garfield, 1970; Code, 1970; Perednia and Allen, 1995; Robb, 1997]. The incorporation of relevant technological innovations into medical practice is an essential part of this reorganization.

Telepsychiatry is the branch of telemedicine that focuses on mental health applications and can be considered to be the use of electronic communication and information technologies to provide or support clinical psychiatric care at a distance [APA, 1998]. Videoconferencing, i.e. the real-time transmission of voice, data, and video images between two or more users at some distance from one another, constitutes the principal, although not the only, communication method in telepsychiatry. Other communication modalities include: phone, fax, email, and the Internet.

Psychiatry appears to be an ideal specialty for the application of telemedicine (i.e. telepsychiatry) for several reasons: most diagnostic and treatment information is garnered through audiovisual communication; there is typically little need for laboratory tests for diagnosis or consultation; and there is a desperate need to extend mental health services to underserved populations in rural and inner-city areas. It is well known that telemedicine applications are of greater relevance in those locations in which the distance, the territorial fragmentation or the shortage of the population limit the availability to health care resources; making difficult the patients' accessibility to general health services and more specifically to the specialized ones [Pedersen and Hartviksen, 1994]. All these conditioners take place in the

Canary Islands. The Canary Islands are an archipelago of the Kingdom of Spain, 1100 km from the mainland, consisting of seven islands of volcanic origin in the Atlantic Ocean. They are located off the north-western coast of Africa (Morocco and the Western Sahara) (see figure 1). They form an autonomous region of Spain with full responsibility for health care. The archipelago has about 2 million inhabitants, 85% of them living on the main islands of Tenerife and Gran Canaria and the remaining 15% of citizens distributed in the other five islands. "El Hierro" (270 km^2; 10700 inhabitants) and "La Gomera" (370 km^2; 21000 inhabitants) are the smaller and less populated islands. Although communications have improved in the last few years, it is still sometimes difficult to travel to "El Hierro" and "La Gomera" islands. There are two daily flights connecting "El Hierro" and "La Gomera" with the main islands. By sea, some express ferries operate several times every day.

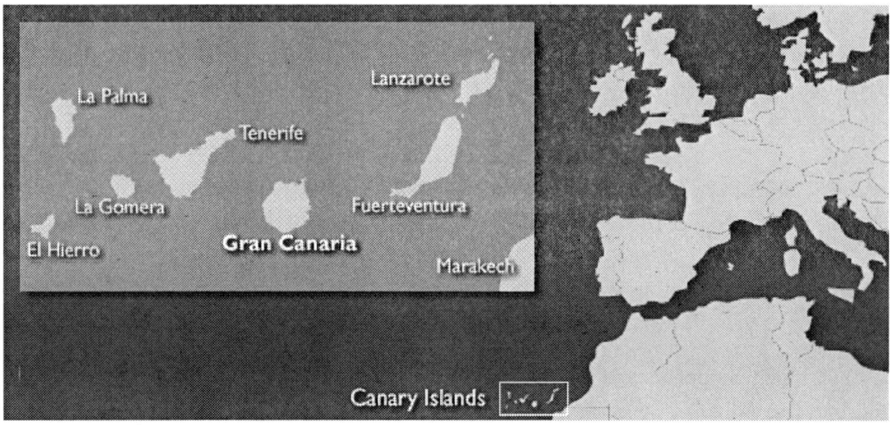

Figure 1. Location of the Canary Islands.

The Canary Islands Health Service developed in 1997 a telepsychiatry program to complement the mental health-care of the citizens living on "El Hierro" and "La Gomera" islands. The main goals were to improve access to specialized health care, reduce costs by reducing the necessity of displacements between islands, reduce isolation and improve the quality of care. Until telepsychiatry became available, the mental health problems of people living on "El Hierro" and "La Gomera" were all dealt with by a community psychiatrist who visits the islands every week. Because of the shortage of medical staff, psychiatric emergencies on the islands were difficult to manage and sometimes necessitated immediate transfer of the patient to Tenerife for assessment by a mental health professional.

Telepsychiatry program was developed as new services in "El Hierro" and "La Gomera" following the success of two six-month pilot projects and the requirements of modern Canary Islands Health Service providing alternatives for care of patients. The telepsychiatry service provides psychiatric consultations to individuals after referral from a general practitioner. A patient living in "El Hierro" or "La Gomera" island with a mental health problem can choose between joining the waiting list to see the visiting psychiatrist or being included in the telepsychiatry program.

The model of service delivery of our telepsychiatry service is based on outpatient therapy; the psychiatrist assesses a patient over videoconferencing and gives guidance to the local health care professionals with regard to the diagnosis and appropriate management of the patient. The consultant psychiatrist is involved in the ongoing direct delivery of patient care. A variety of local supports, eg health care professionals or ancillary staff may be required to assist with managing the equipment, debriefing after a session or, if necessary, to coordinate the transferring to a possible admission for specialist inpatient assessment and treatment. It is the responsibility of the consultant psychiatrist to ensure that such arrangements are made and are adequately documented and followed. We also use videoconferencing for educational support in mental health (via traditional didactic lectures, case discussions or individual supervision) of healthcare professionals, mainly general practitioners. We consider that although telepsychiatry through videoconference can provide an effective means of communication for clinical purposes, it will never be as good as, or preferable to, the clinician being present with the patient. Telepsychiatry should not be advocated as a means of replacing visiting specialists.

We have no particular clinical limitations of our telepsychiatry service. We consider telepsychiatry through videoconference appropriate for the assessment of every patient willing and able to sit in front of a camera and communicate. It is thus more a behavioral and attitudinal consideration, rather than a diagnostic one, when considering the suitability of a clinical situation for telepsychiatry.

After two telepsychiatry pilot projects and eight years of telepsychiatry as a routine service, that involved 256 patients, 1220 teleconsultations and more than 1250 hours of clinical practice, we have learnt some lessons that could be useful for future telepsychiatric developments. While the technology on which telepsychiatry is founded itself is subject to very rapid development, the professional, organizational and institutional terrain on which this technology is set in play is much less amenable to change. So, while the anticipated benefits of telemedicine systems have inspired much trial and demonstration work, there remain very few ‘real’ telepsychiatry services working like ours for more than ten years. According to our experience, we have no doubts about that telepsychiatry is an adequate vehicle for mental health-care that increases access to care and user satisfaction constituting an effective means of delivering mental health services to psychiatric outpatients living in remote areas with limited resources with a clinical efficacy indistinguishable of the corresponding one to face-to-face psychiatric treatment. In the next paragraphs we present the results about acceptability, satisfaction and clinical efficacy of the Canary Islands Telepsychiatry Service along the last decade. The significant technical and interpersonal barriers that discouraged the use of this service delivery method by some psychiatrists working for the Canary Islands Health Service are also described. The extent to which telepsychiatry threatened deeply embedded professional constructs about the nature and practice of therapeutic relationships is analyzed.

The Experience of “El Hierro” Island

The Telepsychiatry Service of the Canary Islands Health Service at “El Hierro” island has been running for one year and its closure was a matter of dying for success. Along the first and unique year of functioning, eighty per cent of the patients to whom telepsychiatry was offered accepted it. During 2001, a total of 40 patients had 40 initial and 126 follow-up teleconsultations. According to the results of a questionnaire survey made [De las Cuevas et al., 2003], patients’ acceptance of and satisfaction with the technology were very high. In their first teleconsultation, about a third of them said that they experienced some initial inconvenience, but this disappeared after a few minutes. Ninety per cent of the patients considered that they received the follow-up care they required and all of those who accepted a teleconsultation indicated that they would use telepsychiatry again in preference to waiting or travelling to see a psychiatrist. The psychiatric consultant agreed that telepsychiatry was an acceptable way of delivering psychiatric consultations and that he could obtain the same information by videoconference as in a traditional consultation. The six referring general practitioners also expressed their satisfaction with the service, although a third of them commented that face-to-face consultations were preferable.

Despite those favorable initial results, after a week's rest at Christmastime 2001, the consultant psychiatrist responsible of telepsychiatry service received a telephone call from the health manager of "El Hierro" island in which he congratulated and appreciated his service delivery and was informed that the telepsychiatry program was considered finished. When requesting an explanation of this decision of no continue with this initiative, the responsible of island' health services commented that the success of the telepsychiatry mean a threat of his claim of having a psychiatrist who continuously lived and worked on the island.

According to the planning criteria of the Canary Islands Health Service at that time (1 psychiatrist for 40,000 inhabitants in consultation in the community) and taking into account the resident population at the island (7.000 inhabitants), "El Hierro" island must have only one day each week consultation.

The patients attended by the telepsychiatry service protested to their health authorities for suspending the service activity but they were convinced by them that in the near future the situation will improve and that it was worth waiting. And so it was, after three years of waiting, which were attended only by the traveling psychiatrist once a week, "El Hierro" island got a psychiatrist who currently resides in the island, passes consultation Monday through Friday, and is on duty every day of the year. This professional must personally seek a replacement for his work every time he wants to leave the island (holidays, attendance at meetings or conferences, etc.)

The Experience of "La Gomera" Island

As a consequence of the results obtained in the first year of introduction of the telepsychiatry service in "El Hierro" island, the Canary Islands Health Authorities decided to expand this healthcare activity to "La Gomera" island. At the same time, and probably as a result of the publications about telepsychiatry activity carried out at "El Hierro" [De las Cuevas et al. 2003; De las Cuevas2005a, 2005b], the Canary Islands Health Service was invited to participate in the project ISLANDS.

ISLANDS (*Integrated System for Long distance psychiatric Assistance and Non-conventional Distributed health Services*) was an European co-funded research project of the thematic area "Quality of Life and Management of Living Resources" (QLRT-2001-01637) belonging to the "Fifth Framework Programme for Research, Technological Development and Demonstration Generic RTD Activities" of the European Union. The overall aim of the project was to develop services to provide modular, non-conventional, remote psychiatric and psychotherapeutic assistance for remote areas. By these means quality of life of the users, quality of mental health care and the economic strength of the region should improve and overweight the costs of implementation and service support. The project pretended to reduce inequalities in mental health services and status among European regions.

The ISLANDS Consortium consisted of 11 companies and organizations with complementary expertise in the areas of information technologies (Fundación Vodafone, ICCS, Maguire and Associates, Interaxon, and Thruth SA) and mental health (Coat Basel and University Hospital Fort de France), as well as medical experts (Canary Islands Health Service) and academic research institutions (Charles University of Prague, University of Innsbruck, University of Athens and Universidad Politécnica de Madrid). They represent 7 European countries (Spain, Greece, Switzerland, Austria, Czech Republic, France and Ireland).

The Canary Islands Health Service was the partner responsible of verification pilots workpackage. In order to validate the reliability, user-friendliness and usefulness of ISLANDS tools in a number of case studies, three different Pilots were realised, in three different European sites (Andros island in Greece; "La Gomera" island in Spain; the overseas departments of Martinique and French Guyana in France), to guarantee the validity and transferability of ISLANDS services across different care systems, cultures and external environments.

As a general overview, the evaluation results of the research project were considered as very positive and encouraging for the sustainability of the tools that were developed under ISLANDS project. What is really true is that as a result of investment in infrastructure carried out in the research project it was possible to consolidate a new telepsychiatry service for "La Gomera" island.

A patient living in La Gomera Island with a mental health problem can choose between seeing the visiting psychiatrist, who travels every Monday from Tenerife Island, or being included in the telepsychiatry program. Telepsychiatry sessions take place every Thursday from 9:00 to 15:00. Emergency access is available from Monday to Friday (8:00 to 15:00). Telepsychiatry service provides psychiatric consultations to individuals after referral from a general practitioner. After the teleconsultation, recommendations are provided directly to the patient's general practitioner via e-mail. Telepsychiatry consultations use commercial videoconferencing equipment (Viewstation 512, Polycom) connected via ISDN lines at up to 512 kbit/s.

The telepsychiatry treatment is conducted by videoconference between the University Hospital de la Candelaria in Santa Cruz de Tenerife (psychiatrist's location) and the Mental Healthcare Centre of San Sebastian de la Gomera (patient's location).

The Community Mental Health Centre team at La Gomera Island consists of one consultant psychiatrist (working on face-to-face modality on Mondays, through videoconference on Thursdays, and available at call during the rest of the week), two clinical psychologists (one full-time and the other part-time), one nurse, two nursing assistants, and one part-time social worker.

The Canary Islands Health Service Telepsychiatry experience at "La Gomera" island was also assessed in terms of user acceptance and satisfaction with very good results [De las Cuevas, 2005a; De las Cuevas, 2005b]. We also evaluated the efficacy of telepsychiatry through videoconference in the treatment of mental disorders by comparing to face-to-face conventional treatment [De las Cuevas et al., 2006]. We carried out a randomized clinical trial where 140 psychiatric outpatients were randomized to either face-to-face treatment or videoconference telepsychiatry treatment. Patients were diagnosed according to International

Classification of Diseases, 10th edition (*ICD-10*) [WHO, 1992] criteria using the Composite International Diagnostic Interview [WHO, 1990]. Treatment involves eight consultations lasting 30 minutes over the 24-week study period. Patients received pertinent psychotropic medication plus cognitive–behavioral therapy during sessions. The same psychiatrist diagnosed and treated all the patients. Change in psychiatric test scores served as the primary efficacy criterion. Efficacy was determined by comparing baseline (visit 1) Clinical Global Impressions-Severity of Illness (CGI-S) and -Improvement (CGI-I) scales [NIMH, 1970] as well as Global Indexes (GSI, PSDI, and PST) from SCL-90R [Derogatis, 1992] with scores obtained at the end of the study period (week 24). Response was defined as a CGI-I score of 1 or 2. Reliable Change Indexes were computed in SCL-90R Global Indexes scores. Of 140 patients randomized, 130 completed 24 weeks of treatment. Only 4 patients dropped out prematurely from the study in videoconference treatment and 6 in face-to-face. The study involves 534 teleconsultations, 522 face-to-face consultations, and more than 500 hours of clinical practice. Significant improvements were found on the CGI and SCL-90-R Global Indexes scores of both treatment groups, showing clear clinical state improvement. No statistically significant differences were observed when the efficacy of videoconference telepsychiatry treatment was compared to face-to-face psychiatric treatment efficacy. This study demonstrated that telepsychiatry treatment through videoconference has equivalent efficacy to face-to-face psychiatric treatment. Telepsychiatry showed to be an effective means of delivering mental health services to psychiatric outpatients living in remote areas with limited resources.

In order to disseminate our experience in the field of telepsychiatry, our research group has participated in several national and international conferences. We made the proposal of three symposia about telepsychiatry to three consecutive Spanish National Congresses of Psychiatry (years 2005, 2006 and 2007, with the attendance of more than 2,000 psychiatrists in each of them) that were warmly welcomed by the scientific and organizer committees of the corresponding congresses and included in the official programs. However, attendance at the organized symposia was absolutely regrettable (never more than five people) implying the low interest aroused by this topic in the Spanish psychiatrists. In the other hand, we also organized two symposia in international meetings including the World Congress of Psychiatry in Cairo (year 2005) that registered a better attendance.

Ten years' experience with the Canary Islands Health Service Telepsychiatry Clinic confirms that telepsychiatry treatment through videoconference has equivalent efficacy to face-to-face psychiatric treatment and that patients and relatives quickly adjust to the new technology and become relaxed and comfortable with this method of providing service. Other lessons from experience with the telepsychiatry program are discussed below.

Lessons Learned

Telepsychiatry Room

We integrated the telepsychiatry videoconference in the same consultation office for face-to-face encounters. In this way we tried that patients who came to face-to-face traditional consultations were familiar with the videoconferencing equipment and get used to its presence once they explained their usefulness and availability for future use, if they wished or needed.

The telepsychiatry room was outfitted in order to obtain the best lighting and acoustic conditions, establishing a relaxed environment. We have designed our Telepsychiatry rooms as one-half of a pair, being each room an extension of the other. This idea was promoted using an interior design that was consistent among telepsychiatry rooms. Telepsychiatry rooms that share the same interior design help all participants feel that they are in the same room. This removes the natural sense of distance and promotes a sense of closeness and privacy, two important factors if the room is to be considered a viable alternative to in-person consultations. This was achieved in our case by placing the same type of chairs at both ends, a curtain of the same color and the color of paint on the wall (see figure 2). The camera should be placed at eye level so that the patient does not have to look up and psychiatrist is not looking down on the patient's head.

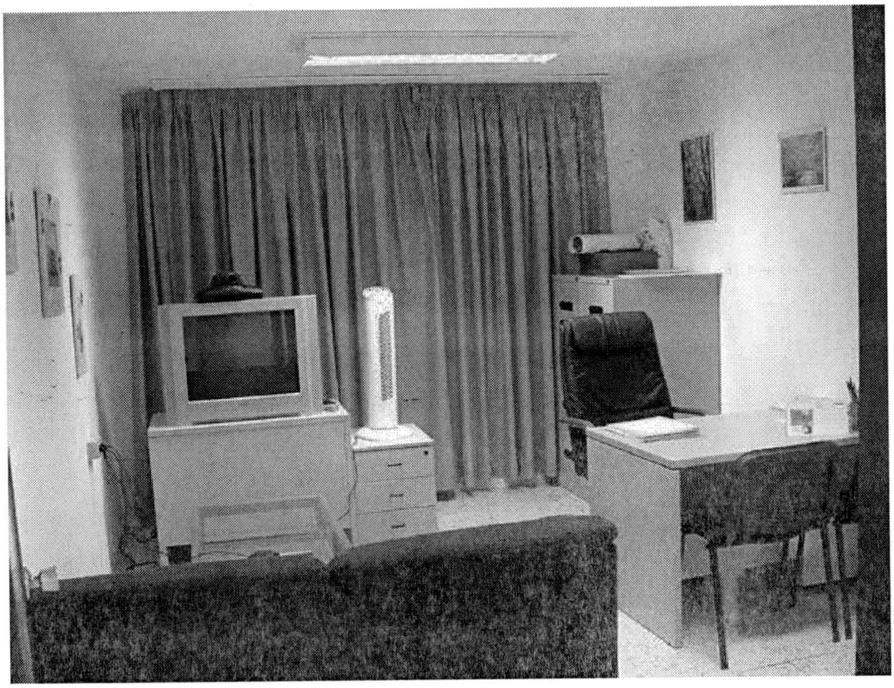

Figure 2. Telepsychiatry room at San Sebastián de La Gomera.

The lighting needs of the telepsychiatry room need to be bright enough and consistent since the psychiatrist needs a clear view of all participants in the room. With our telepsychiatry practice we learnt that the best lighting for telepsychiatry videoconferencing is diffuse fluorescent. It is important to minimize shadows and to create an evenly lit environment. Ideally, the room should not have any exterior windows. If it does, they need to be covered with room darkening drapery/blinds. The best wall color is a neutral non-white color, such as light grey, light blue, or beige.

We consider that audio quality, is one of the most important contributing factors to a favorable telepsychiatry experience, therefore good acoustics are paramount. One item of particular concern is reverberation - the effect of sound reflecting off of hard surfaces. One of the best way to minimize the deleterious effects of reverberation is to coat floors, ceilings, and walls with sound absorbing material. In addition to minimizing reverberation it is also important to isolate the room from external noise sources such as fans and duct work from heating and cooling systems, water pipes, office machines, telephones, and street noise. Microphone placement is also an important factor influencing audio quality. The microphone needs to be placed correctly so that it is at least six feet from the system speakers. The microphone cannot be farther than five feet from the patient to ensure maximum audio quality.

Videoconference System

Our telepsychiatry consultations use commercial videoconferencing equipment (Viewstation 512, Polycom®; Slough, Berks, United Kingdom) providing high-quality enhanced video at 30 frames per second (fps) at 384 to 768 kilobits per second (Kbps) and full-duplex digital audio with noise suppression and echo cancellation. The Polycom Viewstation 512 also has a voice tracking camera and track-to-preset function which automatically focuses on the current speaker.

The equipment and ISDN lines used to transmit the information need to be reliable. We had to change the supplier of ISDN lines. Proper maintenance and immediate attention of any technical difficulty that arises is really important. In the initial pilot projects we had to suspend some consultations as consequence of technical problems. It is really exasperating that a consultation is abruptly interrupted, or where there is no sound or image suddenly. We have no suspension of any consultation by technical difficulties in the past three years.

Working with the Equipment

A critical factor of a telepsychiatry service is the provision of adequate support for the daily operational requirements. The integrity of the telepsychiatry service depends on reliable accessibility of service that ensures continuity of care. This in turn is dependent on the maintenance of high standards of infrastructure support.

The scheduling of telepsychiatry appointments is also an essential part of telepsychiatry service routine: making arrangements for the time and room have to be easy with minimal amount of coordination time; psychiatrists using telepsychiatry need to stay within their appointment times so that other psychiatrists and patients are not delayed; flexibility needs to be built into accommodate patients needs. Scheduling works the best if done in the clinic where the patient is seen.

In our experience, consultations of 30 minutes are enough to work properly, since the same amount of clinically relevant information is usually discussed in a shorter period of time in the telepsychiatry consultations. Another difference—and a possible explanation for the seemingly increased efficiency—is that both the patient and the psychiatrist appear to focus more on the interview during the telepsychiatry clinic.

Activating the telepsychiatry videoconference is almost as easy as making a phone call. For clinicians, only a basic knowledge of common computer software is needed to begin planning the system. Knowledgeable technical assistance is needed in setting up the system and during the early stages of operation. After the telepsychiatry clinic is set up, it can be used by almost anyone. All staff involved, including the remote psychiatrist, should become familiar with the videoconference technology so that care is uninterrupted by alarming situations caused by lack of knowledge of the equipment. New staff must be trained to use the videoconferencing equipment prior to sessions.

New patients and relatives should receive an orientation on what to expect during a telepsychiatry consultation. They should be told how the videoconference operates, what kind of image they can view and what the remote provider will see. Ideally, the patient and provider rooms should be scanned and introductions made to all present.

The camera must be set up so that the consultant clinician can initially view everyone in the room. Before beginning, the consultant should ensure his image is large enough so that his face can be seen clearly. He should sit a few feet away from the camera and zoom in on himself to determine if the size of his image is adequate. It is easier to engage with others when subtleties of facial expression can be seen. It is very useful to memorize, previously to the teleconsultations, the positions in which the patient and relatives may be located. Later, the consultant can easily focus on participants.

It is preferable that the consultant be seated at some distance away from the equipment in order to can look directly at the image on the screen. If the psychiatrist is seated close to the videoconferencing equipment, he should look into the camera. Although it is natural to look at the image on the video screen, the consultant will appear to the other person/people as if staring at their feet. This is because the camera is usually located on top of the video monitor. Eye contact in many cultures is important to establishing rapport so eyes should be kept on the camera rather than on the video screen.

Legal and Ethical Issues

Just as in face-to-face clinical interactions, confidentiality in the context of telepsychiatry needs to be respected and balanced against beneficence and duty of care. It is imperative to ensure the privacy, security and confidentiality of the procedure and to convince patients and relatives of the importance that the providers give to these subjects. The practice of telepsychiatry implies ensuring maximum security of the technical transmission. We considered also important, that the equipment at each connecting site should be located in an area that is suitably soundproof. There should be no audiovisual or audio recording of a telepsychiatry session without written, informed consent from the patient. In our telepsychiatry service the presence of outsiders or non-clinical persons, such as nonclinical technicians, camera operators, and schedulers is in no way allowed. The patient is all the time aware of the persons involved in the telepsychiatry session, and is the responsible for authorizing the presence of another person.

Patient information gathered is routinely stored electronically and physically at each site and is protected as effectively as information used face-to-face encounters. A notation is made in the medical record that indicates that the service was provided via telepsychiatry.

It is important to have a preliminary discussion with the patients regarding expectations concerning the treatment in order to ensure that the consenting process is properly documented. Our telepsychiatry service requires the patient give written consent as a part of standard process.

It is necessary to have emergency procedures in place that allow the psychiatrist could resolve the problems that could arise during teleconsultations. In our telepsychiatry service a telephone line is always available and a nurse and a nursing assistant are ready to intervene at any time. With this design, we consider that patients in crisis can be safely assessed and treated. This meant that if the patient had a crisis, or anxiety or panic attack or much more seriously, threatened self-harm the clinician could intervene, trough his personnel, in a way that secured the patient's safety or that made the 'attack' manageable in some other way.

Lessons Learned Specific to the Psychiatrist's Role

The establishment of this type of healthcare devices is complicated but doable. What it is really hard is to give continuity to these initiatives. The recruitment of staff, especially psychiatrists, is a crucial factor in the success of such services. Applicants should be acquainted with telepsychiatry practice. Many psychiatrists are trained in the more traditional practice or have developed the traditional caseload practice over time. We tried to recruit locally but found any psychiatrist in the area wasn't interested in include telepsychiatry in his/her clinical practice. Although telepsychiatry is actually an aged practice, many psychiatrists are unfamiliar with this communication technology and can be resistant to change. This is true not only of psychiatrists but physicians and other health related professionals as well.

In our experience, the practice telepsychiatry is no different from the traditional face-to-face alternative, only requires certain adjustments to professional communicative behavior and is analogous to the kinds of 'rationalizing' changes to work practices derived from the introduction of clinical protocols [Berg, 1997]. In the same way, videoconferencing requires that the user learn a set of basic rules and etiquette to maximize the equipment's capabilities. However, regardless of telemedicine efficacy, availability and patients desires, if psychiatrists are dissatisfied with telepsychiatry or do not believe in it, they will probably not offer it to their patients [Wagnild et al., 2006].

Many psychiatrists working for the Canary Islands Health Service considered that using telepsychiatry systems placed significant restraints on their capacity to act in what they considered to be the therapeutic interests of patients. They gave priority to accounts of this even when they were the beneficiaries of speedier access to a psychiatric assessment for their patients. They think the telepsychiatry increasingly problematic because it was difficult to 'shoe-horn' their own model of practice into it. Finally, they rejected the system and the continuity of this mental healthcare modality is at the present time threatened by the absence of specialists who believe in this alternative of care and are willing to continue with it.

At the present time we miss the support of the administrators and those responsible of mental health care, which surprisingly on this occasion express an excessive understanding of psychiatrists' worries. Projects that for a previous management team meant a real technological breakthrough that would improve the quality of care for psychiatric patients and to give continuity to their mental health care facilitating accessibility, are questioned by a later management team probably to avoid having to recognize achievements of a predecessor team.

CONCLUSION

New telecommunications technologies promise to profoundly change the spatial and temporal relationship between health professional and patient [May et al, 2001]. Clinical practice in the twentieth century has been characterized by tremendous shifts towards the development of new technologies and treatment modalities. But rapid bioscientific and technological 'advances' in the field of biomedicine seem to be consistently met with contradictory impulses. On one hand, there are demands and expectations for ever more effective medical treatments and interventions; while on the other, there is growing mistrust of the complex of professional and commercial interests that underpins it, and of the potentially iatrogenic form that clinical practices might take [Lupton, 1994, 1997].

Telepsychiatry through videoconference has shown to be, in the Canary Islands, an effective means of delivering mental health services to psychiatric outpatients living in remote areas with limited resources. It has been well received in terms of increasing access to care and user satisfaction and its clinical efficacy was indistinguishable of the corresponding one to face-to-face psychiatric treatment. After telepsychiatry introduction, reductions in unnecessary transferring of patients to the main island, in unnecessary hospitalizations, and in in-patient length of care/stay have been achieved.

Nevertheless, the human factor again is crucial to success. At the present time our main challenge is to change the attitudes of the psychiatrists who consider that their clinical practice could be limited, rather than liberated, by this mental health care technology. Training is important as it pertains to system education and preparation for telepsychiatry care. Interactional problems could perhaps be resolved by more closely attending to communications skills.

It is important that administrators and support staff are reminded of the importance of their in-kind contributions to the program and the value of those contributions to the overall success of the program. We must acknowledge and credit the amount of in-kind contributions from the workers involved in the telepsychiatry program. The time, energy and resources contributed by each of the partners for scheduling, facilities, etc. are absolutely essential to make the program work.

After all these exciting years of telepsychiatry practice we still believe that in the next future telepsychiatry will be considered self-evident. We are confident that promptly the psychiatrists that expressed reluctance toward the use of telepsychiatry change their attitudes and their 'resistance', often rooted in the notion that it would be the videoconference, not the clinician, became the central focus of the consultation, and will adopt telepsychiatry as an effective way to benefit their patients. At the moment some regrettable attitudes have to be overcome for successful implementation of telepsychiatry and it is vital to pay strong heed to issues around change management and the barriers to technology adoption.

REFERENCES

American Psychiatric Association. Telepsychiatry Via Videoconferencing. APA Document Reference No. 980021. Washington, 1998.

Berg, M. (1997). Rationalizing medical work: Decision-support techniques and medical practice. Cambridge, MA: MIT Press.

Code CF. Determinants of medical care: a plan for the future. New England *Journal of Medicine* 1970; 283:679–85.

De las Cuevas C, Artiles J, De la Fuente J, Serrano P: Telepsiquiatría: Utopía o Realidad Asistencial. *Med. Clin.* (Barc) 2003, 121 (4): 149-52.

De las Cuevas C, Arredondo MT, Cabrera MF, Sulzenbacher H, Meise U. Randomized Clinical Trial of Telepsychiatry through Videoconference versus Face-to-Face Conventional Psychiatric Treatment. *Telemedicine Journal and e-Health* 2006, 12(3): 341-350.

De las Cuevas C, Artiles J, De la Fuente J, Serrano P: Telepsychiatry in the Canary Islands: user acceptance and satisfaction. *J. Telemed. Telecare* 2003, 9 (4): 221-224.

De las Cuevas C, Artiles J: Process Quality Analysis of Telepsychiatry. Contributions of Statistical Control Process and Critical Pathway Analysis. *Neuropsychiatrie* 2004, 18 S2: 100-105.

De las Cuevas C, González de Rivera JL: Some considerations about the concept of presence in telepsychiatry. *Neuropsychiatrie* 2004, 18 S2: 112-115.

De las Cuevas C. Telepsychiatry: Psychiatric consultation through videoconference patients' perception and satisfaction . *Cyberpsychology and Behavior* 2005, 8 (4): 313-315.

De las Cuevas C. Clinical Outcomes in Telepsychiatry. World Psychiatric Association Thematic Conference "*Quality and Outcomes Research in Psychiatry*". Valencia, 17-20 de Junio de 2005.

De las Cuevas C. Efficacy of Telepsychiatry. Our experience based on Verification Pilots. *XIIIth WPA World Congress of Psychiatry*, El Cairo, Egypt, September 10-15, 2005.

De las Cuevas C. A review of the first five years of the Canary Islands Health Service Telepsychiatry Programme. *World Psychiatric Association International Congress*, Istanbul, Turquía, July 12-16, 2006.

De las Cuevas C. Is Telepsychiatry a Threat, Challenge or Reality in Mental Health Care? IT and Communications. *Hospital Healthcare Europe 2007/2008, IT27-IT28.* London, Campden Publishing, 2007.

De las Cuevas C. Telepsychiatry: Psychiatric Consultation through Videoconference Clinical Results. *Annual Review of Cybertherapy and Telemedicine* 2005, 3: 159-164.

De las Cuevas C. Telepsychiatry: Psychiatric Consultation through Videoconference Clinical Results. *10th Annual Cybertherapy 2005 Conference. A Decade of Virtual Reality*. Basel, Switzerland, 6-10 de Junio de 2005.

Derogatis LR. SCL-90-R: Administration, scoring and procedures manual—II. Baltimore: *Clinical Psychometric Research*, 1992.

Garfield SR. Delivery of medical care. *Scientific American* 1970; 222:15–23.

National Institute of Mental Health. CGI: Clinical Global Impressions. In: *Guy W, Bonato RR, eds. Manual for the ECDEU Assessment Battery.2*. Rev ed. Chevy Chase, Md: National Institute of Mental Health; 1970:12-1-12-6.

Pedersen S, Hartviksen G. *Telemedicine a review*. Tid SSKr Nor Laegeforen 1994, 114 (10): 1212-4.

Perednia DA, Allen A. Telemedicine technology and clinical applications. *Journal of the American Medical Association* 1995; 273: 483–7.

Robb N. Telemedicine can help change the face of medical care in eastern Canada. *Canadian Medical Association Journal* 1997; 156: 1009–11.

Serrano P, Artiles J, Martínez F, De las Cuevas C, Antolín J, Vázquez C, Suárez J: Telemedicina 2000. Un Proyecto que aproxima los principios de Equidad y Eficiencia en la provisión de Atención Sanitaria en las Islas Canarias. *International Telemedicine* 1999, 12: 12-22.

Sulzenbacher H, Bullinger AH, De las Cuevas C, Meise U. Die Psychiatrie im Internet und das Internet in der Psychiatrie – ein neues Médium und seine Auswirkungen. *Neuropsychiatrie*, 2006 20 (4): 273-278.

World Health Organization. *CIDI core: Composite international diagnostic interview core version 1.0, researchers Copy*. Geneva; WHO, 1990.

World Health Organization: The ICD-10 Classification of Mental and Behavioural Disorders. *Clinical Descriptions and Diagnostic Guidelines* World Health Organization, Geneva; 1992.

In: Perspectives in Psychiatry Research
Editors: Nicole M. Levine and Donna J. Campbell
ISBN: 978-1-61209-236-2

Chapter 2

FEAR EMOTIONAL EXPRESSION IN PSYCHOPATHY AND ANTISOCIAL PERSONALITY DISORDER

Laurent Servais[1], Edith Stillemans[1], Stephan De Smet[2], Bruno Piccinin[3], Pierre Fossion[4], Jérôme Laville[5], Pierre Titeca[1], Jacques Titeca[1] and Elsa Hoffmann[1]

[1]Centre Hospitalier Jean Titeca, Rue de la Luzerne,
11–1030 Bruxelles, Belgique.
[2]Hôpital Militaire Reine Astrid, Service de Psychiatrie, Bruxelles, Belgique
[3]Institution Publique de Protection de la Jeunesse de Fraipont
Liège, Belgique
[4]Centre Hospitalier Universitaire Brugmann,
Place Van Gehuchten, 4–1020 Bruxelles, Belgique
[5]Centre Hospitalier Psychiatrique de Bordeaux, France

INTRODUCTION: PSYCHOPATHY AND THE EMOTIONS

The brain's structure, function and development are the result of the interactions of several factors, including genetic, physiological and experiential variables. At the neurobiological level it has been well demonstrated that the quality of early interaction will determine the structure and wiring of the brain and, therefore, the cerebral functions as well.

As regards the cerebral functions involved in the emotions, the developmental neurosciences have demonstrated the importance of cooperative communication of infant-caregiver attachments for emotional and cognitive development. This gradual emotional and cognitive development is due in no small measure to social interactions in which attachment to the caregivers predominates in the early years of life, subsequently diversifying during infancy and adolescence.

Three stages in the development of the emotional functions can be distinguished. The acquisition of basic emotions (i.e. as inferred from the facial expressions) is the first stage of emotional development, and begins in the first year of life through the infant's early interactions with the mother figure, especially the infant's recognition of the facial expressions of the people in his surroundings in response to certain stimuli as well as the gestures of imitation (Bowlby, 1969).

Subsequently, at the end of the second year, more complex emotions such as shame, envy, guilt and embarrassment emerge (Gordon; in Kaplan and Sadock, 2000).

Finally, empathy – defined as the ability to perceive and, to a certain extent, to experience the emotional responses of others – appears soon afterwards and continues to develop throughout infancy. However, certain less structured and more rudimentary forms of empathy are also found from the age of one year (Gordon; in Kaplan and Sadock, 2000).

To sum up, emotional and cognitive development are inextricably linked. In particular, normal social functioning can only be established via social interactions of high quality in which the emotions act as the basic signals of social regulation. This means that the processing of emotional expressions is fundamental for normal socialisation and interaction.

These findings are of especial interest in the study of what one might call 'the psychopathic disorder', which can be conceptualised as a disability that disrupts the socialisation process. As regards the emotional functions of psychopathic subjects, there is growing agreement that the psychopathic disorder reflects a dysfunction in the systems that process socialisation due to fear conditioning. In other words: in psychopathic individuals, systems that mediate fear (and probably other emotions) are considered to be dysfunctional. From this point of view, psychopathic individuals form an interesting group in which to study the brain structures involved in moral and social reasoning and the emotional process.

This chapter is divided into two parts. First, the nosographical work that seeks to acquire a clearer view of the concept of psychopathy will be discussed both in the adult and in the infant and adolescent. Second, research into the neurophysiological, neurocognitive and neuroanatomical bases of psychopathy will be presented.

PART I: NOSOLOGY AND PSYCHOPATHIC DISORDERS

In this section, the taxonomic work that seeks to better delineate the psychopathological profiles associated with antisocial or asocial behaviour will be discussed, with an emphasis on the profiles' relationship to emotional disturbances. From a developmental perspective, the early manifestations of the psychopathic disorder in infancy and adolescence will also be dealt with.

A precise knowledge of the nosographical categories formulated to acquire a clearer picture of antisocial behaviour, such as the concept of psychopathy, will help us to understand the heterogeneous and sometimes divergent nature of the research findings for this population.

N.B.

Antisocial acts and criminality in general confront our post-modern societies with major challenges.

Decoding criminality and antisocial behaviour from a neurobiological, neurocognitive or psychopathological standpoint is only one way among many of understanding these complex phenomena. So as to avoid becoming embroiled in an enervating reductionism, one should bear in mind that the sociological and criminological points of view are also especially important. Any attempt to understand, prevent or counteract these forms of behaviour must seek to integrate the various existing frames of reference with a view to providing global and coherent responses to these phenomena.

Nonetheless, if one studies the phenomenon of delinquency in any sort of depth one discovers that, from a psychopathological perspective, only one subcategory of delinquency is ultimately ascribable to psychopathological conditions. This will, however, be an important one, because this subset comprises individuals who will persist in their criminal activities.

Moreover, this subcategory is especially important for society as a whole. In fact, in terms of human suffering the repercussions on the victims and their families of these antisocial forms of behaviour cannot be quantified, any more than those that affect the perpetrators themselves and their families. Quite apart from the high fiscal cost to which criminality gives rise (Scott et al, 2001), seeking coherent and ethical responses to this complex problem must be a priority for any society that wishes to consider itself to be democratic. Research in the cognitive sciences can contribute to an understanding of this challenge to society.

1. History and Definition of the Concept of Psychopathy

The sciences of modern psychiatry and criminology gradually emerged during the 19th century. They subsequently differentiated themselves as human sciences as part of a process that had actually begun during the Renaissance. Within this historical framework, in which the first nosographies of mental disturbances gradually saw the light of day, psychopathy as a clinical entity slowly acquired sharper definition alongside other no less important entities, such as melancholia or, later, schizophrenia.

At the very beginning of this process, Benjamin Rush (1786) first put forward the idea that *'moral behaviour is brain based'*. Shortly afterwards, Pinel (1801) described a syndrome characterised by 'blind impulses leading to acts of violence' without interference from the reasoning. He called it 'mania without delirium'. Shortly afterwards, his pupil Esquirol reformulated it as 'instinctive monomania'.

Later, various definitions aimed at more sharply characterising subjects involved in criminal conduct would follow, each reflecting the currently prevailing or fashionable psychological theories. Indeed, throughout history antisocial behaviour has often been considered from two opposing perspectives: as an internal deficit or as an ecological and adaptive response to extremely disrupted, violent and disorganised environments.

Schematically, the nosographical descriptions place the emphasis sometimes on social maladaptation, sometimes on unbalanced an unstable behaviour. In parallel with this, the concept of affective coldness (absence of feelings of guilt, absence of empathy, etc,) gradually emerged as a characteristic trait of psychopathic behaviour.

In 1941, Cleckley published the first edition of his 'Mask of Sanity'. In this standard reference work, the author isolated 16 characteristic traits, among which emotional disturbance is clearly identified. In this connection one can cite in particular lack of remorse or shame, lack of empathy, absence of nervousness, egocentricity and failure to form intimate attachments with others, failure to learn from punishment, and general impoverishment of major affective reactions. Referring to the gulf between the linguistic and the experiential components of emotion, Johns and Quay (1962) wrote that the psychopath knows the 'words' of emotion but not the music (in Patrick et al, 1993).

Shortly afterwards, in his 'Clinical Psychopathology', Kurt Schneider (1950) distinguished, among the different pathological personalities, 'cold psychopaths'[1]. As far as one knows, he was the first author to present affective coldness as a central trait of a personality disorder in which behavioural disturbances are also to be found. Schneider wrote: 'cold psychopaths are people for whom compassion, shame, honour, repentance and conscience simply do not exist... they are often impulsive, brutal and cruel in their actions'.

2. Categorical Nosographical Approaches

At the present time, the two most widely used definitions are the antisocial personality disorder (APD) of the Diagnostic and Statistical Manual (DSM IV) and the Hare Psychopathy CheckList Revised – PCL-R; 1991) (Hare, 1970; 1981; 1986; 1991; Harpur and Hare, 1994).

a) The Antisocial Personality Disorder

Among the criteria laid down for the antisocial personality disorder of the DSM-IV, which is characterised by a pervasive pattern of antisocial behaviour, the flattening of emotional expression is virtually absent. Only the final criterion makes any reference to the impoverishment of the emotional responses, while limiting them to an absence of guilt feelings and indifference to the consequences of the conduct leading up to an action. This diagnostic category, which is in fact almost solely based on behavioural aspects, does not take into account the global emotional impoverishment that characterises the behaviour of the psychopathic personality. In fact, the concept of psychopathy is, *stricto sensu,* distinct from but related to the antisocial personality disorder: impulsivity and antisocial behaviour alone are insufficient to define personalities that fit the construct of psychopathy.

b) Hare Psychopathy Checklist Revised

In the adult subject, the Hare Psychopathy CheckList Revised (PCL-R) is currently considered to be the most effective tool for establishing a diagnosis of psychopathy. The revised version, published in 1991, contains 20 precise, detailed and differentiated items that help identify the presence of the traits that are traditionally regarded as constituents of this syndrome. These items are scored from 0 to 2, and a total equal to or higher than the fixed cut-off of 30 is sufficient for a diagnosis of psychopathy according to PCL-R.

As regards the emotional problems described above, the PCL-R broadly takes these into account through the inclusion of items such as 'need for stimulation/proneness to boredom' (item 3), 'lack of remorse or guilt' (item 6), 'shallow affect' (item 7), 'callous/lack of empathy' (item 8).

The diagnosis of psychopathy as conceived by the Hare Psychopathy CheckList Revised therefore simultaneously takes into account antisocial behaviour and specific personality traits. From this point of view, factor analyses have made it possible to use the Hare

[1] Schneider uses the term 'psychopath' in its true etymological sense, i.e. to mean a personality disorder seen in terms of a deviation from the mean or normal condition, in contrast to the psychoses, which, for this author, correspond by virtue of their somatic basis to the criteria of an illness in its generally accepted sense.

Psychopathy CheckList Revised to isolate two principal factors (Cooke and Michie, 1997; Harpur, Hakstian and Hare, 1988). The first of these factors refers to personality traits, and is composed of the items 'glibness/superficial charm, grandiose senses of self worth, pathological lying, conning/manipulative, lack of remorse or guilt, shallow affect, callous/lack of empathy and failure to accept responsibility for own actions'. It is worth noting that, within this factor, two types of traits can be distinguished, namely traits associated with a problem of narcissism (glibness, superficial charm, grandiose sense of self worth, pathological lying, conning, manipulative) and traits that reflect a disturbance of the affectivity in the sense of deficiency of emotional experience (lack of remorse or guilt, shallow affect, callousness, lack of empathy, failure to accept responsibility for own actions). The second might be considered as an antisocial behaviour factor defined largely by instrumental aggression, which is highly characteristic of psychopathic individuals (Woodworth et al, 2002) and the committing of a wide range of offences. It comprises the items 'need for stimulation/proneness to boredom, parasitic lifestyle, poor behavioural control, early behaviour problems, lack of realistic long-term goals, impulsivity, irresponsibility, juvenile delinquency and revocation of conditional release'.

c) Commentary

The relationship between psychopathy according to the PCL-R criteria and the antisocial personality disorder is asymmetric, since the PCL-R criteria include an assessment of antisocial forms of behaviour as well as personality traits. Predictably, high scores on the second factor are strongly associated with the diagnosis of APD, while high scores on the first factor are less strongly associated. The PCL-R diagnosis is more specific for a subcategory of APD: about 90% of psychopathic offenders meet APD criteria, but only about 25% of those diagnosed with APD meet the PCL-R criteria for psychopathy.

Moreover, whereas scores on the second factor decline with age, scores on the first do not. This stability might reflect the fact that emotional deficit is one of the central features of psychopathy, related to neurocognitive impairment (see below).

3. Dimensional Nosographical Approaches

In a manner complementary to the central definition of psychopathy according to the DSM IV and Hare, other writers have put forward dimensional models rather than categorical ones in their investigation of personality disorders.

Cloninger and Svrakic (1997), for example, suggest that the antisocial personality is characterised by a specific triad, with a high score on the dimension 'novelty seeking' (i.e. the tendency to respond to new stimuli with excitement or exaltation, curiosity, impulsiveness, non-conformism, etc.), a low score on the dimension 'harm avoidance' (i.e. the tendency to respond in a relatively uninvolved manner to aversive stimuli, absence of timidity, pessimism, anxiety, etc.) and a low score on the dimension 'reward dependence' (i.e. the tendency to respond weakly to signals of social and interpersonal gratification, absence of sensitivity, etc.) (Cannon et al, 1993; Cloninger et al, 1995; Sigvardson et al, 1996; Compton et al, 1996; Schmidt et al, 1996; in Pélissolo et al, 1997).

4. Psychopathy as a Developmental Disorder

Psychopathy and antisocial personality disorder are considered to be severe developmental disorders. Many studies, both retrospective (Loeber, 1982, 1990, 1991, 2002) and prospective (Stevenson and Goodman, 2001; Harrington, 2001; Raine, 1996; Caspi, 1996), have shed light on the links between behavioural problems during infancy and adolescence (in particular problems of conduct) and antisocial personality disorder, psychopathy and criminality in adulthood, the first being a very powerful predictor of the second. In parallel with this, confronted with the low level of effectiveness associated with therapeutic approaches to dealing with adult antisocial offenders, more attention has been focused on their early identification in the hope of making effective early interventions and establishing successful prevention programs.

Behavioural problems in infants and adolescents, such as impulsive, oppositional or transgressive behaviour, are, according to the DSM-IV, represented in three different syndromes: the Attention-Deficit Hyperactivity Disorder (ADHD), the Oppositional Defiant Disorder (ODD) and the Conduct Disorder (CD). In parallel, several child and adolescent psychopathy inventories have recently been developed, such as the Psychopathy Screening Device (Frick and Hare, 2001) and the Childhood Psychopathy Scale (Lynam, 1997).

A. CD

A.1. Clinical Features

Clinically, Conduct Disorder (CD) refers to the clustering of persistent antisocial acts of children and adolescents. The symptoms are clustered in four groups: aggression to people and animals, destruction of property, deceitfulness and theft, and, finally, serious violation of rules. All these symptoms with just one exception ('often lies to obtain goods or favours or to avoid obligations' (i.e., 'cons' others') item 11) are descriptions of transgressive behaviour forms. In a manner that is somewhat congruent with that of the APD, the subject's psychological functioning, including the emotional register, is passed over. The absence of a sense of guilt and, more generally, emotional coldness, do not form part of the diagnostic criteria of this problem, any more than does the constant tendency among these subjects to project onto the world around them the blame for their behavioural peculiarities (projection or external attribution). As a result, this quite aspecific diagnosis covers a very wide range of problems.

To sum up: conduct disorder is a heterogeneous problem that 'can best be described as a final common pathway for several initially divergent developmental trajectories' (Steiner, in Kaplan and Sadock, 2000).

A.2. Etiological Factors

From an etiological perspective, twins and adoption studies indicate a large shared environmental (familial) effect, a moderate non-shared environmental effect and a modest genetic effect.

Adoption studies suggest that an interaction between genetic vulnerability and unfavourable family conditions. The importance of the role played by the latter in the genesis of CD is today widely accepted and documented (see introduction). Briefly, poor parenting, rejection of the child, abusive and neglectful behaviour, child maltreatment and parental disharmony with or without violence are obvious risk factors for the development of conduct disorder.

At the neurobiological level, as demonstrated experimentally in the sensory and motors areas, experience plays a fundamental role in the modulation of the synaptic connectivity of areas of emotional and cognitive association. These data are in accordance with the fact that an individual's lifelong emotional abilities reflect an internal representation of the reactions of caregivers in the first years of life.

A.3. Psychopathy Construct in Youth: Callous-Unemotional Traits

The link between conduct disorder in adolescence and the antisocial personality in adulthood has been demonstrated by numerous prospective and retrospective studies. Recently, in a prospective study, J Kim-Cohen et al (2003) confirmed once again that CD (and ODD) are precursors of antisocial personality disorder. Even so, in this study the aspecific and heterogeneous character of CD is underlined by the fact that this diagnosis is also over-represented in the precursors of the main psychiatric adult disorders (anxiety disorder, depression, schizophreniform disorders, eating disorders and mania).

Confronted with the relatively aspecific character of CD as a predictor of APD or psychopathy, some writers, such as PJ Frick and colleagues, have reassigned a central position to affective disturbances, including emotional coldness. In 1994, in a factor analysis of a measure of psychopathy in a sample of 95 clinic-referred children between the ages of 6 and 13, these authors found two dimensions of psychopathic behaviour: one associated with impulsivity and conduct problems (I/CP) and the other associated with the interpersonal and motivational aspects of psychopathy, called callous/unemotional (CU). Scores derived from the CU factor were only moderately associated with measures of conduct problems, and exhibited a different pattern of associations on several criteria that have been associated with psychopathy (e.g., sensation seeking) or childhood antisocial behaviour (e.g., low intelligence, poor school achievement, and anxiety). For these authors, their results suggest that, in youth, psychopathic personality features and conduct problems are independent. In the same way, a one-year follow-up study (Frick et al, 2003) shows that callous-unemotional (CU) traits are predictive of conduct problem severity, severity and type of aggression and self-reported delinquency. In a study of adjudicated youths, these traits, in contrast to behavioural factors (i.e., impulsivity/conduct problems), were also found to be associated with lower emotional distress and a specific social information-processing pattern characterised by an increased focus on the positive aspects of aggression and a decreased focus on the negative aspects of hostile acts (Pardini et al, 2003). This study reinforced the hypothesis of the two-dimensional nature of psychopathy in youths.

Furthermore, a study of juvenile delinquents by Christian et al (1997) found that children with CU traits had more conduct problems with a greater diversity, a stronger history of police contacts, and more familial antecedents of antisocial personality disorder. So, for these authors, CU traits with significant conduct problems seem to designate a subgroup with a very severe pattern of antisocial behaviour who correspond more closely to adult psychopathy.

Finally, Loeber et al (2002) recently published a study about psychopathology antecedents in a clinic-referred sample of young males. These authors found that the best predictors of APD were callous/unemotional behaviour, depression and marijuana use.

B. ODD

B.1. Clinical Features

The central feature of ODD is a recurrent pattern of negativistic, defiant, disobedient and hostile behaviour towards authority figures, which persists for at least six months. The conduct leading up to the heteroaggressive physical act does not form part of the diagnostic criteria for this problem (APA, DSM IV). The subject's provocations and transgressions, even if they do affect his functioning from a social, scholastic or professional point of view, are not sufficiently serious to warrant a reaction from the law enforcement agencies.

B.2. Etiological Factors

The etiological studies of ODD are usually to be found in the body of research on conduct disorder. Briefly, etiological factors of ODD are, like CD, multifactorial (genetic, familial and environmental).

B.3. Psychopathy Construct in Youth

The link between this disorder and the antisocial personality or psychopathy remains unclear and contradictory. The remarks made above regarding CD as a relatively unspecific predictor of problems in adulthood (i.e., psychopathy) are even truer of ODD and could at least partially explain the contradictory data encountered in the literature.

C. ADHD

C.1. Clinical Features

Children with ADHD display early symptoms of hyperactivity, inattention and impulsive behaviour.

C.2. Etiological Factors

It has been consistently observed that ADHD and CD frequently co-occur.

Numerous findings indicate that CD and ADHD share a common genetic aetiology, but that ADHD + CD is a genetically and clinically more severe variant of ADHD alone (Thapar et al, 2001). Clinical prospective studies have largely confirmed that ADHD+CD is a high risk for a worse outcome and that ADHD alone is a low risk for progression to antisocial disorders. For Lynam (1996, 1998), the group of children with the comorbid condition ADHD+CD contains the future psychopathic adult.

C.3. Psychopathy Construct in Youth

From the perspective of the emotions, Barry et al (2000) found that children with both ADHD and a conduct problem diagnosis (ODD or CD) displayed features typically associated with psychopathy, such as a lack of fearfulness and a reward-dominant response style, all the more so when they displayed callous-unemotional traits.

This problem could therefore only have a clear association with APD or psychopathy when it is associated with CD and when the predominant symptomatology is impulsiveness.

PART II: NEUROPSYCHOLOGICAL, NEUROPHYSIOLOGICAL, NEUROCOGNITIVE AND NEUROANATOMICAL BASES

Many studies have sought to shed light on the biological bases of behaviour and antisocial personality disorder. To this end, neurocognitive investigations, evaluations of the functioning of the autonomous nervous system and cerebral imagery (both structural and functional) have been utilised. A synthesis of the relevant data from the literature is presented in this section.

1. Neuropsychological Measures and Antisocial Behaviour

It has been known for some considerable time that frontal lobe damage is associated with emotional and behavioural changes, such as irresponsibility and difficulty in tolerating frustration, frequent impulsivity and increased levels of aggression, shallow affect, lack of empathy and lack of concern for social rules. To some extent, these clinical features mimic the antisocial personality disorder. The term 'acquired sociopathy' was introduced for those individuals who, after lesions of the orbitofrontal (ventral) and medial frontal cortex, presented DSM-III diagnostic criteria for 'sociopathic disorder' (Damasio, 1994). These criteria included 'defective planning', 'lack of remorse' and 'being reckless regarding others' personal safety'. In parallel, the hypothesis was formulated that developmental psychopathy could at least partially be explained by a dysfunction of these cerebral structures.

A. Executive Functions

The literature on neuropsychological measures of executive functions in psychopathic or antisocial disorders is unclear and contradictory. Various factors can explain this confusion:

1. variation in diagnostic criteria (PCL R vs. APD);
2. selection bias associated, for example, with the method of recruitment (samples derived from psychiatric hospital, prisons, forensic settings or community);
3. absence of screening for psychiatric comorbidity, such as substance abuse or psychotic disorders;
4. variation in the inclusion of healthy control comparison groups or, when this is the case, comparison with poorly matched healthy control groups;
5. use of a variety of neuropsychological tasks could have contributed to these conflicting findings.

Thus, Hare (1984) found no evidence of executive function deficits in psychopathic criminals compared with non-psychopathic criminals.

However, in a recent meta-analytic review of 39 studies, Morgan and Lilienfeld (2000) concluded that there was a significant link between executive function deficits and antisocial personality disorder. They also concluded that APD was associated with a broader executive function deficit than was psychopathy.

Dinn and Harris (2000) support the view that a selective orbitofrontal deficit may be associated with psychopathy, as do Lapierre et al (1995), who showed that incarcerated psychopathic subjects were significantly impaired on tasks considered sensitive to orbitofrontal/ventromedial-prefrontal function, including a visual go/no-go discrimination task, Porteus Maze Test and an odour identification task, in comparison with matched control subjects (non-psychopathic inmates). These authors also found that psychopathic subjects did not display performance deficits on measures sensitive to dorsolateral-prefrontal and posterorolandic function.

For Dinn and Harris (2000), the executive function deficits (i.e., dorsolateral) among psychopathic subjects are associated with comorbid psychiatric conditions, while the core interpersonal and affective characteristics associated with psychopathy (egocentricity, callousness, manipulativeness, guile, lack of empathy and remorse) may result from orbitofrontal dysfunction.

More recently, Dolan (2002) found both orbitofrontal and dorsolateral deficits when comparing subjects with APD to healthy controls matched only for age and IQ. In this study, comorbid psychiatric conditions such as psychosis, substance abuse or personality disorders were well controlled.

Further researches are needed to arrive at definitive conclusions. These studies should take into account all the potential biases and limitations described above.

Among infants and adolescents, publications are few and far between and are again contradictory (Raine, 2002a, 2002b; Dery, 1999; Giancola, 1996, 2001; Lahey, 1995; Stevens, 2003).

B. Emotional Processing

Several studies have shown that psychopathic traits are associated with abnormalities in the processing of emotional stimuli.

From an experimental viewpoint, these studies have primarily investigated the ability of psychopathic subjects to recognise and/or identify facial expressions of emotion or tones of voice.

The results show, both in adult subjects (Kosson, 2002; Blair, 2002) and in children (Loney, 2003; Blair, 2001; Stevens, 2001), that subjects with psychopathic traits exhibit deficits in the processing of emotional stimuli, in particular sadness and fear.

2. Psychophysiological Measures and Antisocial Behaviour

Introduction

The psychophysiological measures usually include the electrodermal response, the modulation of the startle reflex and the electromyographic activity of the corrugator muscle.

Schematically, the electrodermal activity is considered as an indicator of emotion arousal though the modulation of the startle reflex as an index of emotional valence. According to Lang (1985; in Patrick, 1993), 'emotional responses to stimuli are defined in terms of two orthogonal dimensions: affective valence and arousal. Valence refers to the directionality of the elicited action disposition, varying from avoidance to approach; arousal refers to the intensity of activation of the response'.

Finally, the measures of the electromyographic activity of the corrugator muscle are regarded as an index of emotional expression.

Adult Studies

From the 1960s onwards, studies have focused on the autonomic nervous responses of psychopathic individuals in punishing and threatening situations.

Several psychophysiological studies have repeatedly found a low autonomic responsiveness in psychopaths with reduced electrodermal responses during anticipation of aversive stimuli related to feelings of fear or threat (Arnett et al, 1997, Hare, 1978, Arnett, 1997; in Herpertz, 2001), or during processing of fearful facial expressions.

Several studies have also shown the same deficit to sad expressions in psychopathic individuals compared with controls (House and Milligan, 1976, Aniskiewicz, 1979, Chaplin et al, 1995, Blair et al, 1997; in Blair et al, 1999).

In a major study, Patrick et al (1993) showed that in psychopaths the startle eye reflex did not show a larger and faster blink during unpleasant visual stimuli than during pleasant stimuli. This impairment of the startle reflex is correlated with a high score in the PCL-R factor 1 (i.e. personality traits). Patrick concluded that 'emotional detachment – defined by factor 1 in PCL-R – appears to be the factor most pertinent to psychopaths'.

These results support the hypothesis that in psychopathic individuals there is a deficit in brain structures governing negative affects (i.e., the amygdala).

Recently, Herpertz et al (2001) used multiple psychophysiological measures (electrodermal response, modulation of the startle reflex, electromyographic activity of the corrugator muscle) to compare emotional responses to pleasant and unpleasant stimuli between criminal offenders with psychopathy or with borderline personality disorder and controls.

The results once again supported the theory that psychopaths display a lack of fear in response to aversive stimuli but also a general deficit in processing affective information whether the stimuli are positive or negative. In contrast to Patrick's results, psychopaths showed no modulation of the startle response in relation to any kind of emotional stimulus. Furthermore, the corrugator muscle response of psychopaths suggested rare aversive facial expressions. The authors add that, although all the psychophysiological data suggest emotional hyporesponsiveness, psychopaths' self-reports of their emotional responses did not reflect this deficiency. This dissociation between self-report and physiological data is paralleled by other studies showing dissociation between the linguistic and experiential components of emotion in psychopaths.

In the same way, Patrick et al (1994) studied low- and high-psychopathic individuals while they imagined fearful and neutral scenes in a cued sentence-processing task. As expected, subjects with a high level of psychopathy showed fewer physiological reactions during fearful imagery, in accordance with the theory of dissociation between semantic and emotional processes in psychopathy.

Youth Studies

Some findings in youth suggest that these deficits (i.e., autonomic arousal or reactivity) appear before adulthood.

For instance, Raine et al (1995), in a 14-year prospective study, found that high levels of autonomic arousal and orientation at age 15 were protective against the development of criminal behaviour at age 29.

Herpetz et al (2001) studied autonomic arousal and electrodermal responses to orienting and aversive stimuli in boys aged 8 to 13 years with Attention Deficit Hyperactivity Disorder (ADHD) + Conduct Disorder (CD) or ADHD alone. As expected, in boys with the comorbid condition they found a decrement of autonomic responses and a faster habituation to orienting and aversive startling stimuli compared with children with ADHD alone. In short, boys with ADHD+CD, who are at high risk for psychopathic evolution, displayed a psychophysiological response pattern very similar to that reported in adult psychopaths.

Psychophysiological Abnormalities as a Sign of Structural Dysfunctions

Like the hypothalamus and limbic system, which are crucial components of the neural circuitry regulating emotions and autonomic functions, the orbitofrontal system also contributes to the regulation of autonomic nervous system activity, including electrodermal activity and the rapid control of arterial pressure (Damasio et al, 1990, Guyton, 1991, Tranel and Damasio, 1994, Tranel et al, 1988; in Dinn and Harris, 2000; Herpertz et al, 2001). Bilateral orbitofrontal lesions in human subjects induce fewer reactive electrodermal responses during exposure to emotionally charged stimuli (Tranel et al, 1988; in Dinn and Harris, 2000). Moreover, patients with amygdala lesions show impoverished aversive conditioning and reduced augmented startle reflexes similar to those seen in psychopaths (Hare et al, 1978, Davis, 1986, Patrick et al, 1993, Bechara et al, 1995, LaBar et al, 1995, Angrilli et al, 1996, LeDoux, 1998; in Blair et al, 1999).

These conclusions among patients with specific cerebral lesions underline the importance of these structures in the autonomic relationships associated with the processing of emotional information.

3. Neuroimaging and Antisocial Behaviour

A. The Cerebral Structures Involved in Emotional Responses: The Supremacy of the Amygdala

There is reasonable agreement concerning the anatomical structure involved in processing expressions of fear, in which the amygdala plays a central role.

This structure, which is a part of the limbic system, displays an extremely complex connectivity with the rest of the brain and is considered as an alarm system when triggered by fear. Anatomically, the amygdala projects to most major areas of the brain: the hypothalamus (release of corticotrophin-releasing hormone – mobilisation of the fight-or-flight reaction), corpus striatum (system of movement), the cingulate, temporal and prefrontal cortices, the locus ceruleus (norepinephrine neurons, which in their turn project to the cortex, the brainstem and the limbic system), the brainstem and medulla (via the nearby central nucleus –

autonomic nervous system). The amygdala, like the nearby hippocampus, receives projections from the thalamus and the temporal, insular, limbic and prefrontal cortices.

Briefly, when triggered by fear the amygdala stimulates the locus ceruleus activity to increase the reactivity of key brain areas and signals the brainstem to fix the face in a fearful expression and initiate autonomic reactions. Furthermore, the direct circuitry between amygdala and thalamus enables the amygdala to act as a repository for partly unconscious emotional impressions and memories. The circuitry between the amygdala, the hippocampus and the prefrontal cortex improves attention and mobilises a wide range of cognitive functions.

It is implicated in fear conditioning, which is recognised as a *sine qua non* for effective socialisation. The amygdala also plays an important role in the modulation of aggressive or submissive behaviours.

Moreover, the amygdala and the limbic system as a whole are highly interconnected with the prefrontal cortex. This is especially highly developed in humans and accounts for 29% of the entire neocortex[2]. As the work of Changeux J-P has underlined, it plays an essential part in the memory functions (especially in the working memory, i.e. the capacity to retain information during a task), the ability to verify the relevance of this information during a learning process and the ability to retain in the mind the objective to be reached during this learning process, deductive reasoning, and the imagination. It also makes it possible to understand the states of mind both of other people and of oneself.

To summarise, the various functions of the cortex are: attention span, perseverance, planning, judgement, impulse control, organisation, self-monitoring and supervision, problem solving, critical thinking, forward thinking, learning from experience and mistakes, ability to feel and express emotions, influencing of the limbic system, empathy, internal supervision.

B. Psychopathy and Structural Imagery

Raine (2000) compared prefrontal grey and white matter volumes using structural magnetic resonance imaging in 21 men with APD, 34 controls, 27 men with substance dependence and 21 psychiatric controls. The APD group showed a subtle structural deficit in the prefrontal grey matter cortex. Indeed, the APD subjects had an 11% reduction in prefrontal grey matter compared with a control group, a 14% reduction compared with a substance-dependent group, and a 14% reduction compared with a psychiatric control group. These results establish for the first time the presence of this kind of structural deficit in APD subjects in a study where confounding factors (i.e., psychiatric comorbidity, psychoactive substance dependence, psychosocial factors) are well controlled.

A second study, by Woerman et al (2000), found significant frontal grey matter reduction, especially in the left anterior frontolateral cortex, in patients with temporal lobe epilepsy with recurrent episodic aggression. These patients were compared with normal controls and non-aggressive patients with the same pathology.

Reductions in the dorsal hippocampal volumes were also found in psychopaths (Laakso et al, 2001), in accordance with experimental results indicating the importance of the dorsal hippocampus in the acquisition of conditioned fear. These data reinforced theories that proposed that 'central features in the birth of psychopathy are due to a deficit in the acquisition of conditioned fear'.

---

[2] By way of comparison, in the chimpanzee, it accounts for 17% of the whole of the neocortex.

C. Psychopathy and Functional Anatomy

In normal subjects, Blair et al (1999) found that neural response to sad and fearful facial expressions had in common left amygdala activation while angry expressions activated the right orbitofrontal cortex. They postulated that there are at least two systems that are implicated in response to different classes of aversive stimuli: the fear- and sad-related system involved in (social) aversive conditioning and the angry-related system that encourages behavioural extinction.

These data reinforced the hypothesis of a dysfunction of the amygdala in psychopathic individuals, since they suggest a selectively reduced autonomic response to fearful and sad expressions.

While several studies have emphasised a selectively reduced autonomic response to sad expressions, there is a limited number of functional neuroimaging studies in APD, psychopaths or violent offenders.

Raine (1994, 1998) found a decreased activation in prefrontal regions (and, more particularly, in the ventromedial regions) in murderers compared with healthy controls matched for age and sex during an auditory activation task. These authors also show that this reduction was primarily manifested in murderers without a history of psychosocial deprivation, suggesting that these deficits could best be explained by genetic rather than environmental influences.

Functional response to neutral and emotional words during a lexical decision task were studied by Intrator et al (1997) using a single photon emission computed tomography in psychopathic and non-psychopathic substance abusers and in community controls. Psychopathic subjects displayed greater relative activation in emotional rather than neutral conditions than the two non-psychopathic groups. This greater activation was interpreted as a reflection of the difficulties in processing emotional information. Furthermore, psychopaths activated more posterior brain regions, suggesting that processing semantic and affective information drew upon an atypical circuitry.

Schneider et al (2000), using an aversive classical conditioning paradigm, found differential effects in the amygdala and in the dorsolateral prefrontal cortex activation. Unexpectedly, psychopaths showed an overactivation of these regions, suggesting a need for an additional effort to form negative emotional associations.

During an affective memory task, functional magnetic resonance imaging (fMRI) of criminal psychopaths compared with criminal non-psychopaths and control subjects revealed a less affect-related activity in limbic structures and an overactivation in the bilateral frontotemporal cortex (Kiehl, 2001).

In a recent functional magnetic imaging study, Muller et al (2003) investigated 6 psychopaths and 6 controls to study the influence of positive and negative affective contents on brain activity. In this design, series of negative and positive pictures were shown while functional imaging was performed. This was of particular interest because this design did not demand the involvement of the higher cortical functions (e.g., attention, language, memory). For the two categories of stimuli, the results displayed multiple differences in hyper- or hypoactivation of the cortical and subcortical structures involved in emotion processing. These results reinforce the hypothesis of a dysfunction of the emotion-related cerebral networks in psychopathy.

Veit et al (2002) compared 4 psychopaths, 4 social phobics (characterised by excessive fear) and 7 healthy controls in differential aversive delay conditioning, with neutral faces as conditioned stimuli and painful pressure as unconditioned stimuli. Functional magnetic resonance imaging revealed brief amygdala activation in psychopaths. In contrast, healthy controls and moreover social phobics displayed differential activation in the limbic-prefrontal circuit (amygdala, anterior cingulate, insula, orbitofrontal cortex).

Neurofunctional imagery sometimes suggested activation deficits, and at other times overactivation of certain cerebral regions involved in the processing of emotional information. In particular, the amygdala displayed variations of this kind depending on the design used, especially according to the stimulation paradigm (e.g., recourse to a memory task or a direct stimulation).

Among psychopathic subjects, different activation patterns were revealed during the processing of positive or negative emotional stimuli.

Abnormal activation patterns have been found in different regions of the emotion-related brain circuit in psychopaths compared with healthy controls. To summarise, there is growing evidence of a disturbed interaction between top-down modulation, in which prefrontal regions play a key role, and bottom-up regulation where the role of the limbic system is central. The neurobiological underpinnings in psychopathy are evidence of a deregulation and a disturbed functional connectivity of the emotion-related area of the brain.

CONCLUSION

The psychopathologic definition of antisocial and psychopathic disorders calls for an improvement in the nosographical frameworks.

The definition of clinical syndromes constructed from behavioural descriptions (e.g. antisocial personality disorder) cover too varied and heterogeneous psychopathologic problems. This lack of specificity is not surprising when one notes that the antisocial behaviours very generally describe any action which transgresses the rules for living in society, in particular legislation, where no act, even an extremely serious one like homicide, is any indicator by itself of any individual psychology.

This non-specificity of antisocial behaviour is even more marked during childhood and adolescence (in children, antisocial acts are overwhelmingly defined by the transgression of family rules) where transgressive behaviours can be the expression of very varied difficulties, underlying irregular or oppositional psychological issues. Recent work indicates that behavioural problems are significantly found among precursors to many psychiatric pathologies in adulthood which again illustrates that the diagnosis of behavioural problems is very unspecific or even aspecific to any subsequent psychopathologic development.

Therefore, from a psychopathological point of view, antisocial behaviours, in addition to their repetitive and diverse nature, must correspond to certain precise criteria assessed by detailed analysis of their modus operandi and contextual elements of committing the act (systematic or non-systematic use of psychoactive substances, transgressions committed alone or in a group etc.). For example, the distinction between planned and unplanned antisocial acts needs to be integrated in a completely non-exhaustive manner into the evaluation of subjects deemed to be psychopaths. Impulsive aggressiveness must be distinguished from actions planned in cold blood.

In addition to antisocial behaviour, from a diagnostic perspective, the assessment of psychological function remains the most sensitive and most specific approach. In particular, emotional coldness is the key element which characterises the psychology of a psychopath. A certain number of other traits can be associated with this coldness as characteristics of this problem. For example, the absence of empathy can be understood as an expression of coldness. It is not actually possible to emotionally identify oneself with others and therefore it is not possible to even partly experience what the other party feels from their own emotional experience even slightly and differently. Likewise, how can the subject experience the feeling of guilt without being capable of experiencing the basic emotions of fear and sadness? In addition to this basic dimension, other specific dimensions are also present and integrated into the diagnostic assessment of the psychopathy, in particular narcissism.

In addition to these behavioural and psychopathological aspects, other parameters must be taken into consideration. For example, it must be possible to take into account the general functioning of subjects described as psychopathic (successful vs. unsuccessful). Similarly, it would be interesting to take into account the latent biographical aspects by making a distinction between psychopathic subjects who encountered major problems during early childhood (physical and sexual abuse, negligence, abandonment, problems in relationships, etc.) and those who experienced few if any early traumas, while controlling for the factors that are experimentally and clinically acknowledged to be risk factors in antisocial behaviour (neonatal problems (Raine, 1996), tobacco abuse during pregnancy (Wachslag, 1997), etc.).

From a neurocognitive, psychophysiological or anatomofunctional perspective, it is increasingly obvious that different parts of the neural network involved in emotion processing are disturbed in psychopathy.

Even if the neurocognitive evaluations remain heterogeneous and contradictory, the data produced by psychophysiological research and investigations of anatomofunctional imagery have revealed several dysfunctions or abnormal patterns. However contradictory the results of this research may be, it has contributed arguments to the two principal explanatory models of developmental psychopathy.

Indeed, the theory of acquired sociopathy proposed by Damasio (1994) implies an impairment in a somatic marker system as the cause of the aberrant social behaviour. This system is, in fact, the link between the subject's internal representations and a somatic marker, i.e. an autonomic nervous system response. These somatic markers are involved in the decision-making processes (the attention paid to the negative consequences to which an action could lead, and the alarm system).

So, according to this theory, psychopathic subjects suffer from a deficit in decision-making that reflects an inability to activate somatic states associated with the anticipation of rewards and punishments.

The theory of VIM (violence inhibition mechanism (Blair, 1995)) suggests that amygdala dysfunction is the main neural substrate involved in emotional deficits in psychopathic subjects. According to this theory, psychopaths fail to display the submission cues that normally inhibit aggressive responses, and this leads to impairments in empathy.

Alongside these models, which implicitly (and, indeed, explicitly) postulate a structural deficit or a deficit in functioning in certain cerebral regions, sight must not be lost of the fact that developmental psychopathy can also be seen as a mechanism of adaptation to especially unpleasant conditions of everyday life. Affective coldness could, in family environments in which extreme violence prevails, constitute the sole means of psychological survival in the child who, one must recall, cannot escape the family system in which he or she is growing up. From this perspective, the results of functional imagery research showing atypical overactivation of certain cerebral regions could reinforce the hypothesis of an adaptative mechanism of this kind.

Hence, it is apparent just how much the early diagnosis of psycho-affective development of children should be made a priority for the authorities when establishing major screening. In the same manner, setting up prevention programmes targeting families and children who display early cognitive or emotional difficulties is extremely important. This preventive approach is probably the only effective way of solving the problems of antisocial behaviour (Scott, 2001), since it is obvious that from adolescence onwards – and even more so in adulthood – therapeutic interventions have a very limited impact.

REFERENCES

Barry CT., Frick PJ., DeShaso TM., McCoy MG., Ellis M., Loney BR., The importance of callous-unemotional traits for extending the concept of psychopathy to children, *J. Abnorm. Psychol.,* 2000; 109(2): 335-40.

Blair R.J., A cognitive developmental approach to mortality: investigating the psychopath, *Cognition,* 1995; 57(1): 1-29.

Blair R.J.R., Neurocognitive models of aggression, the antisocial personality disorders, and psychopathy, *J. Neurol. Neurosurg. Psychiatry,* 2001, 71: 727-731.

Blair R.J.R., Cipolotti L., Impaired social response reversal, a case of 'acquired sociopathy', *Brain,* 2000, 123: 1122-1141.

Blair RJ, Colledge E, Murray L, Mitchell DG, A selective impairment in the processing of sad and fearful expressions in children with psychopathic tendencies, *J. Abnorm. Child. Psychol,* 2001, 29(6): 491-8.

Blair RJ., Mitchell DG., Richell RA., Kelly S., Leonard A., Newman C., Scott SK., Turning a deaf ear to fear: impaired recognition of vocal affect in psychopathic individuals, *J. Abnorm. Psychol.,* 2002; 111(4): 682-6.

Blair R.J.R., Morris J.S., Frith C.D., Perrett D.I., Dolan R.J., *Dissociable neural responses to facial expressions of sadness and anger,* Oxford University Press, 1999.

Bowlby J., Attachment and loss: Attachment, vol 1. *Basic books*, New York, 1969.

Brower M.C., Price B.H., Neuropsychiatry of frontal lobe dysfunction in violent and criminal behaviour: a critical review, *J. Neurol. Neurosurg. Psychiatry,* 2001, 71: 720-726.

Caspi A., Moffitt T.E., Newman D.L., Silva P.A., Behavioral observations at age 3 years predict adult psychiatric disorders. Longitudinal evidence from a birth cohort, *Arch. Gen. Psychiatry,* 1996; 53(11): 1033-9.

Changeux J-P, L'homme de vérité, Ed. *Odile Jacob*, 2002.

Christian RE., Frick PJ., Hill NL., Tyler L., Frazer DR., Psychopathy and conduct problems in children: II. Implications for subtyping children with conduct problems, *J. Am. Acad. Child Adolesc Psychiatry,* 1997; 36(2): 233-41.

Cleckley H, 1982, The Mask of Sanity (rev. Ed.), St. Louis, MO: C.V. *Mosby* (published 1941).

Cloninger C.R., Svrakic D.M., Integrative psychobiological approach to psychiatric assessment and treatment, *Psychiatry,* 1997; 60(2): 120-41.

Cooke D.J., Michie C., Refining the construct of psychopathy: towards a hierarchical model, *Psychol. Assess,* 2001; 13(2): 171-88.

Cooke D.J., Michie C., Psychopathy across cultures: North America and Scotland compared, *J. Abnorm. Psychol,* 1999; 108(1): 58-68.

Damasio AR, Descartes' error: emotion, reason and the human brain. New York, Putnam, 1994.

Dery M., Toupin J., Pauze R., Mercier H., Fortin L., Neuropsychological characteristics of adolescents with conduct disorder: association with attention-deficit hyperactivity and aggression, *J. Abnorm. Child. Psychol,* 1999; 27(3): 225-36.

Dinn W., Harris C., Neurocognitive function in antisocial personality disorder, *Psychiatry Research,* 2000 ; 97: 173-190.

Dolan M., What neuroimaging tells us about psychopathic disorders, Symposium on brain imaging, *Hospital Medicine,* 2002, 63, 6.

Esquirol J. E. D., Des Maladies Mentales considérées sous les Rapports Médical, Hygiénique et Médico-Légal, Paris: *J.B. Baillière,* 1838.

Farrington DP, Ohlin LE, Wilson JQ, Understanding and controlling crime: *Toward a new research strategy.* New York: Springer-Verlag, 1986.

Frick PJ., Cornell AH., Barry CT., Bodin SD., Dane HE., Callous-unemotional traits and conduct problems in the prediction of conduct problem severity, aggression, and self-report of delinquency, *J. Abnorm. Child. Psychol.,* 2003; 31(4): 457-70.

Frick, P.J. and Hare, R.D., The Antisocial Process Screening Device (APSD), 2001, Toronto: *Multi-Health Systems.*

Frick PJ., O'Brien BS., Wootton JM., McBurnett K., Psychopathy and conduct problems in children, *J. Abnorm. Psychol.,* 1994; 103(4): 700-7.

Giancola P.R., Martin C.S., Tarter R.E., Pelham W.E., Moss H.B., Executive cognitive functioning and aggressive behavior in preadolescent boys at high risk for substance abuse/dependence, *J. Stud. Alcohol,* 1996; 57(4): 352-9.

Giancola P.R., Moss H.B., Martin C.S., Kirisci L., Tarter R.E., Executive cognitive functioning predicts reactive aggression in boys at high risk or substance abuse: a prospective study, *Alcohol. Clin. Exp. Res,* 1996; 20(4): 740-4.

Giancola PR, Parker AM., A six-year prospective study of pathways toward drug use in adolescent boys with and without a family history of a substance use disorder., *J. Stud. Alcohol.* 2001 Mar;62(2):166-78.

Hare RD, Performance of psychopaths on cognitive tasks related to frontal lobe function, *J. Abnorm. Psychol,* 1984; 93: 133-140.

Hare R.D., The Hare Psychopathy Checklist-Revised manual, *Multi-Health System,* 1991.

Hare RD, Thorvaldson SA, Psychopathy and response to electrical stimulation, *J. Abnorm. Psychol.* 1970 Dec;76(3):370-4.

Harpur TJ, Hakstian AR, Hare RD., Factor structure of the Psychopathy Checklist., *J. Consult. Clin. Psychol.* 1988 Oct;56(5):741-7.

Harpur TJ, Hare RD., Assessment of psychopathy as a function of age, *J. Abnorm. Psychol.* 1994 Nov;103(4):604-9.

Harrington R., Developmental continuities and discontinuities, *British Journal of psychiatry,* 2001; 179: 189-198.

Herpertz S., Werth U., Lukas G., Qunaibi M., Schuerkens A., Kunert H-J., Freese R., Flesch M., Mueller-Isberner R., Osterheider M., Sass H., Emotion in criminal offenders with psychopathy and borderline personality disorder, *Arch. Gen. Psychiatry,* 2001 ; 58: 737-745.

Intrator J., Hare R., Stritzke P., Brichtswein K., Dorfman D., Harpur T., Bernstein D., Handelsman L., Schaefer C., Keilp J., Rosen J., Machac J., A brain imaging (single photon emission computerized tomography) study of semantic and affective processing in psychopaths, *Biol. Psychiatry,* 1997; 42(2): 96-103.

Kaplan and Sadock, Comprehensive book of psychiatry, Seventh edition, Lippincott Williams and Wilkins, 2000.

Kiehl K.A., Smith A.M., Hare R.D., Mendrek A., Forster B.B., Brink J., Liddle P.F., Limbic abnormalities in affective processing by criminal psychopaths as revealed by functional magnetic resonance imaging, *Biol. Psychiatry,* 2001; 50(9): 677-84.

Kim-Cohen J., Caspi A., Moffitt T.E., Harrington H., Milne B.J., Poulton R., Prior juvenile diagnoses in adult with mental disorder: develpmental follow-back of a prospective-longitudinal cohort, *Arch. Gen. Psychiatry,* 2003; 60(7): 709-17.

Kosson DS, Suchy Y, Mayer AR, Libby J, Facial affect recognition in criminal psychopaths, *Emotion,* 2002, 2(4): 398-411.

Laakso M.P., Vaurio O., Koivisto E., Eronen M., Aronen H.J., Hakola P., Repo E., Soininen H., Tiihonen J., Psychopathy and the posterior hippocampus, *Behav. Brain Res,* 2001; 118(2): 187-93.

Lahey B.B., Loeber R., Hart E.L., Frick P.J., Applegate B., Zhang Q., Green S.M., Russo M.F., Four-year longitudinal study of conduct disorder in boys: patterns and predictors of persistence, *J. Abnorm. Psychol,* 1995; 104(1): 83-93.

Lapierre D., Braun C.M., Hodgins S., Ventral frontal deficits in psychopathy: neuropsychological test findings, *Neuropsychologia,* 1995; 33(2): 139-51.

Loeber R., The stability of antisocial and delinquent child behavior: a review., *Child Dev.* 1982 Dec;53(6):1431-46.

Loeber R., Subtypes of conduct disorder., *J. Am. Acad. Child Adolesc. Psychiatry.* 1990 Sep;29(5):837-8.

Loeber R., Antisocial behavior: more enduring than changeable?, *J. Am. Acad. Child Adolesc. Psychiatry.* 1991 May;30(3):393-7.

Loeber R., Burke JD., Lahey BB., What are adolescent antecedents to antisocial personality disorder?, *Crim. Behav. Ment. Health,* 2002; 12(1): 24-36.

Loney BR., Frick PJ., Clements CB., Ellis ML., Kerlin K., Callous-unemotional traits, impulsivity, and emotional processing in adolescents with antisocial behavior problems, *J. Clin. Child Adolesc. Psychol.,* 2003; 32(1): 66-80.

Lynam D.R., Early identification of chronic offenders: who is the fledgling psychopath?, *Psychol. Bull,* 1996; 120(2): 209-34.

Lynam DR, Pursuing the psychopath: Capturing the fledgling psychopath in a nomological net, *J. Abnorm. Psychol,* 1997, 106, 425-438.

Lynam D.R., Early identification of the fledgling psychopath: locating the psychopathic child in the current nomenclature, *J. Abnorm Psychol,* 1998; 107(4): 566-75.

Morgan A.B., Lilienfeld S.O., A meta-analytic review of the relation between antisocial behavior and neuropsychological measures of executive function, *Clin. Psychol. Rev,* 2000; 20(1): 113-36.

Muller JL, Sommer M, Wagner V, Lange K, Taschler H, Roder CH, Schuierer G, Klein HE, Hajak G., Abnormalities in emotion processing within cortical and subcortical regions in criminal psychopaths: evidence from a functional magnetic resonance imaging study using pictures with emotional content., *Biol. Psychiatry.* 2003 Jul 15;54(2):152-62.

Pardini DA, Lochman JE, Frick PJ., Callous/unemotional traits and social-cognitive processes in adjudicated youths, *J. Am. Acad. child. Adolesc. Psychiatry,* 2003, Mar; 42 (3): 364-71.

Patrick C.J., Emotion and psychopathy: startling new insights, *Psychophysiology,* 1994; 31(4): 319-30.

Patrick C.J., Bradley M.M., Lang P.J., Emotion in the criminal psychopath: startle reflex modulation, *J. Aborm. Psychol,* 1993; 102(1): 82-92.

Patrick C.J., Cuthbert B.N., Lang P.J., Emotion in the criminal psychopath: fear image processing, *J. Abnorm. Psychol,* 1994; 103(3): 523-34.

Pelissolo A, Veysseyre O, Lepine JP., Validation of a computerized version of the temperament and character inventory (TCI) in psychiatric inpatients., *Psychiatry Res.* 1997 Oct 10;72(3):195-9.

Pinel, Traité médico-philosophique sur l'aléniation mentale ou la manie, Paris, Richard, Caille and Ravier, an IX, (1801). 2nd edition, Paris, J. A. Brosson, 1809.

Raine A., Biosocial studies of antisocial and violent behavior in children and adults: a review, *J. Abnorm. Child Psychol,* 2002 Aug; 30(4): 311-26.

Raine A, Brennan P, Mednick SA, Bitrh complications with early maternal rejection at age 1 year predispose to violent crime at ge 18 years, *Arch. Gen. Psychiatry,* 1994 Dec; 51(12): 984-8.

Raine A, Brennan P, Mednick B, Mednick SA, High rates of violence, crime, academic problems, and behavioural problems in males with both early neuromotor deficits and unstable family environments, *Arch. Gen. Psychiatry,* 1996 Jun; 53(6): 544-9.

Raine A., Lencz T., Bihrle S., LaCasse L., Colletti P., Reduced prefrontal grey matter volume and reduced autonomic activity in antisocial personality disorder, *Arch. Gen. Psychiatry,* 2000; 57: 119-127.

Raine A, Meloy JR, Bihrle S, Stoddard J, La Casse L, Buchsbaum MS, Reduced prefrontal and increased subcotical brain functioning assessed using positron emission tomography in predatory and affective murderes, *Behav. Sci. Law,* 1998 Summer; 16(3): 319-32.

Raine A, Venables PH, Williams M, High autonomic arousal and electrodermal orienting at age 15 years as protective factors against criminal behavior at age 29 years, *Am. J. Psychiatry,* 1995 Nov; 152 (11): 1595-600.

Raine A, Yaralian PS, Reynolds C, Venables PH, Mednick SA, Spatial but not verbal cognitive deficits at age 3 years in persistently antisocial individuals, *dev. Psychopathol,* 2002 Winter; 14(1): 25-44.

RidgeàPy D, Hare RD., Sensation seeking and psychophysiological responses to auditory stimulation, *Psychophysiology.* 1981 Nov;18(6):613-8.

Schneider K, CLINICAL psychopathology, MW Hamilton, translator, *Grune and Stratton,* New York, 1959.

Schneider F, Habel U, Kessler C, Posse S, Grodd W, Muller-Gartner HW., Functional imaging of conditioned aversive emotional responses in antisocial personality disorder, *Neuropsychobiology.* 2000;42(4):192-201.

Scott S, Knapp M, Henderson J, Maughan B, Financial cost of social exclusion: follow up study of antisocial children into adulthood, *British. Med. Journal,* 2001, 323: 1-5.

Stevens D, Charman T, Blair RJ, Recognition of emotion in facial expressions and vocal tones in children with psychopathic tendencies, *J. Genet Psychol,* 2001, 162(2): 201-11.

Stevens M.C., Kaplan R.F., Hesselbrock V.M., Executive-cognitive functioning in the development of antisocial personality disorder, *Addict Behav,* 2003; 28(2): 285-300.

Stevenson J. and Goodman R., Association between behaviour at age 3 years and adult criminality, *British Journal of psychiatry, 2001*; 179: 197-202.

Thapar A., Harrington R., McGuffin P., Examining the comorbidity of ADHD-related behaviours and conduct problems using a twin study design, *British Journal of psychiatry,* 2001, 179, 224-229.

Veit R., Flor H., Erb M., Hermann C., Lotze M., Grodd W., Birbaumer N., Brain circuits involved in emotional learning in antisocial behavior and social phobia in humans, *Neuroscience Letters,* 328, 2002, 233-236.

Volavka J, Neurobiology of violence. Washington (DC): *American Psychiatric Press,* 1995.

Wakschlag LS, Lahey BB, Loeber R, Green SM, Gordon RA, Leventhal BL, Maternal smoking during pregnancy and the risk of conduct disorder in boys, *Arch. Gen. Psychiatry.* 1997 Jul;54(7):670-6.

Woermann F.G., van Elst L.T., Koepp M.J., Free S.L., Thompson P.J., Trimb M.R., Duncan J.S., Reduction of frontal neocortical grey matter associated with affective aggression in patients with temporal lobe epilepsy: an objective voxel by voxel analysis of automatically segmented MRI, *J. Neurol. Neurosurg. Psychiatry,* 2000; 68(2): 162-9.

Woodworth M, Porter S, In cold blood: characteristics of criminal homicides as a function of psychopathy, *J. Abnorm. Psychol,* 2002; 111(3): 436-45.

In: Perspectives in Psychiatry Research
Editors: Nicole M. Levine and Donna J. Campbell
ISBN: 978-1-61209-236-2

Chapter 3

FEAR AND ANXIETY IN PSYCHIATRIC DISORDERS, COGNITIVE-BEHAVIORAL CONCEPTS AND TREATMENTS

***A. Velardi*[*1], *R. Willis*[2] *and V. Pomini*[3]**

[1]Unité Hospitalière Médico-psychologique.
Hôpital régional de Delémont.
Fbg. des Capucins 30, 2800 Delémont, Suisse.
[2]Institutions Psychiatriques du Valais Romand,
Rue Saint Guérin 3, 1950 Sion, Suisse.
[3]Unité d'Enseignement des Thérapies Comportementales et cognitives.
Institut de psychothérapie.
Département Universitaire de Psychiatrie Adulte.
Bâtiment des Cèdres, Site de Cery, 1008 Prilly-Lausanne, Suisse

1. INTRODUCTION

Who has never been afraid? No one without a doubt; fear being such an integral part of existence. Fear is essential to the survival of the species because it helps to identify and avoid dangers that can compromise existence. Everyone recognizes the necessity of fear; even if it is an unpleasant experience we prefer avoiding. And when fear no longer has an object, when it is prolonged without any apparent reason and progressively invades an individual's daily life until he can't work, go out or meet other people, it ends up loosing its functional aspect and usefulness: fear then becomes a disease.

Anxiety disorders have the highest prevalence among psychiatric illnesses. Global prevalence per year for all the anxiety disorders oscillates between 8% and 16% according to different studies; the prevalence in a lifetime can be as high as 20% (Bijl, Ravelli, and van Zessen, 1988; Goldberg and Lecrubier, 1995; Magee, Eaton, Wittchen, McGonagle, and Kessler, 1996). However the actual figure is certainly much higher, because there is

* Email: alfredo.velardi@cgh.ch

practically no psychiatric disorder where anxiety doesn't play a role, even if it isn't the primary symptom. Anxiety currently appears as one of the most frequent psychological problems psychiatrists encounter in their practice. Our modern society spends billions of dollars every year on anxiolytic medications (Barlow, 1988), and even more if one counts all forms of therapy, psychotherapy, methods of personal development and also the use of somatic health services (Rees, Richards, and Smith, 1988). Anxiety represents a habitual cause for medical visits, much higher than the rate for colds, coughs, influenza and other minor illnesses (Marsland, Wood, and Mayo, 1976). It also constitutes a frequent source of work absenteeism (Laitinen-Krispijn and Bijl, 2000). Hence, in its sub-pathological and pathological forms, fear represents an important issue for public health and for personal well-being.

As disciplines mainly interested in psychological and mental problems, psychiatry and psychotherapy have developed numerous categorizations and conceptualizations of anxiety disorders. Various types of treatment have also been derived from these theories. Entire volumes have been devoted to this topic, and it would of course be impossible here to synthesize all the various existing approaches used to understand and treat these illnesses. We have therefore chosen to concentrate on one particular psychotherapeutic approach, the cognitive-behavioral therapy (CBT). This treatment has gained so much theoretical and empirical support through the years that it is now recognized as one of the most effective methods to treat this syndrome (Grawe, Donate, and Bernauer, 1994; Kipta, Lueger, Saunders, and Howard, 1999). Let us describe this kind of recommended treatment and its theoretical background.

2. Fear and Anxiety

Fear is one of the basic emotions; other being disgust, joy, sadness, anger and surprise (Ekman, 1994; Ortony and Turner, 1990). Characterized by highly negative affect and physiologic excitation, this emotion appears in situations of danger. It informs of the presence of danger and prepares the organism to face it or to escape (Barlow, 1988).

Fear can vary in intensity: from slight apprehension to extremely intolerable panic. It can take miscellaneous forms where fearful thoughts and bodily reactions are each expressed with more or less intensity. Dangers which produce fear can be real (for example fear experienced during an accident, a catastrophe, an aggression, etc.), but also completely imaginary. In that case fear arouses from the meanings that the individual gives to a situation: fear appears because the person considers the situation as dangerous for him, even though it may not the case. Classically these specific and unfounded fears are called phobias. They most often concern animals (pets, insects), night or darkness, burglars, thunder etc. Simple or multiple phobias are frequent in childhood and have a tendency to disappear with age (Gray, 1991). Phobias of a crowd, open or closed areas (for example public places, restaurants, cinemas, tunnels, elevators, planes, etc.) are grouped under the term agoraphobia. In social phobias the individual is afraid of other people, in particular when the contact with others implies a particular performance (speaking in public, eating at an official dinner, exams, defending one's own rights, making requests, etc.) or the judgement of others. Fear can also be generalized to nearly the entire experience of life. In generalized anxiety disorders indeed preoccupations are no longer focalized on one or a few objects/situations, but can touch upon virtually all domains of existence (social life, social relationships, work, leisure, etc.): mere decisions or routine activities are seen by the person as insuperable obstacles and become instead numerous sources of anxiety. Post-traumatic stress disorders are another pathological form of expression of fear and anxiety. Normally one can experience anxiety and fear during a real traumatizing experience; these emotions can also occur after the trauma (after a few hours, days, weeks or months): compared to phobias, these fears originate from a terrible event that actually happened (violence, sexual abuse, accident, risk of imminent death, etc.). In the case of post-traumatic stress disorder they continue to persist in the absence of any danger. Here, the reasons for fear are no longer a current, future or imaginary danger. On the contrary, they concern the past and they unexpectedly haunt the person during the day as well as the night in the form of flashbacks, nightmares, irritability and anxiety among other symptoms that can last for years.

Even though the phobias evoked up to this point are irrational (because they don't warn of a current or real danger), they remain partially understandable. They can virtually become totally delusional. This is the case for example in psychoses or obsessive-compulsive disorders. Individuals affected by these illnesses sometimes present very strange fears: psychotic patients, for example, can develop the fear that they will be victims of a divine punishment or of a wicked plot against them; in obsessional compulsive disorder, different fears such as being contaminated by filth, being the cause of accidents harming others through negligence, or even committing blasphemies are very current.

2.1. The Distinction Between Fear and Anxiety

It is classic to theoretically distinguish fear from anxiety. This distinction is habitually based on the object that induces the emotion: if the object is concrete we would to refer to fear, if the object is vague, poorly defined or even unidentifiable, we would rather refer to anxiety (fear without object). But other levels can also be taken into account (cf. table 1). One of the major points evoked in favor of this distinction is the fact that fear constitutes a basic emotion, while anxiety cannot strictly be considered to be a pure emotion (Lang, 1984).

Table 1. Classical theoretical distinction between fear and anxiety (according to Barlow, 1988 and Rachman, 1998).

Fear	Anxiety
Concrete object: rational and logical link (shared by everyone) between threat and fear	Source poorly defined, vague: link not clear (not shared by many) between object and anxiety
Limited episode well defined in time	Prolonged duration, persistence, beginning and end not clearly defined
Degree of emergency, imminence of facing a direct and concrete threat	Vigilance, more or less permanent apprehension of future aversive events that are unpredictable and uncontrollable
Physical expression: preparation to act (paralysis, flight or attack)	Cognitive expression: preoccupation, hesitation
Attention directed toward the threat	Attention directed toward oneself
Most extreme expression: panic	Most extreme expression: generalized anxiety

Anxiety appears indeed rather like an indistinct affective state, mixed with fear, but also sadness, anger, or even interest or a feeling of challenge. What seems to make anxiety different from other diffuse affective states such as depression, happiness or shame, essentially lies in two key elements: 1) a certain unpredictability of the feared situation (future), 2) a lack of potential control when facing probable negative events (Barlow, 1988). Every preoccupation is of course focused on the feared situation that may happen: a state of anxious apprehension describes this phenomenon. But a vicious circle can easily set in: the more unpredictable the feared situation proves to be for the person, the more uncontrollable it appears to him, and finally the greater the intensity of preoccupations and anxiety he lives. This state of anxious apprehension develops in pathological anxiety.

Following Barlow's model (1988), one could conclude that panic represents the pathological expression of fear, and that pathological anxiety (for example generalized anxiety) is the pathological clinical manifestation of anxious apprehension states. However, in clinical practice this distinction between fear and anxiety is not always very easy to do, and doesn't prove to be very useful (Rachman, 1998). In fact fear and anxiety do not appear distinct in the patients' eyes, especially when both states are combined with other psychological symptoms, and furthermore, whether we're dealing with well defined fears or with more vague anxious states does not take on a cardinal importance, since in both cases the therapeutic interventions are fundamentally the same.

2.2. Anxiety Disorders in Psychiatry

The two internationally most employed classifications (ICD-10 and DSM-IV) propose a list of anxiety disorders (American Psychiatric Association, 1994; World Health Organization, 1992). These classifications are supposed to be atheoretical and essentially based on the phenomenology of these disorders. They describe a certain number of syndromes which roughly correspond to the different groups of objects that produce anxiety and to the various manifestations of this emotional state. This is probably the reason why these lists are very similar (cf. table 2). One can however observe some differences between both lists. Firstly, anxiety disorders are classified in the ICD-10 among neurotic disorders (F40) that also include disorders induced by stress factors and somatoform disorders, while in the DSM-IV they are grouped in one unique category. Secondly, the ICD-10 classification divides anxiety disorders in a) phobias, b) other anxiety disorders, c) obsessive-compulsive disorders and d) reactions to stress factors. The American manual does not propose such a sub-classification and prefers to make a simple list of disorders, without any grouping and includes moreover anxiety disorders due to a somatic affection or due to the consumption of substances (which are classed in a completely different heading in the ICD-10). Lastly, let's cite that these two systems separate anxiety disorders from hypochondria. Hypochondria, which is the fear of illnesses (fear to become ill or to have an undiagnosed serious illness) is found in each manual in the section dedicated to somatoform disorders, even if anxiety plays a central role in the clinical picture. In the DSM-IV this section is completely separated from the anxiety disorders section, while in the ICD-10 it classed under the heading including all neurotic disorders (along with the anxiety disorders).

Table 2. Classifications of anxiety disorders according to ICD-10 and DSM-IV.

ICD-10	DSM-IV
Phobic anxiety disorders Agoraphobia Social phobias Specific phobias	 Agoraphobia without history of panic disorder Social phobia Specific phobias
Other anxiety disorders Panic disorder Generalized anxiety disorder Mixed anxiety and depressive disorder Other mixed anxiety disorders Other specified anxiety disorders Anxiety disorder unspecified	Panic disorder without agoraphobia Panic disorder with agoraphobia Generalized anxiety disorder Anxiety disorder not otherwise specified
Obsessive-compulsive disorder (OCD) Predominantly obsessional thoughts or ruminations Predominantly compulsive acts OCD mixed form with obsessional thoughts and compulsive acts Other obsessive-compulsive disorders Obsessive-compulsive disorder, unspecified	Obsessive-compulsive disorder
Reaction to severe stress and adjustment disorders Acute stress reaction Post-traumatic stress disorder Adjustment disorders Other reactions to severe stress Reaction to severe stress, unspecified	Acute Stress Disorder Post-traumatic stress disorder
	Anxiety disorder due to a general medical condition
	Substance Induced Anxiety Disorder
Somatoform disorders F45.2 Hypochondrial disorders	*Somatoform disorders* Hypochondriasis

Panic disorder is the repetition of well circumscribed episodes characterized by the sudden presence of fear or terror. The disorder is considered serious when more than four panic attacks occur in one month. Panic often happens unpredictably and is associated with physical symptoms such as pounding heart (palpitations), dizziness, muscle tension, tightness in the chest, choking or a feeling of smothering, sweating, trembling, dry mouth, hot or cold flushes, nausea, blurred vision and "jelly legs" (Andrews, Creamer, Crino, Hunt, Lampe and Page, 2003). Panic attacks are by definition frightening experiences that seem strange and abnormal. Because of the intensity of its physical symptoms, panic is habitually accompanied by ideas of collapsing, dying, losing control or becoming crazy. Some people develop a fear of panic: they tend to restrict their activities and to avoid all places where a panic attack is likely occur. Agoraphobia develops then upon the false premise the person has in mind that his panic is provoked by certain situations (restaurants, cinemas, crowded areas, etc.). Panic and agoraphobia seem therefore to be in a continuum where, after the first experiences of intense fear, people tend to avoid them by limiting their lives to areas of security (Andrews et al., 2003). It is not rare that people explain their agoraphobia indicating that they dread more the judgements of others, if they undergo a panic attack, than the fear itself or its somatic consequences. The social consequences of anxiety appear in this case as the crux of the problem: the nature or object of anxiety is social, and it seems relevant here to take into account the differential diagnosis with social phobia.

Social phobia is a strong persisting fear occurring repeatedly in social situations where social performances are required, such as speaking, giving one's own opinions, defending one's rights, making criticisms, demonstrating an exercise, eating with an important person, etc. Feelings of awkwardness, impression to be criticized by others and fear of losing one's own personal value often accompany theses situations and make them extremely unpleasant for the person. Somet«Ges the contact with others is so aversive that panic attacks and agoraphobic avoidance can develop. Panic and avoidance are clearly related to social situations and limited to them, so that diagnoses of panic and/or agoraphobia are not used.

Generalized anxiety disorder is characterized by excessive worry that is continually present during at least 6 months. Preoccupations concern several domains of daily life (work, finances, health, children, etc.) and can virtually touch upon every minor decision or activity the person has to take and to begin. Physical symptoms are present, but with less intensity than in panic: motor tension (restlessness, trembling or muscle tension, headaches, gastric disturbances) and over-excitement (with irritability and difficulties concentrating) and are more prominent than autonomic symptoms (Brown, Marten, and Barlow, 1995; Marten, Brown, Barlow, Borkovec, Shear, and Lydiard, 1993). It is also important to take note that diagnostic rules for DSM-IV and ICD-10 are not identical: by DSM-IV standards, the autonomic symptoms are excluded from the list of physical symptoms, while the ICD-10 requires the presence of an autonomic over-activity for the diagnosis of this disorder.

Post-traumatic stress disorder consists in a prolonged anxious reaction in response to an extremely threatening or catastrophic event. Distress in such situations is normal, but in post-traumatic stress disorder, recovery from the distressing response does not occur. So during weeks, months and even years after the trauma, anxiety and other pathological symptoms can repeatedly occur, handicapping the person in his daily life, and sometimes having extremely heavy consequences on work, relationships and psychological health. Three types of symptoms are habitually described for this syndrome (Andrews et al., 2003): 1) intrusive symptoms such as distressing memories or images of the traumatic event, nightmares, flashbacks where the person relives the incident, and an emotional disruption when reminded of the event; 2) avoidance symptoms consisting in more or less conscious efforts to forget and to escape any reminders of the event, for example gaps in memory, suppressing thoughts about the event, avoiding conversations, places or activities that can remind the person of the event (in serious cases, this avoidance can lead to emotional distance with others and lost of interest in normal activities); 3) over-stimulation symptoms such as the persistence of a state of hypervigilance, sleep disturbances, difficulties in concentrating or irritability. Depression, guilt, consumption of alcohol and drugs are also often present as related problems to PTSD, but the central feature of the pathology is really the incapacity to integrate the fear and horror experience with the existing view of oneself and the world, with a sort of imprisonment in past painful memories.

Obsessive-compulsive disorder is characterized essentially by obsessions and/or compulsions. Obsessive thoughts are ideas, representations or impulsions that repeatedly invade the person's conscience and induce feelings of distress. They are uncontrollable and against the person's will. They touch upon themes such as violence (harm to self or others), obscenity, contamination (being contaminated or being an agent of contamination), religion (blasphemy), etc. Compared to delusions, obsessions are recognized by the person as products of his own mind and are simultaneously criticized as being senseless. Sometimes however obsessions can be overvalued and considered as if they were part of reality. Compulsive behavior (for example: hand washing, sorting, counting, verification) is repetitive and often ritualized activities that respond to a persistent need or urge to act in this particular way, in order to neutralize obsessions or to decrease the discomfort provoked by a situation or a thought.

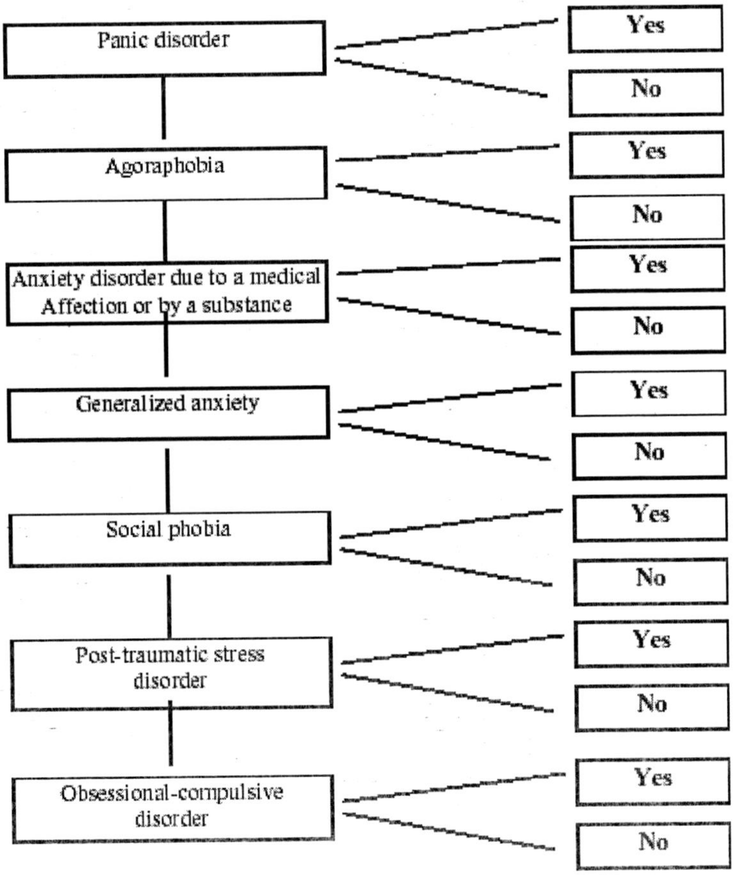

Figure 1. Anxiety disorders investigation guideline.

Rituals serve also a preventive function: verifications for example permit, in the individual's mind, to prevent accidents, fire, fatal errors, etc. If the patient is impeded to perform his obsessions and rituals, anxiety and discomfort increase, which can sometimes lead to aggressive behaviors. Obsessive-compulsive patients often become progressively "tyrants" in their families, where all members have to submit to the increasing number of rituals and rules imposed on them by a patient more and more invaded by his fears (for example, interdiction to sit on the sofas, obligation to change clothes when entering the apartment, impossibility to use the phone without having washed one's hands with soap, etc.).

Flow charts can be used in the diagnostic process. They allow to define each syndrome, in comparison with others. They aid the therapist to identify the elements that are similar in all pathologies and the ones that reveal themselves different from one pathology to another (see for example American Psychiatric Association, 1994). Let us not forget that it is also possible that a person can suffer simultaneously from several anxiety disorders. Guidelines, such as the one depicted in figure 1, represent practical ways to proceed in the diagnostic process. For example, one can ask a person first of all if he has gone through episodes of intense panic. If the answer is positive, the diagnosis of panic disorder must be considered and the existence of agoraphobia must be investigated. If the response is negative, one has to verify the existence of a generalized anxiety disorder. Next, one must exclude or include the presence of social phobia, specific phobia or post-traumatic stress disorder by asking the person to detail the contents of their fears. In every case, investigation necessitates the examination of possible organic or substance abuse that could explain anxiety.

Directive and semi-directive structured interviews exist that permit to elaborate in a rigorous and systematic manner the general psychiatric diagnosis or, more specifically, the diagnosis only for anxiety disorders (Brown, DiNardo, and Barlow, 1994; National Institute of Mental Health Molecular Genetics Initiative, 1992; Robins et al., 2000; World Health Organization, 1993).

3. The Cognitive-Behavioral Model of Fear

The cognitive and behavioral model is essentially based on current scientific knowledge about psychological disorders, integrating results principally coming from neurosciences and experimental psychology. At its origin, this model was based on the learning paradigm, but has been progressively completed by adding other paradigms such as those coming from the cognitive sciences (for example information processing models), studies on emotions, social psychology, neurobiology and neuropsychology. This model also has a clinical counterpart, offering methods of problem analysis and treatment derived from the conclusions of scientific research. These clinical methods of conceptualization and treatment of anxiety disorders vary from a syndrome to another, but are fundamentally the same. What follows is a brief presentation of this basic general approach.

3.1. Cognitive Behavioral Analysis

The cognitive behavioral approach is founded on the functional analysis of psychological problems (Kanfer and Saslow, 1969; Kanfer and Schefft, 1988). This analysis is based on the following key elements: 1) the choice of a pathological behavior (problem), 2) the identification of the external or internal stimuli preceding (and associated with) the problematic behavior (antecedents), 2) the precise description of the behavior at different phenomenological levels (behavior: cognitive, physiological, affective and motor aspects), 3) the observation of consequences following the behavior (positive/negative, immediate and delayed consequences), 4) the estimation of the degree of contingency between antecedents, behavior and consequences, 5) the analysis of the impact of the individual's mental and physical state on this contingency (for example a woman, when she is tired, will perhaps react more rapidly and more frequently to a particular fear stimulus than when she is fit). The SORCK model proposed by Kanfer (Kanfer and Saslow, 1969; Kanfer and Schefft, 1988), represents a classical way to illustrate with simple categories these basic elements of a functional analysis of a behavior (see figure 2).

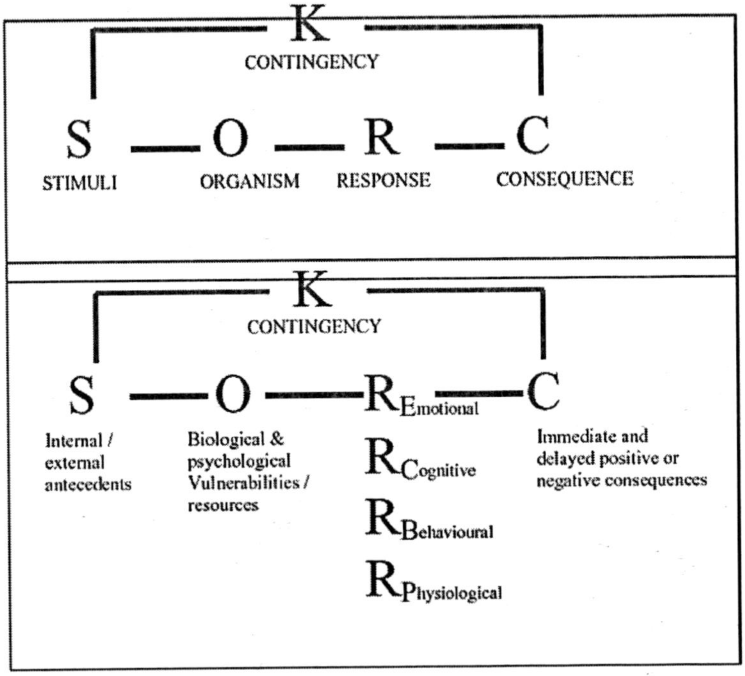

Figure 2. The SORCK model for behavioral functional analysis.

The first step of the functional analysis (S in the SORCK model) is the identification of the antecedent stimuli. Stimuli are all the elements of a situation that can set off a particular reaction. In the case of anxiety, the stimuli are all the objects that produce a person's fear or worry. In a given situation, there are indeed particular stimuli that are specifically associated with the fear reaction, and other elements, in the same context, that don't induce a fear reaction and that are therefore neutral. The cognitive behavior therapist's task is to discover with his patient what are these particular fear stimuli.

The second step concerns the description of the psychological problem in behavioral terms (R in the SORCK model). This description gathers observations made at various levels. For example, the affective reaction called fear (emotional level) often represents the starting point for a clinical description. But this labeling is not sufficient. The therapist must identify the physical and physiological characteristics of anxiety (somatic or physiological level): respiratory problems, abdominal pain, shoulder tension, etc. He must also examine thoughts concomitant with these reactions (cognitive level): "Its unbearable.", "I'll never make it.",

"Here we go, it's happening again! It's horrible! I have to get out of here right away.", etc. Finally motor aspects of behavior are also described, trying to answer this basic interrogation: what does the person do in this situation? Most of the time we will see a reaction of flight from the feared situation or avoidance of confronting himself to this situation (avoidance is habitually present when fear precedes the "danger" itself, that is in the case of anticipatory fears). Other motor behaviors can be attempts to relax, the taking of sedative medication, a phone call to a spouse or companion, a pause in activity, alcohol consumption, etc. The simple emotional label of "fear" can therefore conceal a very large number of different somatic-cognitive-behavioral profiles that this phenomenological description can bring more clearly into the picture.

The third step of this analysis considers the consequences of the behavior itself (C in the SORCK model). On a very short-term basis, the result usually turns out positive: the escape behavior produces a feeling of relief. But the long-term consequences become less advantageous: handicap and social withdrawal (for example agoraphobic persons become isolated and no longer leave their houses alone), the renouncement of a professional activity, marital conflicts, etc. These consequences frequently drive the person to consult a specialist, sometimes after having spent years or decades organizing their lives around their anxiety. Often specialized help is not even sought (Pollard, Henderson, Frank, and Margolis, 1989).

The last two steps of the functional analysis concern: 1) the contingency between the behavioral and the environmental aspects of the problem and 2) the link between the person's global mental and physical state and the frequency and intensity of his problematic behavior (understood in the sense of biological and psychological vulnerabilities). Contingency represents the strength of the association between stimuli, responses and their consequences (K in the SORCK model). Certain stimuli or configurations of stimuli can systematically induce intense fear, while other stimuli provoke this emotion only one out of ten times and at lesser intensities. A big German Shepherd without a leash, barking and chasing after a person will certainly set off in this person a reaction of intense fear, even more if he suffers from dog phobia. Other stimuli connected to dogs will however provoke in the same individual only moderate anxious responses: for example a picture of a dog, a Dachshund on a leash, or a Cocker spaniel eating out of his dish. In the same way, contingency can concern the link between response and consequence. Certain behaviors won't systematically reduce anxiety: for example an attempt at relaxation exercises won't always be totally or even partially effective. In obsessive compulsive disorders, it is not rare that executing the rituals (for example washing one's hands in order to destroy bacterium or to eliminate any trace of filthiness) results in more anxiety than before, as if the person fell in a trap where the behavior that previously relieved anxiety now increases it. The degree of the person's vulnerability (for example state of fatigue, stress, menstruations, personality traits, etc.) indicates that he can be more or less fragile: in a state of vulnerability, less or less intense stimuli can generate fear and have the same effect as stimuli that are a priori more fear inducing (Connor-Smith and Compas, 2002; Friedman, Clark, and Gershon, 1992). This is due to the fact that stress and anxiety are intimately linked (Friedman et al., 1992; Gray, 1991; Robinson, Corbett, and Spurlock, 1996). Vulnerability, in the broad sense of the term, can be a stable biological or psychological trait (indicated by biological or psychological markers) as well as a transient state depending on a particular person's circumstances which in turn can be induced or controlled or not by him (stress induced by a major life event, consumption of coffee or alcohol, etc.). Personal resources represent another form of a stable trait or transient state that can influence the degree of contingency between the antecedents, the behaviors and their consequences (for example a weak tendency to be physically stimulated, coping resources in the face of problems, capacity to seek external help, etc.). These variables determine whether a person will be more or less able to manage their stressful situations. Theses resources and vulnerability states/traits are represented by the organism variable in the SORCK model (O).

The SORCK model leads the therapist to the discovery and precise observation of all the active elements that can influence the behavioral problem under analysis. This model should allow the understanding and even the prediction of anxiety responses in the various situations the patient can go through. The therapist will also be able to verify the role of the immediate and delayed consequences of the various responses the person has when facing his anxiety problem. It appears evident enough that the more meticulous the analysis is, the better the prediction will turn out to be. Nevertheless, it is rarely necessary to attain a very high degree of precision in order to start a treatment. Two to four hours prove habitually to be sufficient to formulate a hypothesis derived from the functional analysis of the patient and this provides the tools that can be used to propose a treatment plan. This hypothesis will be then adapted and corrected according to the newbandata and clinical observations gathered during the treatment. If necessary, this hypothesis can be totally reassessed in the light of new important information or events, and the treatment consequently adjusted. The therapeutic process functions as a constant adaptation of the treatment procedures to the hypothesis elaborated to explain the clinical data.

3.2. The Cognitive-Behavioral Model of Anxiety

In order to explain its origin and its development, the cognitive-behavioral model of anxiety calls upon basic psychological processes. The learning paradigm is principally used through conditioning models (classical-associative and operant conditioning), cognitive information processing models, and the social cognitive learning model.

Historically, the associative learning model was the first explored in studying anxiety. According to this model, fear and phobias often result from the association between a neutral stimulus and one or more stimuli that automatically produced an initial reaction of fear (for example an aversive stimulus or a situation that is really dangerous). These stimuli that automatically cause fear are called unconditioned stimuli, because they are the source of an uncontrollable reflex response of the organism. The classical or associative conditioning links one or more neutral stimuli to these unconditional stimuli that induce the automatic reaction of fear. Neutral stimuli then become conditioned stimuli, because they can now produce fear reactions by themselves, without the presentation of an unconditioned fear stimulus. In this case, fear is a learned response that can be set off automatically by one or more conditioned stimuli that have become themselves fear inducing (Barlow, 1988; Gray, 1991; Rachman, 1978). For example, imagine that just after a small painful bite, a young child develops a fear of goats. He refuses now to pet them while before the incident he indulged in this activity with enthusiasm. Any sudden movements of the animal's head will make him start, because these movements are associated with the painful bite.

We know today that the conditioning of fear is particularly resistant and efficient: sometimes only one association is enough to create a conditioning (Rescorla, 1988). For example, tainted food can cause already after a first experience a definitive aversive reaction, which can be extremely difficult to cancel out: the same food, but fresh, wouldn't even be tasted. Moreover, conditioning can take place even when the two stimuli (the neutral and the unconditional) don't take place at the same time (Mackintosh, 1983). The conditioning seems to appear later after the association between a fear reaction and a neutral stimulus. Let's imagine that the goat's bite is not immediately followed by fear in the child, who, after a short period of crying, continues to pet other goats which have not bitten him. However, after a more or less brief passage of time, the child associates "goat" and "bite" and develops a fear of goats in general (in order to avoid the pain, thinking for example that all goats are in reality unpredictable in their movements). New theories show that even classical conditioning is not a simple reflex reaction: a complex internal information process selectively associates physiological and affective reactions with particular stimuli that are most likely not chosen in a random manner. The conditioning helps to inform the individual about the probable causes of different positive or negative reactions he has had. In this sense conditioning appears as a "mechanical" process as well as a cognitive one (Bandura, 1977; Mackintosh, 1983) that allows the organism to predict his environment (physical and interpersonal) and to adjust consequently its own reactions.

The operant conditioning hypothesis about fear is based on escape/avoidance behavior. This particular behavior reinforces the fear reaction by relieving the subject of his negative consequences (unpleasantness of the negative emotion). This process is called negative reinforcement, because the escape behavior allows the subject to reduce the negative consequences of fear (Mowrer, 1960, Salkovskis, Clark, Hackmann, Wells, and Gelder, 1999). Indeed, escape or avoidance behaviors are central in the maintenance process of anxiety and the development of anxiety disorders. However they can't explain their origin, that is they are not the causes of fear and anxiety. Avoiding or escaping any threat appears completely natural and logical (Gray, 1991): the child will no longer pet the biting goat (avoidance), he will pull his hand away when a goat suddenly moves his head (escape). But by systematically pulling his hand away, the child no longer has the possibility to realize that movements of the goat's head do not always mean that he'll be bitten; on the contrary he will congratulate himself for having escaped from the bite (even if this isn't really true) and learn nothing else than the escape behavior, which will be then reinforced. As he avoids the so called danger, the individual can no longer convince himself that there isn't any real danger. He gets himself into a position where it is for him impossible to learn a new way to deal with the situation (in the present case: how to pet a goat without being bitten!). If the goat example seems a little humorous, analogous situations with a snake (even a non-poisonous one), an hairy spider, an angry and domineering boss, or even the example of a man with a young beautiful woman (or a woman with an handsome young man) are surely much easier to identify with for the reader.

In summary, two forms of conditioning seem to play a key role in the learning of an anxiety disorder: 1) a classical conditioning where neutral stimuli become fear through association with unconditioned stimuli that automatically set off fear; 2) an operant conditioning where avoidance and escape behaviors are reinforced and repeated because they reduce the fear (but without giving the possibility to eliminate it completely). This rather rudimentary model, known as the two factors model (Mowrer, 1960), represents the first historical step in the cognitive-behavioral conceptualization of anxiety disorders. Even though it's dated, it hasn't lost all its pertinence and still constitutes a simple way to explain anxiety problems (Rachman, 1998).

Current models are more complex and use also knowledge derived from cognitive psychology. The role of cognitions has been particularly underlined and studied. In fact the study of cognitions has allowed to understand clinical cases and situations where the conditioning models have proved to be rather limited and unsatisfactory. Cognitive models argue that emotion is mediated by cognition, and that in a given situation the nature of a person's thoughts determines his emotional feelings (Beck and Emery, 1985; Salkovskis, 1996). Beck's model constitutes a key reference for the general cognitive conceptualization of psychiatric disorders (Beck, Rush, Shaw, and Emery, 1979). This author proposes to differentiate beliefs or schemas from automatic thoughts. Schemas (or beliefs) represent a sort of interpretative reality filter that can be activated or not in certain situations. When it's activated, a schema will promote the production of thoughts congruent with it (in competition with alternative thoughts which could challenge it). These thoughts are called "automatic" because the individual can hardly control them: they furnish a first and immediate interpretation of reality which gives a particular sense to it. These automatic thoughts can next colour the emotional experience in a positive or a negative way depending on their contents. It is actually hard to know if thoughts have preceded emotions or not; but in any case, their mutual relationships and the parallelism in the contents are always quite obvious: fear is very often related to threatening thoughts, sadness or depression can accompany gloomy and pessimistic thoughts. Automatic thoughts can often take an absolute and nuance-deprived character. Their imperative, timeless and generalizing aspects (thoughts are applied to any circumstance, without any consideration of a situation's particularity), often make up veritable cognitive tyrants against whom it is frequently very difficult to resist.

Beck's work demonstrates that anxious and depressive automatic thoughts are distorted views of reality: they don't resist to logical analysis. The premise of cognitive therapy is then to get the patients to progressively realize that they suffer because they do not correctly treat information received from their environments (when for example they consider as threatening something which is actually innocuous). Challenging theses cognitive distortions can bring new thoughts about the feared situations and favourably influence their anxiety. Table 3 synthesizes the habitual cognitive distortions observed in therapy by anxious and depressive patients. The reader will be aware of the importance of the words themselves used or of the subtle deviations from a pure logical analysis of a situation (in the anticipations, inferences, pseudo-logical conclusions, etc. made by the patients). Cognitive distortions are a normal part of human thinking. They are deeply discussed in therapy only because certain are hypothesized to have lead to emotional disorders. The idea is not to suppress all forms of cognitive distortions but to reduce the impact of the ones that are directly connected to psychological disorders.

Beck theorizes that behind automatic thoughts, there exists a great variety in beliefs and schemas. These schemas are progressively constructed during childhood. They reflect an individual's vision of the world and of himself, which has been forged through his developmental history, the influences of his surroundings, his education and his more or less traumatizing life events (Ingram, Miranda, and Segal, 1998). Beliefs explain why the automatic thoughts are provoking thoughts. According to their types of beliefs, the world will be considered as threatening and dangerous, the self as vulnerable and the future as unpredictable and incontrollable by subjects suffering from anxiety disorders (Beck and

Emery, 1985). In comparison a depression-provoking schema will lead the person to interpret his world as negative, without worth, himself as useless and helpless, and his future as lost or without hope (Blackburn and Davidson, 1990). If cognitive schemas don't change even after psychological treatment, they constitute one of the aspects of the individual's vulnerability towards anxiety or depression (Ingram et al., 1998; Rachman, 1998).

Other forms of cognitions and cognitive processes have also been studied in anxiety disorders. One of them is self-efficacy beliefs, a sort of expectation, that Bandura (1986) conceptualized in his social cognitive model of human behavior. Self-efficacy beliefs reveal the individuals' perception of their capabilities to perform effectively and to achieve specific results.

Table 3. Definitions and examples of the most frequent cognitive distortions (Blackburn, 1992; Blackburn and Davidson, 1990).

Cognitive distortion	Definition	Example
Selective abstraction	To consider only a part of reality to give meaning to a situation. To draw a conclusion only from one or two details (often of poor significance)	Surprised by a difficult question, an orator says to himself " I must really be a bad speaker; he will tell to all others that I'm a stupid man. Then everyone will make fun of me ".
Arbitrary inference	To make conclusions without proof or even to insist upon a conclusion in the presence of contradicting facts	" My boss didn't say anything about my being late with Mr Muller's file, I'm sure he's going to fire me "
Overgeneralisati on	To apply one unique form of reasoning for all possible situations.	" Everyone thinks I'm stupid " " All dogs bite " " Every physical symptom announces a sudden and serious illness "
Minimisation or maximalisation	To evaluate in an erroneous way the intensity or the importance of a reaction/event (exaggeration of suffering and minimalization of success).	" I can't stand it " " Anyone can do what I did "
Personalization	To refer independent events only to oneself; to attribute the cause of an event only to oneself.	" The new supervisor hasn't talked to me yet, I must not be smart enough for her. " " It's my fault if ... "
Dichotomic thought	To interpret situations only in extreme categories (black or white, all or nothing, good or bad) without any possibility of a shade of grey between two opposites	" Either I'm a courageous man who can confront any dangerous situation, or I'm a looser and a coward. " " Either I have success with this woman, or I'll never attract any woman . "

Self-efficacy is a cognition that precedes action, because it influences the choice of an individual to begin or not a particular activity or behavior. If the person thinks 1) that the behavior he wants to adopt will help him to achieve his desired goals (outcome expectations) and 2) that he's able to perform effectively this behavior (personal competence or self-confidence), then he will adopt it. The answers to both questions are naturally dependent on the pursued goals and the current and particular context where the person is (affective state, social and environmental conditions, past history, etc.). But if the individual responds negatively to one of these two questions, the probability that he doesn't behave in this way increases.

According to Bandura's (1986) social cognitive theory, self-efficacy is a key element of to motivation. It is a part of a self system that enables to exercise self-regulation of behaviors, thoughts and feelings. Through this self control system individuals possess the capability to influence their own thoughts and actions. Self-efficacy beliefs influence these motivational and self-regulatory processes in several ways: a) by acting on the choices to do something and to pursue this action, b) by determining how much effort will be expended on an activity, c) by deciding how long an effort will be persevered when obstacles appear. Efficacy beliefs also influence the amount of stress experienced by individuals as they engage in a task. Strong self-efficacy beliefs clearly enhance feelings of personal accomplishment and well-being. On the other hand, people with low self-efficacy may believe that things are more difficult than they really are; a belief that fosters stress and feelings of helplessness. In the case of anxiety, this model is particularly useful to predict if a person will expose himself to his proper fears, and to what extent he will agree to be confronted with his anxiety-provoking situations (Bandura, 1988).

Another important cognitive aspect reported in anxiety concerns the attentional processes. It seems in fact that one can observe during anxious episodes a double movement of attention: 1) a global scanning in search of threatening elements in the environment (vigilance or hypervigilance), 2) during the experience of fear itself, a focalization on what is internally felt (attentional self-focus). These movements of attention favor the development of fear and even panic. Self-focused attention appears indeed as an important maintaining factor in anxiety disorders because it increases access to negative thoughts and feelings, interferes with performance, and prevents the individual from observing external information that might disconfirm his or her fears (Clark and Wells, 1995).

Hypervigilance, by maintaining the organism prepared for danger, favours physiological excitation and cognitive stress. Cognitively, the individual directs his attention toward all potential threats (those of course that depend on his own cognitive schemas, personal phobias, and negative expectations); physiologically his organism is in a state of tension necessary for immediate and rapid action. This state of hypervigilance probably results from a cognitive fear schema (for example: the world is dangerous and I'm vulnerable to any possible attack), as we've seen before in Beck's model. Barlow (1988) proposes to call this type of schema an apprehensive hypervalent cognitive schema which roughly corresponds to the predisposition of an individual to detect in a given situation all sources of negative affect, in order to avoid it. It appears clearly that in this state of cognitive and physiological tension, the occurence of a stress or anxious reaction becomes more probable even in less demanding contexts.

When a stress reaction is started, the focalization on one's internal experience increases this reaction through the salience of perception. Because the person is more concentrated on what's internally happening than on the outside world or on the activity that has to be accomplished, he will be highly receptive to his internal stimuli: consequently the emotional experience is intensified and the habituation to fear stimuli reduced (Scheier, Carver, and

Matthews, 1983). Furthermore, the direct consequence of this dysfunction in attention is a possible reduction in the performance quality during a task, or even its failure: the individual feels paralysed by emotion, he can't find his words, he doesn't remember even obvious things, he can no longer organize or plan out his activity, simple gestures are executed awkwardly, etc. This decline in performance troubles in turn the person who will associate the situation with his anxiety and failure or incompetence. From now on he will fear the return of this emotion that will be equal to him as a return of incompetence. On a long term basis, individuals can abandon their activities because they are afraid of being invaded by anxiety when performing.

Conceptualizations of anxiety have varied and been refined over time. Researchers have elaborated more and more complete models, or have orientated themselves towards different and new or poorly investigated aspects of these disorders. We have described here three or four various learning paradigms and cognitive models which were applied to anxiety. From these multiple visions it is now central to try to find out the essential points that might constitute a global psychological model of anxiety disorders as a basis for the explanations given to patients or to the general public.

1. We can consider fear and anxiety as alarm reactions that are more or less intense. Fear's function is to warn the individual of a danger, and to prepare the organism to affront it or to flee. Because of this, fear is a negative reaction: it is perceived as unpleasant for the individual, and therefore avoided. These alarms can be justified (in front of real danger) or not (in phobias). In this last case, we talk of false alarms, because they don't warn of real dangers. Real or false alarms aren't pathological in themselves. Pathology derives from the fact that these alarms are inadequately and repetitively set off in non threatening situations.
2. People apparently show specific individual predispositions to develop anxious reactions (physiological vulnerability or higher sensitivity to stress, cognitive vulnerability in the form of fear cognitive schemas). According to the "diathesis-stress" model the interaction between personal vulnerability and stress factors can favour the development of anxiety disorders, particularly in contexts when the subject's capacities of adaptation and stress management are overwhelmed.
3. Anxiety disorders most likely result from learning. Initial alarms (real or false) become learned alarms that inappropriately occur in innocuous situations. The origin of the disorder is not always all that clear. One can suppose in some cases that a naturally phobogenic stimulus has favored a conditioning: stimuli that are associated to those that cause the initial reaction of fear can in turn become fear. However it is not always easy to find out what the initial conditioning was and in what context it appeared. In any case, because of the negative value of anxious affect, the individual rapidly learns the behaviors that relieve him from anxiety. These are essentially escape (flight) or avoidance. They are reinforced by their positive consequences on a short term basis (relief from anxiety), but they have a negative effect on a long term basis. Avoidance actually favours the maintaining of anxiety in three ways: 1) it blocks the processes of natural habituation to fear stimuli and to physiological reactions of anxiety, because each time the stimuli are perceived and anxiety is felt, the whole process is stopped by the escape behavior which brutally interrupts the negative emotion, 2) it doesn't permit the individual to have the concrete experience

that the feared situation doesn't contain any real danger, and to thusly modify his internal representations and interpretations, 3) it impedes the development of anxiety management strategies that are more constructive and less handicapping. Therefore flight and avoidance are at the same time natural and automatic behaviors in the face of anxiety, but also big contributors to the processes that maintain anxiety as a pathological state.

4. Different cognitive processes mediate anxiety reactions and can install a vicious cycle of anxious apprehension (Barlow, 1988). The existence of these processes permits to distinguish normal anxiety (where they are absent) from pathological anxiety. Three types of cognition are implied: 1) attentional processes, 2) outcome and self-efficacy expectancies, 3) cognitive schemas and automatic thoughts.

At the attentional level, we first observe hypervigilance in people suffering from anxiety disorders. These subjects are in a state of anxious apprehension that is more or less permanent. Hypervigilance is particularly present in situations where there's a high probability of occurrence of feared events. Attention is focalized here on the external environment, to detect every probable danger, in order to avoid it or to reduce its impact. But in the case where negative affect is set off, attention is then directed toward the internal experience. This in turn increases emotion even more (which therefore favors the escape behavior!). Moreover, the redirection of attention on the internal experience does not allow good task performances because the attentional resources are no longer allocated to the right place. This results in an effective decrease in the quality of activity that in turn plays a role in the subject's interpretation of the situation (lowering of self-esteem, feeling of loss of control, incapacity to face things, negative expectations, etc.). These movements of attentional processes play therefore a role in the vicious circle of anxiety, Fear of failure nourishing avoidance behaviors (which impede habituation to fear and innocuous feared stimuli) is itself justified by real failures due to fear! If this process is highly adaptive in the case of real danger (where failure can mean serious wounds or death), it becomes pathological in phobias by maintaining the fears rather than by diminishing them.

Hypervigilance is naturally concomitant with anticipative thoughts and negative expectations. Anxious expectations tend in their contents to consider the world as threatening and unpredictable and to see the individual as weak and incapable to deal with his problems or to control the course of events. These characteristics of unforeseeability, personal vulnerability and uncontrollability seem by the way to constitute the specific traits that allow distinguishing anxious individuals from others (Barlow, 1988). With negative self-efficacy and outcome expectancies, the individual will be less inclined to begin courageous attempts to confront his feared situations. That maintains him in an avoidant attitude which doesn't allow the reduction of the anxious apprehension process.

These negative expectations have without a doubt their substrate in thought schemas that are profoundly anchored in man's persona. Schemas are beliefs about oneself and the world that act as interpretative filters of reality. They can be activated or not in certain situations through hypothesized associative processes and neurocognitive nodes in the brain. The activation of such cognitive schemas will in difficult situations produce automatic thoughts that provide the individual with a key to immediate interpretation of what's happening. These thoughts guide him toward the attitude to follow. Unfortunately these interpretations are often biased. They communicate a series of cognitive distortions that end up rendering the person weakly adapted and weakly adaptable. Automatic thoughts, congruent with the underlying cognitive beliefs, tend to exaggerate the severity and the dangerousness of the situation and the person's weaknesses in a way that they negatively color affect.

In summary cognitive, behavioral and physiological processes contribute to the maintaining of anxiety. The adaptive reasons are obvious: a habituation that is too rapid and a disinterest in front of real dangers would quickly drive our species toward extinction. We can therefore affirm that the processes in themselves do not allow to judge if anxiety is pathological or not. Anxiety will be considered pathological when it's maintained by the vicious cycle of anxious apprehension favouring the importunate production of anxious episodes in situations that are not dangerous for the person (Barlow, 1988). Pathology therefore lays more in the contents or objects of anxiety, in the suffering and handicap that's follow, than in the implicated psychological processes, which are in a certain sense normal and adaptive but displaced. Changing anxiety reactions apply then to almost identical methods used to modify any old bad habits! We will briefly review in the next section some of the habitual methods employed in the cognitive behavior therapy of anxiety disorders, without entering in the details and the variants developed specifically for every particular disorder.

4. Methods of Intervention in Cognitive-Behavior Therapies for Anxiety

The different facets of anxiety and the processes that are implicated represent as many entry points for therapeutic intervention. In fact, behavioral and cognitive approaches have provided for therapists a large arsenal of methods that aim to modify one or another aspect of the anxious reaction (cf. table 4). Behavioral interventions focus on flight and avoidance behaviors that they attempt to decrease. They favour the development of alternative coping strategies that don't have the disadvantages of flight or avoidance. Cognitive interventions target automatic thoughts and underlying beliefs, attentional processes, and negative expectations. The goal is to aid the patient to regain a certain degree of control on these cognitive processes and positively modify their role in the vicious circle of anxiety. Interventions on a physical level try to reduce the physiological impact of anxious reactions. If he succeeds, the subject will feel to a lesser degree the physical signals of anxiety. He will consequently concentrate his attention less on them, and therefore will not be overwhelmed by the intensity of his emotional reactions. In general, treatment strategies combine various specific techniques.

For example, the emotional reprocessing, which is certainly a central feature of any psychotherapy, is the combination of behavioral and cognitive techniques, because for emotional processing to occur, exposure has to be done with cognitive restructuring that allow the corrective experience necessary for change (Barlow, 1988; Foa and Kozak, 1986; Rachman, 1980). The separation of techniques is relatively artificial; clearly separate categories of interventions are generally made only for pedagogical purposes. In practice the therapists tend to use them conjointly and to integrate them in individualized strategies elaborated for every patient or group of patients.

Table 4. Goals and methods of intervention in behavioral cognitive approach to anxiety.

Dimension	Goal of treatment	Possible interventions
Behavior	To eliminate escape and avoidance behaviors	Exposure with response prevention and development of alternative anxiety management strategies (coping strategies)
Affect	To accept the experience of anxiety and to favour the emotional reprocessing of anxiety	Emotional reprocessing: exposure to the full emotional experience (at all levels: behavioral, cognitive and physiological) that allows the learning of corrective information (especially: anxiety will not last indefinitely, the real probability of harm and danger is low, the emotion itself is not unbearable).
Thought	To reorient attention towards the task	Self-instructions (in the hope of regaining control of attentional processes that guide the reorientation towards the task). Learning and use of problem solving techniques.
	To modify expectations of negative self-efficacy	Discussion and reflection about the relevance of the negative expectations; prospective comparisons between expectations and what really happens; experience of success in difficult situations; observation and imitation of successful models.
	To modify automatic fear thoughts and replace them by more realistic ones	Cognitive restructuration (by Socratic interviewing methods); identification and correction techniques of automatic thoughts ; psychopedagogical intervention.
	To modify the basic cognitive schemas that produce fear automatic thoughts	Cognitive restructuration through Socratic interviews, evaluation of the relevance and the usefulness of different schemas of thought (intervenes later in treatment).
Physical	To reduce the physiological intensity of excitation and stress concomitant with the experience of anxiety	Relaxation, breathing exercises, vaso-vagal techniques for reduction of heart rate, biofeedback.

Paradoxically the first goal of cognitive behavior therapy for anxiety is not the total elimination of any anxiety reaction (that would be catastrophic for the individual's survival). It rather proposes a relearning procedure, where the patient will progressively understand his own emotional functioning, accept it and try to master its different aspects. He will learn to isolate the cognitive and behavioral automatisms that maintain anxiety in inadequate contexts. According to Barlow (1988), three targets are essential to the success of anxiety treatments: 1) the modification of action tendencies associated with anxiety (avoidance, escape, but also hypervigilance), 2) the development of a feeling of control towards the environment (in spite of the presence of emotional signs of anxiety: events are not totally out of control, one can do something active to change the current situation), 3) the reorientation of attentional processes towards the task (instead of maintaining a self-focused attention on the internal experience). Other targets or goals of treatment (such as modification of automatic thoughts or reduction of physiological arousal) appear useful but according to this author remain secondary: these aspects modify themselves when the emotional reprocessing has been successfully done.

4.1. Behavioral Interventions

Methods of behavioral intervention have as a goal to reduce or even eliminate avoidance and escape in situations where they shouldn't be present. This is in fact one if not *the* key points in any anxiety therapy. The principal technique of behavioral intervention is exposure with response prevention. Multiple variants have been developed of which the guiding rule is always the same: "anxiety will decrease if you stay in the innocuous feared situation. If you let yourself completely live the anxious reactions that the situation induces, without turning to avoidance or any safety behaviours, this could reassure you without totally convincing you that the situation and its related anxiety are not dangerous and unbearable".

The efficiency of durable exposure has been understood for a long time through processes of cognitive and physiological habituation or extinction of the anxious response. Figure 3 is often presented to patients as a simple explanatory model and as a justification of the regular practice of this technique.

The model predicts that if the person fully experiences anxiety, without escaping the situation, without being wounded in any way, and becoming more and more aware that the dangers and other catastrophic scenarios are only the products of his imagination, his emotional reaction will tend to disappear with time. It can take hours before the first panic progressively resolves to become a sensation of weak tension, and only the rehearsal of exposure exercises will provide the necessary confidence to approach with tranquillity that which before produced intense fear. The organism gets used to anxiety evoking stimuli just as someone gets used to the noise of a train that regularly goes by their window, to the point where they don't even hear the express rushing by each hour to the next station. As with the train, feared situations (the noise of the trains) attract attention, but little by little the organism recognizes them automatically, concluding that there is no danger, and no longer directs its attention towards them.

After a period of being exposed to feared situations, the individual ends up learning that the negative consequences he feared do not occur. In these conditions, the strength of the link decreases and the stimuli from their anxiety-provoking state return to a sort of neutrality state.

Habituation and extinction are two major facets of the process of anxiety reduction (Barlow, 1988). Habituation refers to the natural reduction of the response's intensity (often measured on a physiological level); it is in relation with biological processes that are controlled on a primary neurological level. Extinction refers to the reduction of the strength of the conditioning when the fear stimuli are not followed by real negative consequences. It is the equivalent of unlearning the link between stimulus and response. In this way, habituation corresponds to a form of exhaustion of the biological response to anxiety, while extinction can happen only if the exposure is not followed by negative consequences (Barlow, 1988).

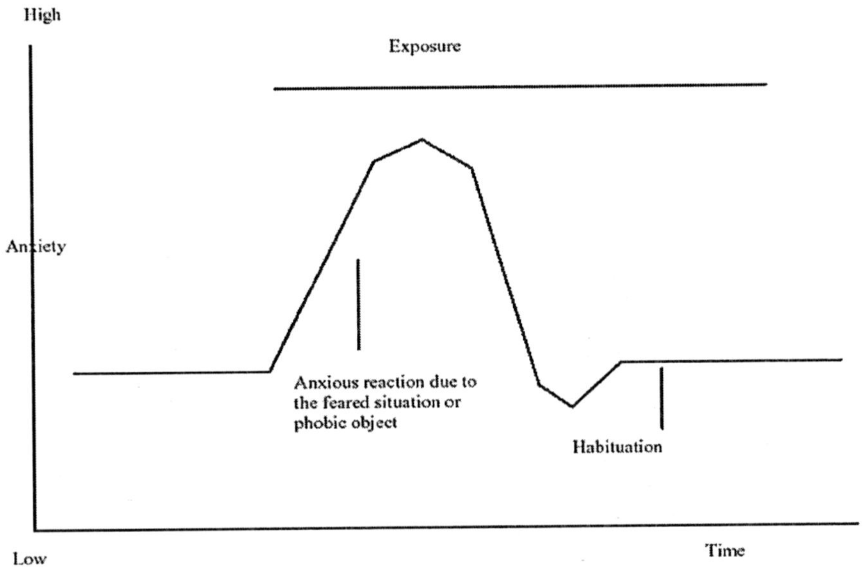

Figure 3. Processes of anxiety and habituation responses in feared situations.

Given this, extinction deals more with cognitive processes while habituation seems rather a physiological phenomenon. With the habituation process, the individual learns that the anxiety response does not indefinitely persist and that it naturally ceases with time, while in extinction he understands that the situation is in reality not dangerous and that therefore the alarm reaction has no reason to be triggered off. A cognitive invalidation of the negative expectations would therefore exist that could mediate the process of anxiety reduction, even if behavioral methods are used as primary therapeutic techniques (Seligman and Johnston, 1973).

Exposure can be gradual or massive, done in imagination or in vivo (Leahy and Holland, 2000; Marks, 1987). Graded exposure is based on a hierarchy of fear stimuli previously established with the patient. It indicates the intensity of the anxiety for each item, ranging from the weakest to the most intense. The person progressively exposes himself to the anxiety-evoking situations, respecting this hierarchy: only when he has successfully mastered the weakly feared items, he then confronts himself with the items that are more delicate to manage. Before he carries out the in-vivo exposure, the person does it in imagination, thinking about the fear stimuli (and not directly confronting them). Once a person is capable of mentally coping without fear with his perilous situations, he will more easily be able to dare to expose himself to the real situations. Massive exposure is a lot more direct and doesn't bother itself with a complicated preparation: the individual is plunged from the beginning into the worst situation for himself and he must face it until habituation occurs. Compared to graded exposure, in vivo massive exposure (flooding) or implosion procedures (massive exposure in imagination) requires more time in the situation, but assuredly shortens the length of therapy. Massive exposure unfortunately presents the major defect of enticing very few patients to adopt it as treatment; the drop out rate in this therapy is significantly higher than the 12% habitually described in graded exposure therapies (Emmelkamp and Wessels, 1975; Jannoun, Munby, Catalan, and Gelder, 1980; Matthews et al., 1976). Furthermore, a brutal change in a person's behavioral habits can directly affect the interactions with the surroundings, bringing the risk of a negative destabilisation for the patient or his family

(Himadi et al., 1986; Peter and Hand, 1988). In most cases and in particular with very anxious patients, the therapist will therefore prefer to adopt a progressive strategy, that is maybe slower, but generally more easily accepted.

Exposure treatments are conducted in four steps. The first consists of a socialization to treatment: the patients are informed about the behavioral model of anxiety where the role of escape/avoidance is especially stressed. The rationale of the exposure therapy is clearly explained and the steps of the treatment described. To help more anxious clients to accept this treatment, the preparatory phase can be extended to the learning of some coping strategies (relaxation training, self-instructions, etc.). Clients can in this way feel more confident to entry the exposure phase of the therapy, which induces often great apprehension.

In the second step, patients create with their therapists a hierarchy of items including the major cues that provoke anxiety. Theses cues are ranked from least to most difficult in an anxiety-scale (in 8 or 10 points, from tranquillity to panic). Habitually lists of 10-15 items are generated with the preoccupation that every point of the anxiety scale corresponds with at least one specific item. If the items are ranked either at the bottom or at the top of the scale graded exposure cannot be easily conducted, because it is impossible to program exposure exercises with a real graduation of the difficulty. This work is also an occasion to identify more precisely the various cues that can produce anxiety and sometimes to deepen the understanding of various facets of the disorder. With flooding strategies (massive exposure), a list of fear stimuli is also collected in order to identify all fear cues and to determine what could be a very difficult exposure situation to confront with. The more massive the exposure is, the more time the therapist must dedicate to it: habitually 40 to 120 minutes are sufficient to complete the procedure, but with massive exposure or with some serious cases (such as obsessive-compulsive disorders) durations can be much longer and last more than 4-5 hours. In this case, graded exposures are often preferred both by patients and by therapists (increasing also compliance to the treatment), because they are less difficult to conduct and are also less time consuming; it is however not proved that they are more effective than massive exposures (Fiegenbaum, 1988).

Thirdly an initial exposure is prepared and worked through during a therapy session. This exposure can be an in vivo exposure or an imaginary exposure (depending on the therapeutic strategy negotiated with the patient). In graded exposure, this step begins with an item that is at the bottom of the list, so that the exercise doesn't trigger too much anxiety. The patients have the opportunity here to make a first positive and successful experience in confronting himself with anxiety. Therapist should be aware that, although the first items are perhaps relatively easy to confront with, anxiety symptoms should appear during exposure and the patients should go through this emotional experience without avoiding it or trying to reassure themselves with any safety signals or behaviors. This is the reason why it is often recommended to cease pharmacological treatment before the exposure intervention: clients should not attribute their successes to the anxiolytic drug or other talismans or hidden self-protection measures… For the first exposure to be a successful experiment, patients should have experienced the increase in anxiety and the habituation process where tension and symptoms progressively decrease (if they not completely disappear). Exposure mustn't be terminated before the entire process of habituation has been completed. The risk is then more the result of a sensitization to anxiety with an avoidance strategy than a real habituation/ extinction process.

Finally the last step consists of the rehearsal of the exposure exercise through the entire hierarchy of items. These repeated exposures are generally done outside the therapy session, as homework done by the patients between sessions. This is then discussed and guided during the encounters with the therapists. Patients normally become more and more independent and autonomous, understanding through their own experiences what works for them in the exposure therapy and how they can use these strategies in other feared situations. Practice of in vivo exposure outside the therapeutic sessions is a key element for the success of the therapy. Habitually at least two to three exposure sessions are programmed with the patients: but the more frequent the exercises are, the more effective and rapid is the therapy. Situational exposures vary in accordance with the anxiety-provoking cues and the diagnostic of the patients. Table 5 describes some of classical exposure exercises for various anxious states.

4.2. Cognitive Interventions

Cognitive interventions can also take multiple forms and be based on various intervention techniques. Beck's approach, most likely the best known, organizes the therapeutic work around automatic thoughts, schemas and cognitive distortions (Beck and Emery, 1985; Beck et al., 1979). Using the Socratic dialogue (Taylor, 2000), the therapist identifies the automatic thoughts and progressively interrogates their logical distortions, before he brings to light the underlying beliefs and discusses their probable origin and their rationality or utility for the current circumstances.

Table 5. Examples of exposure exercises for various types of anxiety disorders.

Anxiety disorder	Exposure exercises
Panic	Running up and down stairs. Turning on a chair to the point of dizziness.
Agoraphobia	Taking the bus from one station to the next. Walking through a supermarket and buying something.
Social phobia	Speaking in a group of persons. Asking for information at a desk.
Obsessive compulsive disorder	Leaving the apartment without verifying if all the lights are switched off. Touching a piece of dirty laundry without washing one's hands.
Post-traumatic stress disorder	Exposure to the memories of the traumatic event (emotional reliving of an accident, a funeral, scenes of violence during childhood). Exposure to objects and situations that are avoided, even if they do not represent any current danger.
Generalized anxiety disorder	Thinking of a problem that happens during a trip (automobile break down). Thinking of losing one's job.

The key message upheld by the therapist is that the catastrophic interpretations of a situation (more than the situation itself) render it unpleasant and worsen the anxiety (Clark, 1986). It is possible through careful discussion about them and through corrective exercises to change the way the patient thinks about his feared situations and consequently to modify his feelings towards and during them. The basic idea of cognitive interventions is to challenge the distorted thoughts and beliefs through discussion or various forms of exercises / experiences, in order to replace them with more realistic and adaptive ones that can relieve from anxiety and give sufficient self-confidence.

Cognitive restructuring follows three to four major steps. Firstly the patient is informed about the assumptions of cognitive therapy through simple examples taken from ordinary life and from his own experiences. Once he is convinced of the link between thoughts and emotions, particularly in the sense that thoughts can influence emotions, the second step consists in identifying the automatic thoughts related to the feared situations. The patient evokes here all the catastrophic interpretations running through his head when he feels anxious or panicky. The therapist tries to discover what the antecedent stimuli are and especially what dangers do they represent for his client. This allows to understand the reasons for fear in the client's mind.

These interpretations are then questioned with the aim to stress the cognitive distortions they manifest. Through logical reasoning, therapist and client should conclude that the thoughts are in fact misinterpretations of the situation, and that they must be corrected, because they induce a lot of suffering and because alternative explanations also exist. The patient learns here to relativize the pertinence of his thoughts. He's invited to systematically ask himself if his anxious thoughts reflect reality or can they be challenged by alternative interpretations that could also correspond to the situation. It is absolutely necessary that the patient is intimately convinced of the logical errors present in his thoughts. He should agree for example with the idea that he exaggerates certain points and minimizes others, that he draws conclusions without veritable proof, or that he filters certain details of a situation to uphold his affirmations while forgetting other elements that could prove the contrary or support a different interpretation. This act of looking for alternative thoughts that are simultaneously more realistic and reassuring has a therapeutic impact by reducing tension and anxiety. But it also favours a sort of metacognitive process, where the patient progressively learns to criticize himself when he observes himself having dysfunctional attitudes. The individual becomes little by little able to identify his dysfunctional thoughts that provoke anxiety. He interiorly discusses them (or puts them on paper), and replaces them with anxiolytic thoughts. Different cognitive procedures exist, more or less standardized and more or less original and creative for realizing this work (McMullin, 2000). As the cognitive intervention progresses, the basic beliefs and the cognitive schemas are identified and discussed. At this point some authors make a distinction between maladaptive assumptions and dysfunctional schemas (Leahy and Holland, 2000). Assumptions are at a deeper level than automatic thoughts but not at the same fundamental level such as the schemas are. Assumptions are often expressed with "if... then..." or "I should..., to..." statements. Schemas or beliefs, as we have already said, represent more basic ideas about oneself, the others and the world. Statements are often affirmative and simple; they do not give rules or guides as the assumptions do. Table 6 gives some examples of automatic thoughts, assumptions and schemas. Such a distinction is however not always easy to grasp by patients (and sometimes by the therapist too!). It is our opinion that this distinction is not of fundamental importance for the success of the therapy. It seems nevertheless clear that the work on beliefs is very useful to favour a more fundamental change (helping perhaps by relapse prevention and self-management) that the transitory learning of compensatory coping strategies cannot do.

Table 6. Automatic thoughts, maladaptive assumptions and dysfunctional schemas by various types of anxiety disorders.

Fear stimulus (activating event)	Automatic thought	Maladaptive assumption	Dysfunctional schemas
Panic she feels a slight sensation of dizziness while she is standing in line at a supermarket checkout	Here we go again! I need to go out immediately or I'll go insane.	If I don't control my anxiety, I will become psychotic and finish my life at the asylum.	The frontier between normality and madness is really tenuous.
Agoraphobia she's coming in the store	People see that I don't feel good.	I should never be weak, especially in normal situations such as going out to do some shopping.	People make fun of the ones that are weak.
Social phobia a man remains indifferent to her	He doesn't like me.	If I'm not an attractive woman for the men around me, I will remain alone.	I'm an unlovable woman.
Obsessive-compulsive disorder in front of a door of the medical office	Someone ill could have touched this door.	I should protect myself perfectly from any germ, especially AIDS, or I will die.	The world is full of invisible dangers. I could be very easily be contaminated by AIDS viruses.
Post-traumatic stress disorder image of one's dead son in a car accident	I'm guilty; I should be dead instead of my son.	I cannot be happy again without my son.	A guilty man must pay for his errors.
Generalized anxiety disorder before a dinner she's organizing	Everything will go wrong.	If I'm not completely prepared, I will fail.	I'm incompetent.

With the modification of basic dysfunctional schemas, the individual certainly reduces his psychological vulnerability to anxiety and regains the necessary self-confidence to manage better stressful events and to maintain control over his physiological and emotional responses. Numerous books display lists of distorted thoughts, categories of logical distortions, and frequent or typical dysfunctional beliefs (Andrews et al., 2002; Babior and Goldman, 1997; Kozak and Foa, 1997; Leahy and Holland, 2000; White, 1999). Such books propose various targeted cognitive exercises too, which help the reader to modify his cognitive habits. They can be used as self-management guides for therapy or as a bibliotherapy tool completing the work done in sessions with a psychotherapist.

Other cognitive approaches appear more directive than cognitive restructuring. They propose one or another type of cognitive anxiety management methods to the client, by inviting him to take control again of his attentional and cognitive processes. These methods are essentially based on self-instructions, mental training and problem-solving skills. They are often elaborated and exercised in the office with the client before they are used in reality, during exposure exercises or during problematic situations. Table 7 summarizes such mental instructions, derived from the stress inoculation training method (Meichenbaum, 1977; Meichenbaum and Turk, 1976) that aims to improve the way one copes with one's anxiety.

Table 7. Self-Instructions Used to Cope with Anxiety-Inducing Situations.

1. Preparation
What do I have to do?
I can prepare a plan of action.
I can succeed.
No negative comments! Think in a rational manner!
It is useless to worry too much. Worry will not improve anything; on the contrary it will worsen my present state.
Remember that avoiding fear only worsens it!
Don't do more or less than you've planned to do: it has to be a little difficult but not too much. It can't be too easy either; otherwise I won't make any progress.
I know I can do it, even if maybe it won't be perfect: what counts is that I do it.
2. Confrontation (exposure)
One step at a time, I'm putting myself to the test.
Try to not think too much about fear. It's better to concentrate on what you have to do.
Stay in contact with reality, don't close up on yourself.
What do you see around you? Is it really dangerous for you?
I can manage the situation; I am able, even if I feel intense fear.
3. Management of negative feelings
I can take a break if I feel too scared. But I mustn't leave the situation.
Remember what the therapist said: fear is nothing other than an emotion like any other, maybe more unpleasant, but certainly not unbearable or mortal. This is not the worst thing that can happen to me.
If I stay long enough in this situation, anxiety will go down. I will have won my bet and succeeded at my challenge.
If I evaluate my fear on a scale from 0 to 10. Where am I at now? Has it gone up or gone down? Why? Anyway, once 10 is reached my fear can't go any higher.
4. Reinforcements
Ok, well done. You did well. You're a champion!
It wasn't as bad as I thought it was going to be. I can do positive things even if I'm scared.
Was it really worth it to make such a fuss for this fear?
This experience will help me a lot for the future. Now I've understood that fear decreases with time as long as I stay in the situation.
The more I repeat this type of exercise, the better things will get.

Stress inoculation training takes place in three phases (Meichenbaum, 1996). 1) In the first phase (conceptualization phase) pedagogical work is done with the patient, during which he broadens his knowledge about fear and elaborates his own model in accounting for the specificity of his personal anxious problems. During the exchanges with his therapist, the patient is gently encouraged to view his fears and their triggering events as problems to be solved and not as unchangeable fatalistic events. 2) In the training phase the patient learns various methods of anxiety management: relaxation or breathing techniques, self-instructions, emotional self-soothing techniques, problem solving, interpersonal communication skills, etc. He also learns to use these different methods by applying them mentally (for example by imagining that he is going through the stressful situation) or even by facing minor problems that are treatable in the therapist's office. The in-vivo training is gently introduced and tailored to the current competencies. 3) In the last phase (application phase), various opportunities to apply the new skills in real situations are searched for, according to a program which takes into account a gradually increasing level of skills needed to manage the situation. Personal experiments are carefully designed and prepared in order to be successfully coped with by the patient. Rehearsal, generalization procedures and relapse prevention interventions are also included in this phase. Stress inoculation training aims at providing the patient with an accessible and mastered repertoire of cognitive and behavioral skills that help him to cope with either various types of stressors or a particular specific difficulty.

4.3. Interventions at Physical Level

Methods of intervention acting on a physical and physiological level complete behavioral and cognitive methods. These methods are employed essentially for counteracting the physiological responses of anxiety. They provide the patients with simple and portable coping strategies to rapidly reduce or control tension and other physical symptoms. Diverse relaxation techniques can be applied. Passive methods, for example Schultz' autogenic training (Luthe and Schultz, 1969), often necessitate a quiet place, lying down or being seated, and generally require an auditory support that is verbal or musical. The individual is placed in a comfortable position and attentively listens to the therapist's instructions, with a soft agreeable music in the background. Progressively he will attain a state of tranquillity and relaxation, by simply following the given suggestions (for example "your arms become heavy and warm", "your body attains a state of relaxation", "the wrinkles on your forehead disappear", etc.). It is not even a rare event that the subject falls asleep when practising relaxation: in this case, the objective of total relaxation is perhaps certainly reached but it is then difficult to work with the person!

Active relaxation methods are at less risk of putting clients to sleep and are less demanding concerning the context: they can be practised virtually anywhere and at any time. In these methods, of which Jacobson's progressive method (1938) is a famous prototype, the individual learns to feel sensations of relaxation by differentiating them from feelings of tension (Barlow and Cerny, 1988; Leahy and Holland, 2000; Öst, 1987). The following sequence is habitually applied to various muscular groups: 1) during a few seconds the patient contracts as hard as possible the concerned group of muscles (for example: the hand, the forearm, the shoulders, etc.), 2) he releases the contracted muscles so that they loosen up progressively; during this phase he focuses his attention during 10 to 20 seconds on the physical sensations that emerge. Afterwards he can take a pause with a deep sigh, before repeating the sequence on the same or on another group of muscles. Specific movements are proposed in order to allow the individual to correctly contract the muscular group that he's working on: for example squeezing one's fist, shrugging one's shoulders, pushing one's tongue against the palate, etc. Once the patient has understood the different exercises and correctly recognizes the sensation of relaxation, he can simply associate these sensations to a word (for example "relax", "calm", etc.). This last phase is called the cue controlled relaxation, because the releasing of the muscles is associated with a particular cue (in this case a word). Through conditioning, these words will be able by themselves to set off calming reactions that were previously attained through the tension-relaxation exercises. Leahy and Holland (2000) propose for example a six-steps relaxation technique that brings the patients from a global relaxation to more focused relaxation and finally to a cue controlled relaxation (table 8).

Table 8. Six-Steps Relaxation Procedure For Coping With Anxiety and Tension (Leahy and Holland, 2000).

Step	Exercise
Twelve-muscle-group-relaxation	Application of the tense-relax technique to 12 groups of muscles: 1) lower arms, b) upper arms, 3) lower legs, 4) thighs, 5) stomach, 6) upper chest and back, 7) shoulders, 8) back of the necks, 9) lips, 10) eyes, 11) eyebrows, 12) upper forehead and scalp. The tense-relax technique follow this sequence: a) let the patient focus on breathing during two or three breaths; b) let tense a group of muscles during 5 seconds (counting from 1 to 5 is possible; it helps patients and therapists to give the rhythm of the exercise); c) let release the muscles and focus during 15-20 seconds on the sensations in these muscles (with helping instructions); d) repeat the procedure a-c for all groups of muscles; e) count down from 5 to 1 and give for every number a new relaxation suggestion; f) focus on breathing during 1 minute; g) count up from 1 to 5 while inviting the client to become alert again; h) let practice at home 2 times a day during 1-2 weeks (with and without audiotaped instructions).
Eight-muscle-group-relaxation	Same tense-relax procedure but limited to the eight following groups of muscles:1) whole arms, 2) whole legs, 3) stomach, 4) upper chest and back, 5) shoulders, 6) back of the neck, 7) face, 8) forehead and scalp. Time of the releasing period should be increased to at least 30 seconds.
Four-muscle-group-relaxation	Same tense-relax procedure but limited to only four groups of muscles: 1) whole arms, 2) upper chest and back, 3) shoulders and neck, 4) face. Vary the positions and the settings for the practice (waiting for the bus, during a pause at the office, walking, etc.).
Release-only relaxation	Relaxation of the same four-muscle-group as in the precedent step, but without the phase of tension: a) let the patient focus on one group of muscles (with noticing any tension), b) let the patient recall the sensation of relaxation and then release the tension (during 30-45 seconds), c) if the tension is totally absent, proceed to the next group of muscles, d) when the person is fully relaxed, proceed as usual with the counting down and counting up procedure.
Cue controlled relaxation	1. Application of the release-only relaxation When relaxed let the patient take deep breaths and say "relax" at each exhalation while releasing any tension that could be detected. 2. Application of the breathing and saying "relax" phase without the release-only procedure. 3. Application of the cue controlled relaxation 10-15 times each day
Practice in stressful situations	Apply the relaxation technique in more and more stressful situations, especially when first signs of anxiety appear.

Relaxation methods are very useful and often highly appreciated. They frequently improve the sensation of well-being. Nevertheless they require rigorous training during 2 to 4 weeks, before being able to self-control them and to benefit fully from their effects. Some patients are incapable, especially in a state of anxiety or in crisis situations, of learning or practising them. It is not rare to observe that relaxation techniques even have a paradoxical effect by inducing anxiety in patients who practise it (Heide and Borkevec, 1984). This is why briefer methods, that are simpler forms of relaxation, have been proposed as a physical adjuvant to the management of anxiety. We can mention here in particular different breathing methods and vaso-vagal techniques that permit to lower heart-rate (Bannister, 1983; Satory and Olajide, 1988). The individual can in this way control the frequency and amplitude of his breathing: he can thusly learn to regulate its frequency (by counting for example from 1 to 3 at each inspiration and each expiration), to block it a few seconds after inspiration, or to find an agreeable rhythm (Leahy and Holland, 2000). It is important here to make a clear understandable difference between "chest breathing" and "diaphragm breathing" and to help the patient to learn a diaphragmatic breathing (Taylor, 2000).

5. Effectiveness of Cognitive-Behavioral Treatements: A Brief Overview

Cognitive behavior therapies have achieved very good results in controlled outcome studies. Numerous literature reviews and meta-analyses have synthesized a large amount of studies. Specific phobias were historically the first disorders that behavioral therapies treated. The results have always been positive and encouraging: exposure to phobic stimuli (with the corresponding processes of habituation and extinction) has been widely demonstrated as an effective way to reduce such phobias (Andrews et al., 2002). A debate has been devoted to the question of the usefulness of cognitive elements in therapy. Do they improve the results of the behavioral interventions? No definitive answer can be made, because some empirical results have contradicted this view, while the theoretical model and some other studies have tended to support it (Andrews, 2002; Beck et al., 1985).

For panic and agoraphobia the meta-analytic reviews conclude that cognitive behavior therapies are well tolerated, moderately to highly effective, and certainly represent the most effective treatment amongst psychological interventions (Taylor, 2000). However other psychotherapies seem to have been insufficiently studied to seriously conclude to the superiority of cognitive behavior therapy for panic disorder and agoraphobia. But in the current situation of incomplete knowledge about the effectiveness of other forms of psychotherapy, cognitive behavioral treatment appears as the treatment of choice for these syndromes. This is particularly true for new treatment packages specifically designed for panic disorder and agoraphobia (often called the second generation of cognitive behavior therapy or CBT2). Such therapeutic programs focus their interventions on the panic processes, by correcting the cognitive catastrophic misinterpretations of internal stimuli and by offering exposure to body sensations rather than exposure to external fear stimuli (Barlow and Cerny, 1988; Clark and Salkovskis, 1987; Craske, Meadows and Barlow, 1994). Chambless and Gillis (1993, 1994) find in their meta-analytic study that such treatment packages have lower attrition rates (8%) than applied relaxation alone (12%) or in-vivo exposure alone (16%). Moreover, 88% patients having had CBT2 were free of panic at the end of treatment (61% for applied relaxation group, 54% for the exposure group and 12% for the waiting list group). In comparison with pharmacological treatments, CBT2 interventions do not clearly appear superior at posttreatement, but their strength lies in the long-term effects. In fact long-term follow-up studies (from 2 to 6 years) show that exposure treatments and cognitive-behavior therapies of the second generation maintain their gains through the time and are thus likely to be more effective than short-term pharmacotherapies (Taylor, 2000). These results are easy to interpret: psychological treatment favours cognitive and emotional restructuring and give coping strategies and management techniques that medication cannot offer! If drug treatment is conducted without these psychological adjuvants, nothing is learned by the patient, and the emotional problems are more likely to reappear once the pharmacological intervention is stopped.

For social phobics, cognitive behavior therapies have proved also to be superior to placebo treatments or waiting lists. Combined treatments including cognitive interventions and subject's exposure to social situations with social skills training seem to be more effective than treatment offering only isolated components (Taylor, 1996), especially if the outcome at follow-up (3 to 6 months) is taken into consideration. Few studies have assessed the impact of cognitive behavior therapy on a long-term basis. Heimberg and colleagues reported at 4.5 to 6.5 years after treatment, superior results for cognitive behavior interventions in comparison with a therapeutic package composed by education and supportive psychotherapy (Heimberg, Dodge, Hope, Kennedy, and Zollo, 1990; Heimberg, Salzman, Holt, and Blendell, 1993). The group format can be preferred to individual therapy: the group itself realizes an intrinsic exposure to social contacts. Such an exposure is not always easy to create, because of the often unexpected or brief nature of social situations and interpersonal interactions (Butler, 1989): the group situation therefore appears as a good opportunity to do it. However there is no definitive scientific evidence that the group format results in better outcomes than the individual format (Gould, Buckminster, Pollack, Otto, and Yap, 1997). Needless to say that the economic and intrinsic advantages of the group format habitually make the therapists prefer it.

There is again wide agreement that cognitive behavior therapies provide substantial relief and clinically and statistically significant improvement for patients suffering from generalized anxiety disorders (Borkovec and Whisman, 1996; Fisher and Durham, 1999; Gould, Otto, Pollack, and Yap, 1997). This active approach is clearly superior to non treatment conditions and to nondirective therapies (Durham, Fisher, Treliving, Hau, Richard, and Stewart, 1999; Durham, Murphy, Allan, Richard, Treliving, and Fenton, 1994). Cognitive interventions aim for better tolerance of uncertainty and the correction of erroneous beliefs about worry or cognitive avoidance while behavioral techniques use in particular relaxation methods and problem solving skills training. Both methods have proved to be effective (Borkovec and Costello, 1993; Ladouceur, Dugas, Freeston, Léger, Gagnon, and Thibodeau, 2000; Öst and Breitholtz, 2000). As with specific phobias or social phobias, the debate about the question of the active components of the therapy, here expressed in the comparison between relaxation procedures and cognitive behavioral oriented programs, remains open. If for theoretical reasons cognitive behavior therapies seem to be preferred to purely behavioral interventions, empirical evidence doesn't support such an affirmation (Andrews et al., 2002). Data are nevertheless lacking that could allow to pose a clear differential indication for every sort of treatment.

Various treatment options can be offered to patients suffering from post-traumatic stress disorder. These options combine cognitive and behavioral components in various ways, stressing on anxiety management techniques, exposure to traumatic memories or cognitive restructuring. Anxiety management techniques are mostly derived from the Stress Inoculation Training (Meichenbaum, 1985): they try to provide the patients with coping strategies for the physical (relaxation and breathing training), behavioral (various skills training to improve assertiveness and to help patients to resume the disrupted daily activities) and cognitive domains (such as thought stopping or distraction techniques to gain control over unexpected and distressing memories). Prolonged exposure treatments have been demonstrated in controlled trials as marginally superior to anxiety management programs, especially at follow-up measures (12 months), with around 60% of improvement in severity of the disorder for (Foa, Dancu, Hembree, Jaycox, Meadows, and Street, 1999, Foa, Rothbaum, Riggs, and Murdock, 1991). Resick and Schnicke (1993) have proposed and evaluated a more cognitive oriented therapy, called Cognitive Processing Therapy: cognitive restructuring techniques focus on five primary themes in post-traumatic stress problems: safety, trust, power, self-esteem and intimacy. Results are encouraging (with 40-55% improvement at post-treatment), but perhaps not as effective as exposure treatments, where very good results have been more recently found with improvement rates varying between 65 to 80% (Resick, and Schnicke, 1992; Richards, Lovell and Marks, 1994; Thompson, Charlton, Kerry, and Lee, 1995). Controlled studies have then provided favourable results for the cognitive behavioral treatment of post-traumatic stress disorder. However it appears relatively difficult to differentiate between programs, because studies did not always have targeted the same population (i.e. suffering from similar traumatic events). As a rule of thumb, Andrews et al. (2002) propose that cognitive behavior therapy for post-traumatic stress disorder improves around two thirds of the patients, with 30% doing very well after a follow-up period of one year.

Behavioral therapies based on the prolonged exposure to obsessional cues with response prevention of the rituals have been largely documented and considered as the recommended treatment for obsessive compulsive disorders. One can expect at posttreatment until 60% to 70% of improvement in the severity of rituals by half the patients who complete the treatment (Foa, Steketee, and Ozarow, 1985). We can expect improvements to be maintained at 3 years, with an approximate dropout rate of 10%: in a follow-up study 78% of the patients who completed the treatment remained improved after a period of 3 years, with an average of 60% of improvement in the targeted rituals (O'Sullivan, Noshirvani, Marks, Montiero, and Lelliot, 1991). However we have to keep in mind that around a quarter of patients may refuse treatment, because of time commitment and fear of being confronted to obsessions without being able to cope with anxiety (Greist, 1998). Motivational adjunctions and carefully elaborated hierarchies of cues can overcome the problem of accepting the treatment, but they increase the treatment duration. Cognitive procedures have also been under empirical investigation. Van Oppen and colleagues found for example that cognitive therapy and self-controlled exposure led to similar results: significant improvements were observed in both groups, with perhaps a tendency to do better by the cognitive intervention group (van Oppen, de Haan, van Balkom, Spinhoven, Hoogduin, and van Dyck, 1995). Finally psychosocial therapies including cognitive-behavioral interventions and pharmacotherapy are also considered by clinicians as a good treatment strategy, because of probable synergetic effects of medication and psychological interventions for the symptom reduction and the relapse prevention. However there aren't any definitive results about a possible additive effect: current studies indicate that both strategies are equally effective but that the combination of the two does not significantly improve the results of the therapies alone (Kobak, Greist, Jeffersen, Katzelnick, and Henk, 1998). Therefore the choice of a treatment remains clearly in the hands of the therapists (and theirs clients) who have access to cognitive, behavioral and pharmacological interventions in order to administer the different therapies they propose to their patients.

CONCLUSION

Fear is a central feature in human emotional life and this emotional state is perfectly normal. The psychophysiological process of anxiety tends naturally to maintain this emotion through avoidance mechanisms that reinforce it. The mechanisms of fear are particularly efficient in the case of real danger, because they help the organism to be rapidly prepared and immediately react in front of a real danger. Fear becomes pathological when it appears in non dangerous situations, when it is maintained by these normal psycho-biological mechanisms, impeding the person the overcome his emotions, and creating suffering and handicaps that can be invasive and insuperable.

The cognitive-behavioral models of fear and anxiety disorders are based on the classical syndromes described by international classifications of psychiatric disorders, such as the DSM-IV or the ICD-10. Using learning paradigms (associative learning and operant conditioning) they stress the role of the environmental and the behavioral components of the fear process: they show how association between fear and situations can transform neutral stimuli in anxiety-provoking stimuli; they also show how escape and avoidance behaviors reinforce the anxiety response. The cognitive part of these models stresses the role of efficacy and outcome expectancies in the behavioural choices, the impact of the attentional processes in the anxiety response, and the link between automatic distorted thoughts, their underlying beliefs and the emotions they can trigger.

These theoretical models, issued essentially from experimental psychology, social psychology and neuropsychology, have provided new insights of the phenomenon and have brought new ideas for treatment methods. Today, therapists have a relatively vast arsenal of intervention methods. Techniques of cognitive behavior therapy can be classified in three broad categories: 1) behavioral interventions which essentially include exposure with response prevention techniques, 2) cognitive interventions which can be subdivided in cognitive restructuring (working on automatic thoughts and underlying beliefs), self-instructional training (to modify coping strategies and attentional processes), and working on self-efficacy expectancies, 3) physical interventions such as breathing retraining or relaxation methods. Currently, treatments for anxiety rarely use in fact one type of intervention at a time. They rather combine diverse ingredients. It is up to the therapist to adjust as well as possible these diverse interventions to the characteristics of the patient and to formulate a pertinent and efficient sequence therapeutic strategy.

Therapeutic plans usually align themselves with the following structure (according to Andrews et al., 2002; Barlow and Cerny, 1988; Leahy and Holland, 2000): 1) investigation and assessment (including diagnostic, functional analysis of fear □gimuli, behaviors, affect, cognitions, and consequences), 2) information about the disorder and its treatment, 3) proposal of treatment, 4) application of treatment (where its components are defined in phase 3), 5) evaluation of the efficiency of the interventions, 6) end of treatment (with work on relapse prevention, eventual "booster" sessions, and final evaluation). From now on the models of the general conception of anxiety and the intervention methods can be adapted to each specific anxiety disorder, with the goal of ameliorating their pertinence and efficiency.

Numerous manuals and self-help books have been edited to aid therapists and patients to structure their therapy (Andrews et al., 2002; Babior and Goldman, 1997; Barlow and Cerny, 1988; Kozak and Foa, 1997; Leahy and Holland, 2000; White, 1999). They generally present the current models of anxiety in a didactical way, often with simple words so that anyone can understand the theoretical background of the therapy. With this in mind, they display tables with lists of symptoms, avoidance behaviours, distorted thoughts, their related categories of logical distortions, and classical dysfunctional beliefs. Therapeutic interventions are described step by step, and various charts, diagrams and working sheets complete these descriptions and give to the reader all that is necessary to begin self-therapy.

In more classical psychotherapy, the therapist guides his patient during the treatment process. He helps to diagnose the anxiety disorder; he elaborates with his client the therapeutic hypothesis and proposes what could be the treatment of choice for him. In behavioral and physical interventions the therapist adopts the role of a coach training his client in correctly making the exposure and in adequately learning the relaxation method. In cognitive interventions, he appears more as a gentle conversation companion, bringing to light the relationships between thoughts and emotions, and questioning the relevance of some automatic thoughts and beliefs. He never imposes his modes of thinking; he rather helps his client to discover new beliefs that appear more appropriate to him. He functions like a philosophical guide, searching more, like Socrates, to reflect upon thought processes that intervene in the anxiety problem, instead of giving recipes for positively thinking. This humble attitude of collaboration that characterizes the cognitive-behavior therapist isn't the only attitude he adopts. In fact, in order to correctly achieve his work he must equally present–beyond his qualities of listening, collaboration, warmth, empathy and flexibility–a professional attitude. He has to show his mastering of the theoretical knowledge and techniques in the pathologies he treats, and his capacity to structure a treatment in a coherent way, for an individual session as well as for the length of an entire treatment (Blackburn and Davidson, 1980).

If most of the anxiety disorders can be treated with cognitive behavior therapies with reasonable positive expectancies regarding the outcome, some limitations have to be mentioned here.

First of all, we need more long-term outcome studies that prove permanent achievement of the gains years after the treatment. The aim of the cognitive behavior therapy is to develop self-management skills by the patients, so that they can use in the future what they have learned in therapy to prevent the relapse or the recurrence of the disorders. If relapse is impossible to avoid, previous therapies should lead the patients to need less therapy and professional help in this occasion. Such results still have to be demonstrated.

Secondly, we need to better our knowledge of what the really the active components of treatment are. Today the comparisons between cognitive and behavioral interventions have not allowed clinicians to reach any definitive conclusion in this debate: often isolated elements are equally effective, and the combination of therapies does not always prove to be better than the interventions alone.

Thirdly, we also need more results about the outcome of other forms of therapy for anxiety disorders. Only pharmacological and cognitive behavioral treatments have been scientifically studied. That's also the reason why they are the treatments of choice today in modern psychiatry. Nevertheless a panacea does not exist for the treatment of anxiety disorders. Cognitive behavior therapies are surely the current treatments of choice, but progress can still be made to improve not only the clinical outcomes for patients, but also the theoretical knowledge about this central emotion in the life of human beings.

REFERENCES

American Psychiatric Association. (1994). *Diagnostic and Statistical Manual of Mental Disorders (4th edition).* Washington DC: Author.

Andrews, G., Creamer, M., Crino, R., Hunt, C., Lampe, L., and Page, A. (2002). *The treatment of anxiety disorders. Clinician guides and patient manuals.* Cambridge: Cambridge University Press.

Babior, S., and Goldman, C. (1997). *A 10-week recovery program for overcoming panic, anxiety and phobias.* La Jolla, CA: Whole Person Press.

Bandura, A. (1977). *Social learning theory.* New York: Prentice-Hall.

Bandura, A. (1986). *Social foundations of thought and action. A social cognitive theory.* Englewood Cliffs, NJ: Prentice-Hall.

Bandura, A. (1988). Self-efficacy conception of anxiety. *Anxiety research, 1*(2), 77-98.

Bannister, R. (1983). *Autonomic failure.* Oxford: Oxford University Press.

Barlow, D. H. (1988). *Anxiety and its disorders. The nature and treatment of anxiety and panic.* New York, NY: The Guilford Press.

Barlow, D. H., and Cerny, J. A. (1988). *Psychological treatment of panic.* New York, NY: The Guilford Press.

Beck, A. T., and Emery, G. (1985). *Anxiety disorders and phobias: a cognitive perspective.* New York: Basic Books.

Beck, A. T., Rush, J., Shaw, B., and Emery, G. (1979). *Cognitive therapy of depression.* New York: Guilford Press.

Bijl, R. V., Ravelli, A., and van Zessen, G. (1998). Prevalence of psychiatric disorder in the general population: results of The Netherlands Mental Health Survey and Incidence Study (NEMESIS). *Social Psychiatry and Psychiatric Epidemiology, 33*(12), 587-595.

Blackburn, I.-M. (1992). *Coping with depression* (reprinted ed.). Edinburgh: Chambers.

Blackburn, I.-M., and Davidson, K. (1990). *Cognitive therapy for depression and anxiety.* Oxford: Blackwell Scientific Publications.

Borkovec, T. D., and Whisman, M. A. (1996). Psychosocial treatment for generalized anxiety disorder. In M. R. Mavissakalian and R. F. Prien (Eds.), *Long-term treatments of anxiety disorders* (pp. 171-199). Washington, DC: American Psychiatric Press.

Brown, T. A., DiNardo, P., and Barlow, D. H. (1994). *ADIS - Anxiety Disorders Interview Schedule for DSM IV. Adult and Lifetime combination kit.* Boulder, CO: Graywind Publications Incorporated.

Brown, T. A., Marten, P. A., and Barlow, D. H. (1995). Discriminant validity of the symptoms constituting the DSM-III-R an DSM-IV associated symptoms criterion of generalized anxiety disorder. *Journal of Anxiety Disorders, 9*, 317-328.

Butler, G. (1989). Issues in the application of cognitive and behavioral strategies in the treatement of social phobia. *Clinical Psychology Review, 9*, 91-106.

Chambless, D. L., and Gillis, M. M. (1993). Cognitive therapy of anxiety disorders. *Journal of Consulting and Clinical Psychology, 61*, 248-260.

Chambless, D. L., and Gillis, M. M. (1994). A review of psychosocial treatments for panic disorder. In B. E. Wolfe and M. J. D. (Eds.), *Treatment of panic disorder: a consensus development conference* (pp. 149-173). Washington, DC: American Psychiatric Press.

Clark, D. M. (1986). A cognitive approach to panic. *Behavior Research and Therapy, 24*(4), 461-470.

Clark, D. A., and Salkovskis, P. M. (1987). *Cognitive therapy for panic attacks: therapist's manual*. Oxford: Departement of Psychiatry, University of Oxford.

Clark, D.M., and Wells, A. (1995) A cognitive model of social phobia. In R.G. Heimberg, M. Liebowitz, D. Hope, and F. Scheier (Eds) *Social Phobia: Diagnosis, Assessment, and Treatment* (pp 69-93). New York: The Guilford Press.

Connor-Smith, J. K., and Compas, B. E. (2002). Vulnerability to social stress: Coping as a mediator or moderator of sociotropy and symptoms of anxiety and depression. *Cognitive Therapy and Research, 26*(1), 39-55.

Craske, M. G., Meadows, E. A., and Barlow, D. H. (1994). *Mastery of you anxiety and panic II and agoraphobia supplement: therapist guide*. San Antonio, TX: Psychological Corporation.

Durham, R. C., Fisher, P. L., Treliving, L. R., Hau, C. M., Richard, K., and Stewart, J. B. (1999). One year follow-up of cognitive therapy, analytic psychotherapy and anxiety management training for generalized anxiety disorder: Symptom change, medication usage and attitudes to treatment. *Behavioural and Cognitive Psychotherapy, 27*(1), 19-35.

Durham, R. C., Murphy, T., Allan, T., Richard, K., Treliving, L. R., and Fenton, G. W. (1994). Cognitive therapy, analytic psychotherapy and anxiety management training for generalised anxiety disorder. *British Journal of Psychiatry, 36*, 101-119.

Ekman, P. (1994). *The nature of emotion: fundamental questions*. New York: Oxford University Press.

Emmelkamp, P. M. E., and Wessels, D. H. (1975). Flooding in imgination vs flooding in vivo: a comparision with agoraphobics. *Behavior Research and Therapy, 13*, 7-15.

Fiegenbaum, W. (1988). Long-term efficacy of ungraded versus graded massed exposure in agoraphobics. In I. Hand and H. U. Wittchen (Eds.), *Panic and phobias. Treatments and variables affecting course and outcome* (pp. 83-88). Berlin: Springer-Verlag.

Fisher, P. L., and Durham, R. C. (1999). Recovery rates in generalized anxiety disorders following psychological therapy: an analysis of clinically significant change in the STAI-T across outcome studies since 1990. *Psychological Medicine, 29*, 1425-1434.

Foa, E. B., Dancu, C. V., Hembree, E. A., Jaycox, L. H., Meadows, E. A., and Street, G. P. (1999). A comparison of exposure therapy, stress inoculation training, and their combination for reducing posttraumatic stress disorder in female assault victims. *Journal of Consulting and Clinical Psychology, 67*(2), 194-200.

Foa, E., and Kozak, M. J. (1986). Emotional processing of fear: exposure to corrective information. *Psychological Bulletin, 99*, 20-35.

Foa, E. B., Rothbaum, B. O., Riggs, D. S., and Murdock, T. B. (1991). Treatment of posttraumatic stress disorder in rape victims: a comparison between cognitive-behavioral procedures and counseling. *Journal of Consulting and Clinical Psychology, 59*(5), 715-723.

Foa, E. B., Steketee, G. S., and Ozarow, B. J. (1985). Behaviour therapy with obsessive-compulsives: from therapy to treatment. In M. Mavissakalian and S. M. Turner and M. Michelsen (Eds.), *Obsessive-compulsive disorder: psychological and pharmacological treatments*. New York: Plenum Press.

Friedman, E. S., Clark, D. B., and Gershon, S. (1992). Stress, anxiety, and depression: Review of biological, diagnostic, and nosologic issues. *Journal of Anxiety Disorders, 6*(4), 337-363.

Goldberg, D. P., and Lecrubier, Y. (1995). Form and frequency of mental disorders across centres. In T. B. Ustun and N. Sartorius (Eds.), *Mental illness in general health care: An international study* (pp. 323–334). New York: John Wiley and Sons.

Gould, R. A., Buckminster, S., Pollack, M. H., Otto, M. W., and Yap, L. (1997). Cognitive-behavioral and pharmacological treatment for social phobia: A meta-analysis. *Clinical Psychology Science and Practice, 4*(4), 291-306.

Gould, R. A., Otto, M. W., Pollack, M. H., and Yap, L. (1997). Cognitive behavioral and pharmacological treatment of generalized anxiety disorder: A preliminary meta-analyis. *Behavior Therapy, 28*(2), 285-305.

Grawe, K., Donati, R., and Bernauer, F. (1994). *Psychotherapie im Wandel. Von der Konfession zur Profession*. Bern: Hogrefe.

Gray, J. A. (1991). *The Psychology of fear and stress* (2th ed. reprinted with corrections ed.). Cambridge: Cambridge University Press.

Greist, J. H. (1998). The comparative effectiveness of treatments for obsessive-compulsive disorder. *Bulletin of the Menninger Clinic, 62*(suppl. A), A65-A81.

Heide, F. J., and Borkovec, T. D. (1984). Relaxation-induced anxiety: Mechanisms and theoretical implications. *Behavior Research and Therapy, 22*(1), 1-12.

Heimberg, R. G., Dodge, C. S., Hope, D. A., Kennedy, C. R., and Zollo, L. J. (1990). Cognitive behavioral group treatment for social phobia: Comparison with a credible placebo control. *Cognitive Therapy and Research, 14*(1), 1-23.

Heimberg, R. G., Salzman, D. G., Holt, C. S., and Blendell, K. A. (1993). Cognitive-behavioral group treatment for social phobia: Effectiveness at five-year followup. *Cognitive Therapy and Research, 17*(4), 325-339.

Himadi, W. G., and et al. (1986). The relationship of marital adjustment to agoraphobia treatment outcome. *Behavior Research and Therapy, 24*(2), 107-115.

Ingram, R. E., Miranda, J., and Segal, Z. V. (1998). *Cognitive vulnerability to depression*. New York: The Guilford Press.

Jacobson, E. (1974). *Progressive relaxation: A physiological and clinical investigation of muscular states and their significance in psychology and medical practice*. Chicago, IL: University of Chicago Press.

Jannoun, L., Munby, M., Catalan, J., and Gelder, M. (1980). A home-based treatment program for agoraphobia: Replication and controlled evaluation. *Behavior Therapy, 11*(3), 294-305.

Kanfer, F. H., and Saslow, G. (1969). Behavioral diagnosis. In C. M. Franks (Ed.), *Behavior therapy: appraisal and status* (pp. 417-444). New York: MacGraw Hill.

Kanfer, F. H., and Schefft, B. (1988). *Guiding the process of therapeutic change*. Champaign, IL: Research Press.

Kobak, K. A., Greist, J. H., Jeffersen, J. W., Katzelnick, D. J., and Henk, H. J. (1998). Behavioral versus pharmacological treatments of obsessive-compulsive disorder: a meta-analysis. *Psychopharmacology, 136*, 205-216.

Kopta, S. M., Lueger, R. J., Saunders, S. M., and Howard, K. I. (1999). Individual psychotherapy outcome and process research: challenges leading to greater turmoil or a positive transition? *Annual Review of Psychology., 50*, 441-469.

Kozak, M. J., and Foa, E. B. (1997). *Mastery of obsessive-compulsive disorder. A cognitive-behavioral approach*. Boulder, CO: Graywind Publications Incorporated.

Ladouceur, R., Dugas, M. J., Freeston, M. H., Leger, E., Gagnon, F., and Thibodeau, N. (2000). Efficacy of a cognitive-behavioral treatment for generalized anxiety disorder: evaluation in a controlled clinical trial. *Journal of Consulting and Clinical Psychology, 68*(6), 957-964.

Laitinen-Krispijn, S., and Bijl, R. V. (2000). Mental disorders and employee sickness absence: the NEMESIS study. Netherlands Mental Health Survey and Incidence Study. *Social Psychiatry and Psychiatric Epidemiology, 35*(2), 71-77.

Lang, P. J. (1984). Cognition in emotion: concept and action. In C. Izard and J. Kagan and R. Zajonc (Eds.), *Emotions, cognition, and behavior*. New York: Cambridge University Press.

Leahy, R. L., and Holland, S. J. (2000). *Treatment plans and interventions for depression and anxiety disorders*. New York: The Guilford Press.

Luthe, W., and Schultz, J. H. (1969). *The autogenic Therapy. Vol 1. Autogenic methods*. New York: Grune and Stratton Inc.

Mackintosh, N. J. (1983). *Conditioning and associative learning*. New York: Oxford University Press.

Magee, W. J., Eaton, W. W., Wittchen, H. U., McGonagle, K. A., and Kessler, R. C. (1996). Agoraphobia, simple phobia, and social phobia in the National Comorbidity Survey. *Archives of General Psychiatry, 53*(2), 159-168.

Marks, I. M. (1987). *Fears, phobias and rituals: panic, anxiety and their disorders*. New York: Oxford University Press.

Marsland, D. W., Wood, M., and Mayo, F. (1976). Content of family practice: a data bank for patient care, curriculum and research in family practice. *Journal of Family Practice, 3*, 25-68.

Marten, P. A., Brown, T. A., Barlow, D. H., Borkovec, T. D., Shear, M. K., and Lydiard, R. B. (1993). Evaluation of the ratings comprising the associated symptoms criterion DSM-III-R generalized anxiety disorder. *Journal of Nervous and Mental Disease, 181*, 676-682

Matthews, A. M., Johnston, D. W., Lancashire, M., Munby, M., Shaw, P. N., and Gelder, M. (1976). Imaginal flooding and exposure to real phobic situations: treatment outcome with agoraphobic patients. *British Journal of Psychiatry, 129*, 362-371.

McMullin, R. E. (2000). *The new handbook of cognitive therapy techniques*. New York: W.W. Norton and Company.

Meichenbaum, D. (1977). *Cognitive-behavior modification. An integrative approach*. New York: Plenum Press.

Meichenbaum, D. (1985). *Stress inoculation training*. New York: Pergamon Press.

Meichenbaum, D. (1996). Stress inoculation training for coping with stressors. *The Clinical Psychologist, 49*, 4-7.

Meichenbaum, D., and Turk, D. (1976). The cognitive-behavioral management of anxiety, anger and pain. In P. Davidson (Ed.), *The Behavioral Management of Anxiety, Depression and Pain*. New York: Brunner/Mazel.

Mowrer, O. H. (1960). *Learning theory and behavior*. New York: Wiley.

National Institute of Mental Health Molecular Genetics Initiative. (1992). *Diagnostic Interview For Genetic Studies (DIGS) - version 2.0*. Bethesda: National Institute of Mental Health.

Ortony, A., and Turner, T. J. (1990). What's basic about basic emotions? *Psychological Review, 97*(3), 315-331.

Öst, L.-G. (1987). Applied relaxation: Description of a coping technique and review of controlled studies. *Behavior Research and Therapy, 25*(5), 397-409.

Öst, L. G., and Breitholtz, E. (2000). Applied relaxation vs. cognitive therapy in the treatment of generalized anxiety disorder. *Behaviour Research and Therapy, 38*(8), 777-790.

O'Sullivan, G., Noshirvani, H., Marks, I. M., Montiero, W., and Lelliot, P. (1991). Six year follow-up after exposure and clomipramine therapy for obsessive compulsive disorder. *Journal of Clinical Psychiatry, 52*, 150-155.

Peter, H., and Hand, I. (1988). Patterns of patient-spouse interaction n agoraphobics: assessment by Camberwelle Family Interview (CFI) and impact on outcome of self-exposure treatment. In I. Hand and H.-U. Wittchen (Eds.), *Panic and phobias 2. Treatments and variables affecting course and outcome* (pp. 240-251). Berlin: Springer-Verlag.

Pollard, C. A., Henderson, J. G., Frank, M., and Margolis, R. B. (1989). Help-seeking patterns of anxiety-disordered individuals in the general population. *Journal of Anxiety Disorders, 3*(3), 131-138.

Rachman, S. (1978). *Fear and courage*. San Francisco: W.H. Freeman.

Rachman, S. (1980). Emotional processing. *Behavior Research and Therapy, 18*, 51-60.

Rachman, S. (1998). Panic and anxiety. In S. Rachman (Ed.), *Anxiety* (pp. 87-113). Hove: Psychology Press.

Rees, C. S., Richards, J. C., and Smith, L. M. (1998). Medical utilisation and costs in panic disorder: a comparison with social phobia. *Journal of Anxiety Disorders, 12*(5), 421-435.

Rescorla, R. A. (1988). Pavlovian conditioning. It's not what you think it is. *American Psychologist, 43*(3), 151-160.

Resick, P. A., and Schnicke, M. K. (1992). Cognitive processing therapy for sexual assault victims. *Journal of Consulting and Clinical Psychology, 60*(5), 748-756.

Resick, P. A., and Schnicke, M. K. (1993). *Cognitive Processing Therapy for sexual assault victims: a treatment manual*. Newbury Park, CA: Sage Publications.

Richards, D. A., Lovell, K., and Marks, I. M. (1994). Post-traumatic stress disorder: evaluation of a behavioral treatment program. *Journal of Traumatic Stress, 7*, 669-680.

Robins, L. N., Cottler, L. B., Buchholz, K. K., Compton, W. M., North, C. S., and Rourke, K. N. (2000). *Diagnostic Interview Schedule for the DSM-IV (DIS-IV)*. St. Louis, MO: Washington University School of Medicine.

Robinson, E. L., Corbett, M. O., and Spurlock, H. (1996). The effects of physical and mental stress on cardiovascular reactivity in a group of African American female college students. *Journal of Anxiety Disorders, 10*(6), 543-553.

Salkovskis, P. M. (Ed.). (1996). *The frontiers of cognitive therapy*. New York: Guilford Press.

Salkovskis, P. M., Clark, D. M., Hackmann, A., Wells, A., and Gelder, M. G. (1999). An experimental investigation of the role of safety-seeking behaviors in the maintenance of panic disorder with agoraphobia. *Behavior Research and Therapy, 37*(6), 559-574.

Sartory, G., and Olajide, D. (1988). Vagal innervation techniques in the treatment of panic disorder. *Behavior Research and Therapy, 26*(5), 431-434.

Scheier, M. F., Carver, C. S., and Matthews, K. A. (1983). Attentional factors in the perception of bodily states. In J. T. Cacioppo and R. E. Petty (Eds.), *Social psychophysiology: a sourcebook.* New York: Guilford Press.

Seligman, M. E. P., and Johnston, J. (1973). A cognitive theory of avoidance learning. In J. McGuigan and B. Lumsden (Eds.), *Contemporary approaches to conditioning and learning*. New York: Wiley.

Taylor, S. (1996). Meta-analysis of cognitive-behavioral treatments for social phobia. *Journal of Behavior Therapy and Experimental Psychiatry, 27*(1), 1-9.

Taylor, S. (2000). *Understanding and treating panic disorder. Cognitive-behavioral approaches*. Chichester: John Wiley and Sons.

Thompson, J. A., Charlton, P. F. C., Kerry, R., and Lee, D. (1995). An open trial of exposure therapy based on deconditioning for post-traumatic stress disorder. *British Journal of Clinical Psychology, 34*, 407-416.

van Oppen, P., de Haan, E., van Balkom, A. J., Spinhoven, P., Hoogduin, K., and van Dyck, R. (1995). Cognitive therapy and exposure in vivo in the treatment of obsessive compulsive disorder. *Behaviour Research and Therapy, 33*(4), 379-390.

White, J. R. (1999). *Overcoming generalized anxiety disorder - Client manual: a relaxation, cognitive restructuring, and exposure-based protocol for the treatment of GAD*. Oakland, CA: New Harbinger Publications.

World Health Organization. (1992). *The ICD-10 Classification of mental and behavioral disorders: diagnostic criteria for research*. Geneva: World Health Organization.

World Health Organization. (1993). *Composite International Diagnostic Interview - Version 1.1*. Geneva: World Health Organization.

In: Perspectives in Psychiatry Research
Editors: Nicole M. Levine and Donna J. Campbell
ISBN: 978-1-61209-236-2

Chapter 4

ON THE POSSIBILITY OF DIRECT MEMORY

Stephen E. Robbins
Center for Advanced Product Engineering, Metavante Corporation
10850 West Park Place, Milwaukee, WI, USA 53224

ABSTRACT

Is experience stored in the brain? The answer to this question is critical, for it strongly constrains possible theories of the nature and origin of consciousness. If the answer is "yes," conscious experience *must* be generated from stored "elements" within the neural structure. If the answer is "no," Searle's principle of neurobiological sufficiency, as one example, carries no force. On the other hand, a theory of direct perception can be construed to actually require a "no" answer, but then would require a theory of memory not reliant on brain storage. Perception research is reviewed which describes the invariance laws defining the elementary, time-extended, perceived events that must be "stored" and which speaks simultaneously to the nature of the qualia of these events. To support this description of perceived, external events, a model of "direct memory" is described, wherein the brain is viewed as supporting a modulated reconstructive wave passing through a holographic matter-field. The modulation pattern is determined or driven by the invariance laws defining external events. The model is applied to several areas of memory theory in cued-recall, to include verbal paired-associate learning, concreteness and imagery, subject performed tasks and priming. Some implications are reviewed for cognition in general, mental imagery, eye-witness phenomena and the question of whether everything experienced is "stored." The model is predictive and at the very least holds its own relative to current theory without appealing to storage of experience within the brain.

INTRODUCTION

How is experience stored in the brain? The question is intimately related to our theory of consciousness. An embodiment of the point is Searle's (2000) "principle of neurobiological sufficiency." This states, in essence, that a material (neurobiological) framework is entirely sufficient to support a theory of consciousness, i.e., it is a framework sufficient to support a solution to the hard problem (Chalmers, 1995). By implication, neurobiological storage must be entirely sufficient to account for the retention of this experience. Therefore, and somewhat circularly, if neurobiological storage is sufficient to account for memory, then the experiences of remembering, of memory images, of dreams insofar as memories contribute to this phenomenon, of illusions insofar as memories are a contributing factor - all must be accounted for by some form of "generation" from neurobiologically stored elements or structures.

It is not necessary to *start* with Searle's neurobiological principle. We need simply note the near universal assumption that the retention of experience is totally accounted for by storage in the neurobiological brain. This demands "neurobiological sufficiency" in and of itself. Again it is implied that dreams, memory images, imagistic thought and aspects of illusions must be pure, generated end-results of this neurobiological storage. If we add in the standard concept that input from the external world must be at least temporarily stored (e.g., in "iconic" stores) and processed as part of the perceptual process, then the perceptual image of the external world itself must be such a generated end-result. Where one stands on the question of the brain-storage of experience, just as Bergson (1896/1912) argued, is crucial. The implications of each side of the bet must be clear: If we hold that neural storage is sufficient to account for the retention of experience, it must be understood that this answer absolutely constrains all theories of the origin and nature of consciousness. Images, dreams, even perceptual images and perceptual experience must somehow be generated from stored elements within (or modifications of) the neural substrate. With this, there is the requirement to show (at least) how memory *images* or memory *experiences* arise. To refuse neurobiological sufficiency is to at least imply that memory may not be stored in the brain, with the requirement to show what a model of memory retrieval would look like.

There is a massive weakness here. The entire neurobiological framework of supposition assumes we know what experience is! That is to say, it presumes we have a theory of perception. It assumes that we have solved, for example, how the coffee cup being stirred on the table surface out in front of us is perceived as precisely this – a dynamically transforming *image* of a coffee cup with liquid surface being stirred by a spoon, external to us, in space. If we cannot solve this problem, if we have no true theory of perception, and therefore of experience, we have no certainty of what is it we are trying to store. This entire suppositional framework on neurobiological storage, then, must be seen for what it is – it can only be an *hypothesis*, nothing more. Its truth-status is inextricably linked to the unresolved (hard) problem of consciousness.

Let me be, quite literally, direct. Suppose, for the moment, that perception is indeed, direct. This is to say that the neural processes are simply *specifying*, to use Gibson's (1966) term, a past form of the motion of the matter-field, and that the image of the coffee cup therefore is precisely where it says it is – within the external matter-field. As such, perception, aka experience, is not occurring solely within the brain. If this is so, experience cannot be exclusively stored within the brain. But then we require a model of the retrieval of experience that supports this.

My purpose here is to introduce a quite different model of memory into the realm of concepts populating the sphere of the debate on consciousness. It is a model which does not rely on the hypothesis that the brain is the storehouse of experience. It is a model of *direct* memory. It does not see the brain, save in a precisely limited sense, as the encoder and recorder of experience. In its most succinct form, it sees the brain as supporting a reconstructive wave passing through a holographic matter-field. I will lay out the properties of the model and implications for several areas of memory research. Whether the model is powerfully predictive of new results is certainly one criterion for judgment, and limitations here may be simply due to the author's lack of imagination. I think the case will be made, at minimum, however, that the model is at least as explanatory as any current general conception of memory relying on the concept of storage, and further, it at least accounts for the remembered image of an *event* – something no current model successfully addresses. If so, it introduces an important alternative to one of the underlying, implicit concepts (neural storage of experience) in the consciousness debates.

Experience, Perception and the Coding Problem

The problem of memory begins with the problem of conscious perception. Experience, which the brain must store, can only be perceived events. What is the "problem of conscious perception" that must be solved? In this, there is perhaps no more stark and concise a painting than that of Crooks' (2002) verbal-diagrammatic presentation. In Figure 1 (top), the square represents an external object (or distal stimulus), the circle is the brain, and the arrows represent the light rays reflecting from the object to the brain (or proximal stimulus).

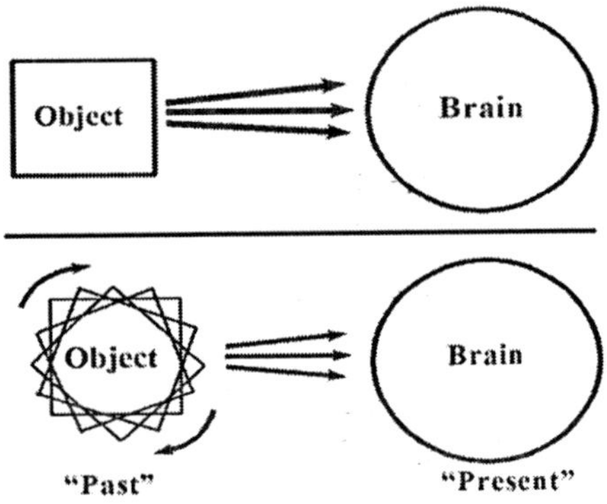

Figure 1. Perception of a Square (Top: Crooks' description. Bottom: The added dimension of time and the dynamic).

This is perception from a scientist's eye view. The rays continue through the retina, the photic energy is transduced and encoded within the central nervous system (CNS) of the observer perceiving the square into a neurally-based representation of the object. As Crooks notes, the processing of the physical energy ends in the relevant sensory cortex. *There is no return of vision to the square*. All perception then, even though of an *external* object, is occurring within the CNS. This is the undeniable finding of neuroscience.

The paradox is clear: we cannot actually see into physical space or directly observe the distal stimulus, yet our experience, our everyday phenomenology, is that of actually doing so. The object appears located externally to the brain, in depth, in volume, in space. It is a disturbing, counterintuitive paradox. We are virtually wired to believe otherwise, to hold that perception is direct. But Figure 1 stands in eloquent contradiction. All perception, all experience of the external world must be *indirect*, occurring, somehow within the dark world of the brain and its neural processes.

The Coding Problem

Though this picture is the "undeniable finding of science," science has no theory today on how the *image* of the square, external, in depth, arises from these processes "within the circle." The essence of the dilemma can be termed the "coding problem" (Cf. Bickhard and Ritchie, 1983; Bickhard, 2000). What is the coding problem? The light patterns or sound patterns of the external matter-field are being translated to the brain's own form of "code." The external world is "encoded" in the form of neural firing patterns. I am picking "neural" as a level here, but this could be quantum states, resonating water molecules, chemical flows, etc. This encoding resides in the strange, dark, "internal world" of the brain. How, we can ask, can a code, which is supposed to stand in for something known, i.e., for the external world, itself be the means by which the external world is known? Three dots, "..." (a code), encoded in your neural matrix so to speak, can stand for an "S" in Morse code, the number 3, the three blind mice, or Da Vinci's nose. How is the domain of the mapping specified? How is a code unfolded as the external world without already knowing what the external world looks like?

Chalmers (1995) famously framed the problem as the "hard problem." How, argued Chalmers, after describing your neural firing patterns, or your changing bit patterns, or your functional architecture, or whatever model you are building, do you account for qualia – the look and feel of the external world? How, when all is said and done, do white, steaming coffee cups arise, or the singing sounds of a violin spring forth from some data processing architecture (which all rests on changing patterns of bits) or from some neural net architecture (with its firing patterns) which you are perhaps describing?

Theorists of consciousness have tended to emphasize this "qualia" formulation of the problem. One seldom if ever sees the problem discussed in terms of accounting for the "external image." But when the hard problem is phrased exclusively as "trying to account for the qualitative feel of the world," we unfortunately disguise the coding problem which constitutes a major dimension of this difficulty. The problem of the external image has been the subject of the theory of perception for 2000 years (cf. Lombardo, 1987, for an historical overview). Its submergence under the question of qualia, while emphasizing an aspect of the problem of the external image, has been perhaps to our detriment. It is the *image* of the external world we are trying to account for. The image, we feel, is somehow coded in the neural flows of the brain. How is the code unfolded as the image of the external world – the steaming coffee cup with surface swirling while being stirred?

Innumerable theorists have claimed to solve the hard problem while failing to recognize the coding problem untouched at the core of their theory. We cannot take the neural-encoded information, apply an "integrating" magnetic field (e.g., McFadden, 2002), and claim we have explained the experience of the coffee-cup-being-stirred when we cannot explain how this integration unfolds the code. We cannot expect a higher order thought (HOT) or concept (Rosenthal, 2002; Gennaro, 2005) to unfold the neural code as the external image without a theory as to how a "thought" could possibly do this. We cannot expect RoboMary (Dennett, 2005), a theoretical robot who does not perceive color, to overcome this lack simply by self-programming the range of "color codes" in her "color registers." Dennett simply misses the coding problem. We cannot encode the world holographically within the brain, in neural holoscapes, as Pribram (1971, 1991) attempted, and think we have solved the problem when we cannot explain how holographic neural processes now unfold the coded information.

Why is the problem of conscious perception the very beginning of the problem of the storage of experience? Add time and the dynamic to Figure 1 (bottom): let the square be a "rotating" square. We are perceiving the *past*. To perceive a motion – a square "rotating" – we are perceiving some *extent of time*. Perception - the external image - is already a memory. This is true even for Crooks' static square. If we are unable to explain not only the origin of our experience as the external image, but this external image as an ongoing memory or image of the past, how can we begin to explain the storage of experience?

Holography – Unfolding a Code

Holography, despite the above mini-critique of Pribram, is in fact a very concrete method of unfolding a code, and unfolding it as an image. A brief explication of holography serves as an object lesson for how nature solves a coding problem, and is required to understand a theory of direct perception or "direct specification" such as Gibson's (1966, 1979). As indicated earlier, it is, after all, the possible directness of perception that has the possibility of changing our view of how the brain stores experience.

Technically, we know that a hologram is the recorded interference pattern of two waves (Figure 2). The *reference* wave is usually emitted from a source of coherent light such as a laser. The *object* wave arises from light reflected from the object for which we intend to make a hologram. The object wave is complex. Each point of the object can be visualized as giving rise to a spherical wave, spreading towards and over the plate. The information for each point is thus spread across the entire hologram plate. Conversely, then, the information for the entire object is found at any point of the hologram – each point reflects or carries information for the whole. Any portion of the hologram is thus sufficient to reconstruct the image of the entire object. The plate is the recording/encoding of this complex interference pattern (where crest meets crest, or crest meets trough, etc.). It is itself a complex code. The pattern looks nothing like the original object.

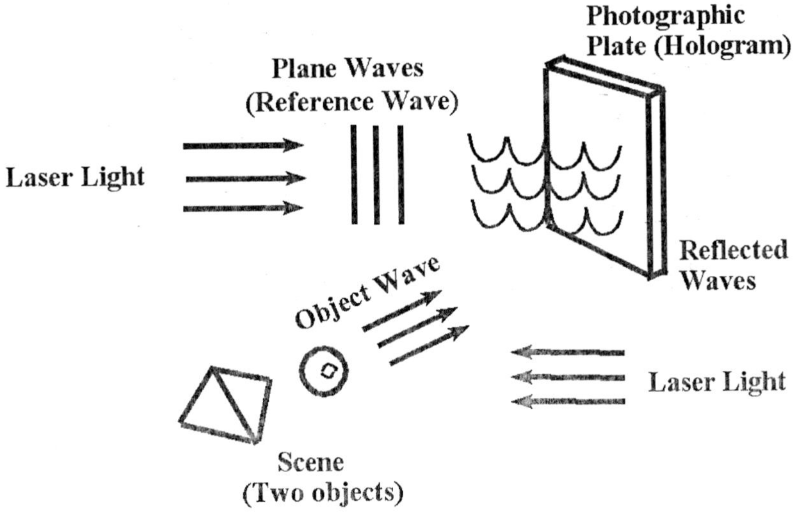

Figure 2. Construction of a hologram. The hologram is the record of the interference pattern formed by the reference wave and the object wave.

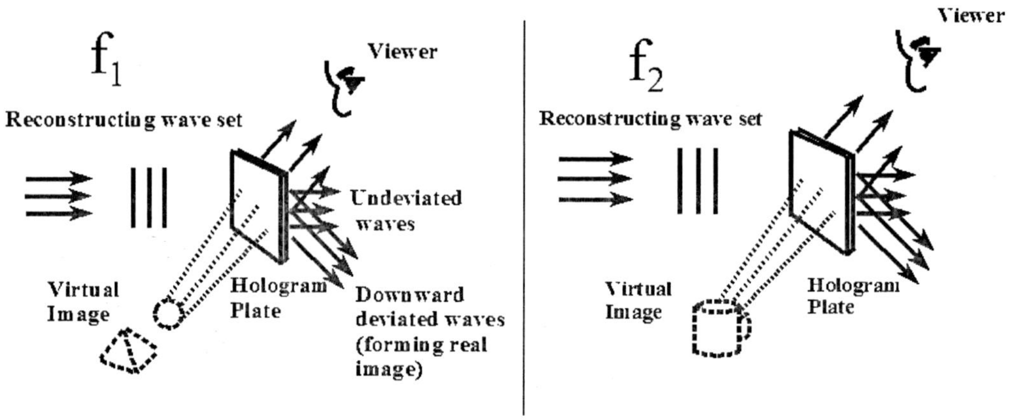

Figure 3. Holographic reconstruction. The reconstructive wave, modulated to frequency 1, reconstructs the stored wave front (image) of a pyramid/ball. The reconstructive wave, modulated to frequency 2, now reconstructs the wave front of the cup.

Figure 3 (left) shows the process of image, or more precisely, wave front reconstruction. A reconstructive wave - a wave with the same frequency as the original reference wave - is beamed through the hologram plate. The wave is diffracted (as waves of water passing through and around barriers in a harbor) as it passes through the interference fringes recorded on the plate. A viewer, placed in the path of the upward traveling wave set, believes himself to see the source of the original wave set located behind the hologram plate, in depth, in volume. This wave set specifies what is termed the "virtual image."

For a series of n wave fronts (events) w_i, each wave front can be stored using a different reference wave frequency, f_i. If a reconstructive wave is modulated to each precise frequency successively, each wave front is successively reconstructed (Figure 3, left/right). But if the reconstructive wave consists of a composite set of frequencies, f_1 thru f_n, a composite wave front or image is reconstructed.

Holography, then, is a powerful method of solving a coding problem, and, of course, for retrieving information. But can it be applied in the context of the brain and experience? Better applied, that is, than simply treating the brain as a "hologram?" Gibson's theory contains a possible approach. In the course of reviewing it, we will inevitably obtain a view of the information defining the external events – "rotating" squares and coffee being stirred in cups - that must be "encoded," to include a view of the nature of the qualia of these events.

Gibson and the Invariance Structure of Events

Gibson's (1950) fundamental insight came in recasting the problem of depth perception. When considered from the viewpoint of Newtonian space, as stated by the bishop/philosopher Berkeley, a single static eye could not give any information about the third dimension since the latter consisted of the line of sight itself, a line represented by only a single point on the retina (Figure 4, line ABCD). There is nothing to indicate whether the point is near or far, for the point remains invariably the same on the retina. Thus, according to Berkeley, "distance of itself, and immediately, cannot be seen." This led to a history of attempts to account for the perception of distance in terms of "depth cues," and ultimately then to "judgments" and mental operations for inferring depth.

Gibson turned to the notion of the "ground," and the problem was reformulated such that it became how the continuum of distance across the ground in all directions is visually perceived. Thus the problem became how the different distances, w,x,y,z on the ground line G_1G_2 are perceived (Figure 4). Note that when the eye is put in motion, something varies on the retina in this situation, while in the older formulation the distances always project to the same point. Note also that the relative distances zyxw are preserved under the projective transformation indicated, i.e., they are projectively invariant.

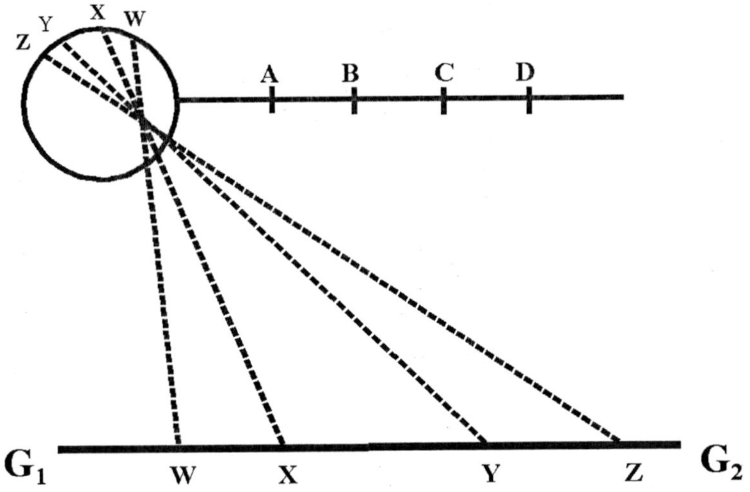

Figure 4. The "Ground" (After Lombardo, 1987).

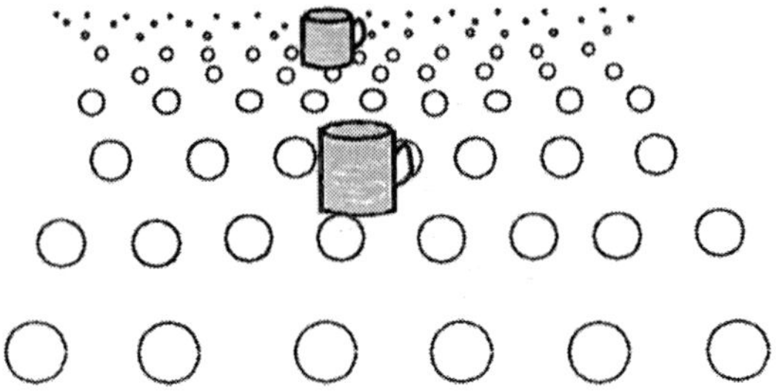

Figure 5. Texture density gradient (Gibson, 1950). The horizontal separation, S, is proportional to the distance, or $S \propto 1/D$, the vertical separation as $S \propto 1/D^2$. The cups on the gradient can be viewed as the same cup in two different positions.

The "ground" contains a great deal of mathematical relations, extremely useful for organisms usually engaged in locomotion across it. Gibson (1950) would introduce the notion of texture density gradients. A typical example of such a gradient can be a tiled floor, a rug, a beach, a tiled table top, or a surface strewn with rocks (see Figure 5). The rocks or tiles are our texture "units" and have a decreasing horizontal separation (S) as a function of the distance, $S \propto 1/D$, and vertically as $S \propto 1/D^2$. This gradient of increasing density of texture units on the retina should produce a perception of continuous distance in all directions across the surface.

It is external *events* that are perceived. Let us cast further discussion in terms of a simple event, for example, "stirring coffee." Suppose our coffee cup rests on a table top. In Figure 6, the cup is shown in two successive positions as it moves across a gradient towards an observer. The size constancy of the cup as it moves is being specified, *over time*, by the invariant proportion, $S \propto 1/N$, where S is the (increasing) vertical size of the rod on the retina, N the (decreasing) number of texture units it occludes ($SN=k$). When the gradient itself is put in motion, as in driving down a road, it becomes an optical flow field – a gradient of velocity vectors where there is an increasing point velocity as the distance from the eye decreases, $v \propto 1/d^2$, all radiating from a single point, the point of optical expansion (Figure 6).

Let us suppose further that the cup is cubical in structure. If the cup is rotated, then as a side rotates into view, an expanding flow gradient is defined, and as the side rotates away, a contracting flow gradient is defined (cf. Domini et al., 2002). The top surface becomes a radial flow field. The cup's edges are sharp discontinuities in these flows. If the cup is static (it can never truly be so given the saccadic motion of the eye), and the spoon is stirring the coffee, another form of radial flow field is created over the liquid surface. There are other symmetry or invariance laws supporting the *form* of the cubical cup; the form is a function of its symmetry period (cf. Robbins, 2004a).

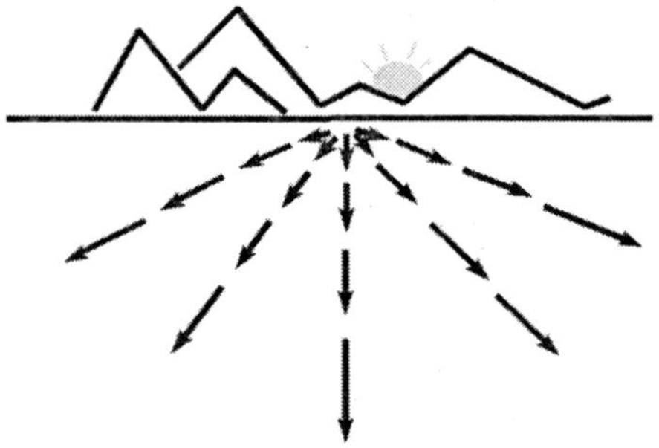

Figure 6. Optical flow field (left). A gradient of velocity vectors is created as an observer moves towards the mountains. The flow field "expands" as the observer moves. The velocity of each vector is inversely proportional to the distance from the observer, $v \propto 1/d^2$.

In this case, since it is carried into itself every 90 degrees, it has a period of four. When we poured the coffee into the cup, the rate of increase of the pitch of the sound as the cup fills with liquid is an invariant specifying the (visual) time it will take for the cup to fill to the brim (Cabe and Pittenger, 2000).

The stirring motion of the hand is a complex of forces. The use of the spoon is a form of "wielding." This is described (cf. Turvey and Carello, 1995) under the concept of the "inertia tensor." A rigid object's moments of mass distribution constitute potentially relevant mechanical invariants since they specify the dynamics of the object. The object's mass (m) is the zeroth moment, while the first (static) moment is mass (m) times the distance (d) between the point of rotation and object's center of mass. The second moment is conceived as the object's resistance against angular acceleration. In three dimensions, this moment is a 3 x 3 matrix called the inertia tensor. The diagonal elements I_1, I_2, I_3, are eigenvalues and represent the object's resistance to angular acceleration with respect to a coordinate system of three principal axes (cf. Kingma et. al, 2004). There will be an inertia tensor (invariant), I_{ij}, specific to spoon-stirring. Over the periodic motion of the stirring spoon, there is likewise a haptic flow field defined, and within this, there is an adiabatic invariant – a constant ratio of the energy of oscillation to the frequency of oscillation (Kugler and Turvey, 1987):

$$\frac{\text{Energy of oscillation}}{\text{Frequency of oscillation.}} = k$$

This is a mere beginning of what we can term the *invariance structure* of an event. The invariance structure of an event can be defined thus: a specification of the transformations and structural invariants defining an event and rendering it a virtual action. The transformations define the information specifying the form of the change – rotating, swirling, flowing. The structural invariants define the information specific to that undergoing the change – a cup, a liquid, a field of grass or stretch of gravel. When stirring our cup of coffee, we are involving multiple areas of the brain – visual areas, motor areas, auditory areas, haptic areas. Even the action-goal of "stirring" must be supported by the pre-frontal areas. Over these, we have a resonant feedback from the multiple re-entrant projections between all areas which supports a dynamical pattern occurring over time. For practical purposes, we have a near-global, time-extended pattern (or attractor) supported over the brain. The pattern itself, in some form, must support the ongoing invariance structure of the coffee-stirring event being specified in perception.

Invariance and Action

Having mentioned virtual action, let us relate invariance to action. Over this flow field and its velocity vectors a value, τ, is defined by taking the ratio of the surface (or angular projection) of the field at the retina, r(t), to its velocity of expansion at the retina, v(t), and its time derivative. This invariant, τ (or tau), specifies time to impending contact with an object or surface, and has a critical role in controlling action (Kim et al., 1993). A bird, for example, coming in for a landing, must use this τ value to slow down appropriately to land softly. As the coffee cup is moved over the table towards us, this value specifies time to contact and provides information for modulating the hand to grasp the cup.

Turvey (1977) has asked how such information is transduced to the muscles. Let us suppose that the cup is being moved laterally across the table in front us. We wish to reach out and intercept the cup as it moves. In this context, Turvey described a "mass-spring" model of the action systems, where, for example, reaching an arm out for the cup is conceived as in releasing an oscillatory spring with a weight at one end. "Stiffness" and "damping" parameters specify the end-point and velocity of such a system. Turvey argued that the needed muscle-spring parameters must be realized *directly* in the coordinative structures via properties of the optic array, e.g., the texture density gradient across which the cup moves and the quantity of texture units it occludes. Turvey termed these parameters, which must be realized directly in the dynamical pattern supported by the brain, "tuning" parameters for the action systems.

Bergson (1896/1912) captured the implications most succinctly: perception is *virtual action*.

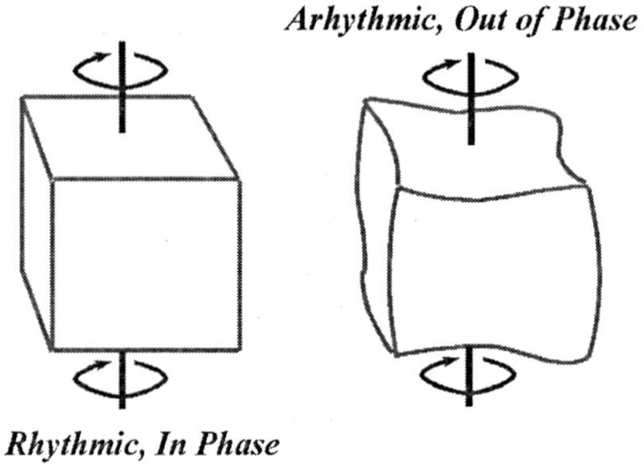

Figure 7. Rotating cubes, strobed in phase with, or out of phase with, the symmetry period.

[Objects] send back, then, to my body, as would a mirror, their eventual influence; they take rank in an order corresponding to the growing or decreasing powers of my body. The objects which surround my body reflect its possible action upon them. (1896/1912, pp. 6-7).

In the direct perception model, it is the information (invariants) relevant to action that are selected from the wealth of information in the environment – the external image is simultaneously a specification of possible action.

There is a large set of findings pointing to the general concept that the objects and events of the perceived world are in a real sense mirrors of the biologic action capabilities of the body (Cf. for example Viviani and Stucchi, 1992; Viviani and Mounoud, 1990; Glenberg, 1997; O'Regan and Noë, 2001; Cisek, 2001; Cisek and Kalaska, 2002; Thelen et al., 2001; Clark, 1999). Churchland et al. (1994) express the importance to visual computation of re-entrant connections from motor areas to visual areas, and these connections, in the context of virtual action, may carry an implication deep enough to incorporate - as Weiskrantz (1997) has discussed on the findings of Nakamura and Mishkin (1980; 1982) - the reasons blindness can result simply from severing visual area connections to the motor areas.

Form, Velocity Flows and the Time-Extent of Events

A rotating, wire-edged cube, strobed in phase with its symmetry period, appears indeed as a rigid cube in rotation (Figure 7). Strobed out of phase, it becomes a wobbly, distorted, plastic-like object (Shaw and McIntyre, 1974). The out-of-phase strobe is destroying the symmetry (invariance) information defined over time, which specifies the form of the cube.

This is clearly a question of dynamics. Beneath the perception of form, the very powerful energy models (Weiss and Adelson, 1998; Weiss et al., 2002) envision a neural-based array of filters tuned to extract motion information from velocity flow fields. These models have specifically eschewed addressing the "correspondence problem" of standard, feature-based approaches to form. This problem is highly manifest if we imagine a movie frame filled with random dots, all of which change position on the next frame, and give ourselves the problem of tracking them. This problem, and the feature "matching" models that attempt to overcome it, soon prove to be intractable. The energy model specifically bypasses the need to track changing "features." The energy model does not use position (or the change of some feature from position to position) to compute motion. Motion is treated as "spatiotemporal orientation," and the model consists of a network of "spatiotemporal filters." The Reichardt (1959) filter of Figure 8 is a precursor with significant formal relations.

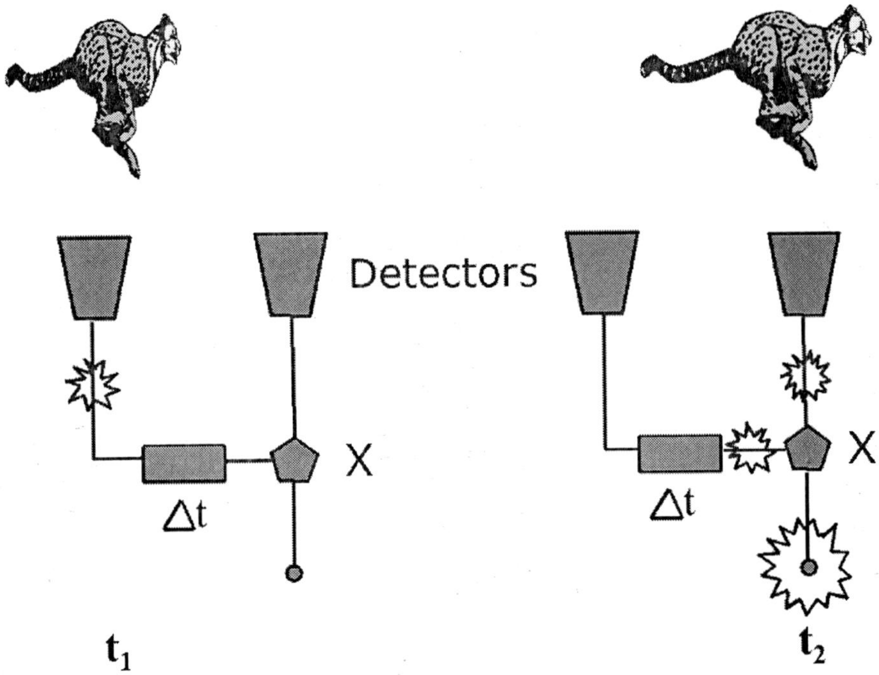

Figure 8. Reichardt filter or correlation model (Reichardt, 1959). It has two spatially separate detectors. The output of one of the detectors is delayed over a period of time (Δt) and then the two signals are multiplied. The output is tuned to speed. Many detectors tuned to different speeds are required for the true speed of a pattern, and the difference of pairs of detectors tuned to different directions is taken. (Robbins, 2004a).

Due to the aperture problem arising from the limited scope of the receptive fields of these filters, this velocity information is inherently *uncertain*, therefore probabilistic (Bayesian) constraints must be employed (Figure 9). The constraint employed by Weiss et al. is "motion is slow and smooth." Used as a Bayesian constraint applied to velocity fields, the principle explains a wide array of illusions of perception, for example Mussati's (1924) illusion wherein a narrow ellipse in rotation becomes wobbly (non-rigid) and distorted while a wider ellipse in rotation maintains its form (Figure 10). From this perspective, given the inherent uncertainty of information, form is always an optimal percept – even so-called "illusions" are optimal percepts.

The apparently intrinsic "static" features of objects – edges, corners, straight lines – are all ephemeral creatures of time and these velocity fields. A Gibsonian cube in rotation is a partitioned set of these flow fields, where we have an expanding field as a face rotates into view, a contracting field as the face rotates away from view, a circular flow field at the top surface, and the edges and corners merely sharp discontinuities in these flows.

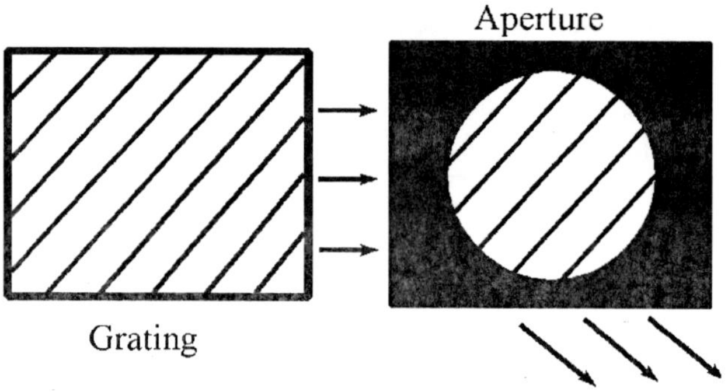

Figure 9. The aperture problem. The card with the grating is moving to the right, and passes beneath the card with the circular aperture. The ends of the moving lines are now obscured, and only the downward motion of the lines is seen in the aperture.

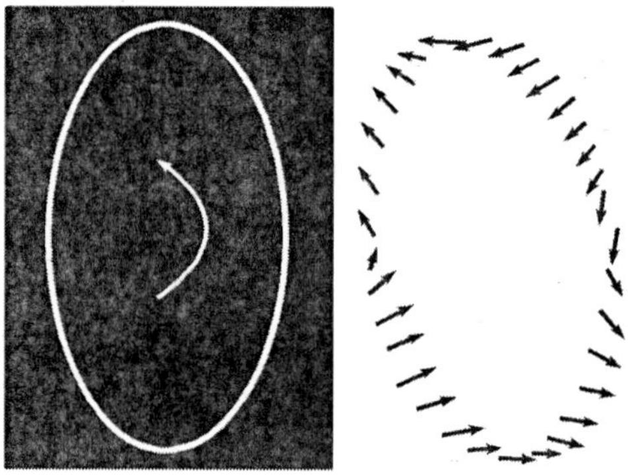

Figure 10. The normal velocity vector components (right) of the edge of the rotating ellipse (left). These tend to induce non-rigid motion. (After Weiss and Adelson, 1998).

In the case of Shaw and McIntyre's wobbly, plastic-like, virtually non-cube which has lost its rigid edges, it can be argued that a yet higher order temporal symmetry constraint has been disrupted by the out-phase strobe, causing the dynamical specification of the non-rigid wobbly cube (Robbins, 2004a). As the strobe rate changes, from in-phase to out-of-phase, we are conscious of the two different (successively specified) forms. The forms being specified are functions of the application of constraints on flowing fields. The structure of the forms reflects invariants existing over these time-extended flows.

Qualia, Flows and the Scale of Time

The slowly rotating cube is a certain quality. The wobbly non-cube is certain quality. A cube spinning swiftly enough to appear as a cylinder surrounded by a fuzzy haze is another quality. Forms themselves are "qualia." Just as for color, there are no simple properties in the matter-field that correspond to form. Just as matter is commonly held to have no intrinsic color, color being considered a "secondary property" of matter (cf. Byrne and Hilbert, 2004, for discussion), so we would be equally forced to hold the same for form. There has been an almost implicit theme that qualia are akin to tiny, non-material atoms (cf. Goguen, 2004, for a critique), for example atom-like color qualia which would account for the color of our rotating cube. This implicit theme is taken to absurdity in the case of form. What could form qualia possibly be? What, other than the forms themselves? While consciousness theorists have designated qualia as "ineffable, the "ineffable" of form is this: invariance over the time-extended, flowing field.

One cannot have perceived invariance over a flow without simultaneously perceiving the flow. Thus we have initially arrived at the reason that the "primary memory" that supports the perception of "rotating" cubes, i.e., all time-extended perceived events, has primacy over the problem of qualia. But to fully appreciate the problem, we need to enter upon some considerations of the scale of time in defining the events that are perceived, and which therefore must be equally intrinsic to the events that are remembered.

The external matter-field in which the brain is embedded is a scale-less field in terms of time. If we regard a fly in the external field from this "null-scale" perspective, at best we might visualize it as an ensemble of atoms with their electrons slowly, extremely slowly, working their way around their orbits, or as quarks slowly changing state, or as an ensemble of vibrations very slowly developing in a vast vibrational sea. The brain is imposing a scale of time upon this matter-field. The fly "buzzing" by, his wings a-blur at 200 beats/sec, is an index of the scale of (perceived) time. This is also a function of the dynamics of the brain, ultimately of the chemical velocities supporting its computations. In principle, the chemical velocities can be changed via some catalyst or set of catalysts, even raising the temperature will accomplish this (cf. Hoaglund, 1966). At higher chemical velocities underlying the neural processes, the fly would become perhaps a "heron-like" fly, slowly flapping his wings. We have altered the dynamics and changed the perception. The time-scale has changed. The brain's "code" has changed.

The scale of time is an integral aspect of the quality of the event. i.e., of qualia. The "heron-like" fly is a different quality than the "buzzing" fly, the "rotating" cube a different quality than the "wobbling" cube, or at a different scale, a different quality than a rapidly spinning cylinder with fuzzy edges (once the slowly rotating cube), the "red" of normal scale is a different quality than the slightly more vibrant red (where the electromagnetic field oscillations develop more slowly) that would be experienced at the scale where the fly is heron-like. (Would we have qualia "atoms" for each possible scale?) Each of these cases simultaneously involves different time-extents taken over the history of the evolution of the matter-field – the "buzzing" fly is a perception summing a far greater history of the matter-field than the heron-like fly.

The timescale of the perceived world is therefore an intrinsic aspect of the brain's neural "code." The energy-dynamics of the brain with its underlying attractors is clearly involved in the specification of scale – and the time-scale of the events that must be stored.

Invariance Laws and Space-Time Partitions

If we can change the perceived scale of time by adjusting underlying chemical velocities, we have effected a transformation roughly analogous to the relativistic change of the "space-time partition." If this is possible in principle, we must ask how nature deals with it. In the relativistic framework, in such a transformation, it is the form of the law (d=vt, d'=vt') that remains invariant to the motions of various observers. This is one significance of invariance laws defining perceived events – the event can be specified by the same law across partitions.

The growth of the facial profile (Figure 11) is defined by a strain transformation upon a cardioid. This law holds and defines the event, whether it is sped up to a very rapid event (as in a time-lapse movie) or remains the very slow event it is in our normal time-scale.

If we take our slowly rotating cube – a figure of 4-fold symmetry - and gradually speed up its rotation, it passes through a series of perceived forms (Figure 12) with multiple serrated edges, each of 4n-fold symmetry, until eventually it becomes a cylinder surrounded by a fuzzy haze – a figure of infinite symmetry. Rather than speeding up the cube, were we to effect this same transformation by slowly retarding the chemical velocities of the brain underlying the attractor supporting the form, the same 4n-fold symmetry law holds across the changing "space-time partition." Kugler and Turvey (1987) note, referencing Feynman (1965), laws are but "secret ways" of talking about conservations. Invariance (or conservations) under scale transformations is termed *gauge* invariance. In essence, what we are discussing here is a fundamental symmetry operation to which these laws should be expected to be invariant, namely, transformation of the scale of time.

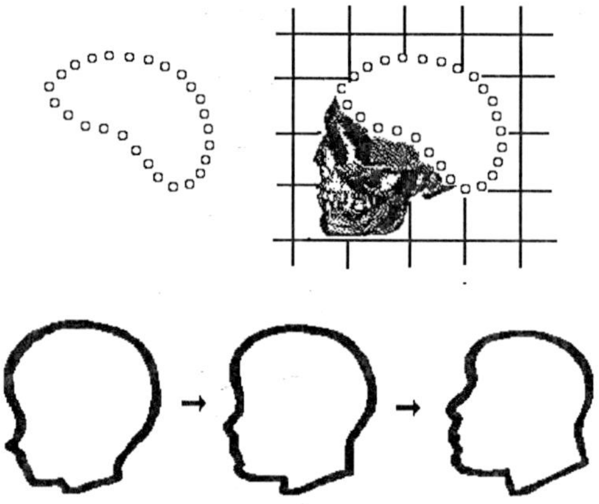

Figure 11. Aging of the facial profile. A cardioid is fitted to the skull and a strain transformation is applied. (Strain is equivalent to the stretching of the meshes of a coordinate system in all directions.) Shown are a few in the sequence of profiles generated. (Adapted from Pittenger and Shaw, 1975).

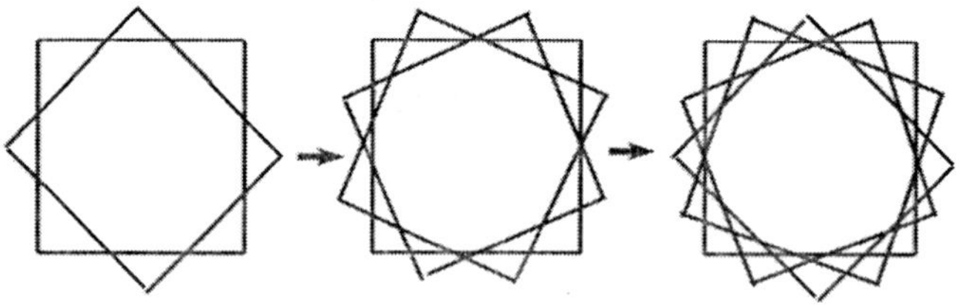

Figure 12. Successive transformations of the rotating cube (2-D view) through figures of 4n-fold symmetry as angular velocity increases. (Robbins, 2004a).

The dynamics of the brain must "encode" the invariants defining the event. The invariants exist only over time-extended transformations – the code somehow represents time-extent. And it represents scale. I have already noted that one cannot have perceived invariance over a flow without simultaneously perceiving the flow. This simple fact leads to the problem of the nature of the "primary memory" that supports the perception of "rotating" cubes and all time-extended perceived events.

Primary Memory

I am appropriating the term "primary memory" here. I mean a form of memory even more fundamental than the sense in which James (1890) used the term. The question is critical, in fact, again, has primacy over that of qualia: no qualia can exist without some extension in time. But what is the origin of this extension?

Let us place the question more concretely in terms of the brain: how does the brain support the perception of a rotating cube? It is a natural theoretical tendency to model this in terms of samples or snapshots of the event, where the snapshots are stored in a short-term or immediate memory medium, or "iconic" store, etc., allowing the motion to be reconstructed. The event of the rotating cube would be parsed into a series of slices, each consisting of a frozen, static snapshot comprised of the static features of the cube – its edges, vertices, surfaces - at some position along the imagined circle of the rotation.

The "sampling model" of the memory supporting the perceived event is inherently flawed. Each sample is only a static state. A series of such states is simply a series of static states. We have lost the motion. Do we introduce some sort of "scanner" within the brain to scan the stored samples? Then we must explain how the scanner perceives motion. We begin an infinite regress.

There are other practical difficulties. Let us remember the implications of Shaw and McIntyre's wobbly non-cube. A strobe in-phase with the cube's symmetry period allowed the brain to specify a cube in rotation. But a strobe out-of-phase ended in a specification of a plastic, wobbly object. The strobe flash is equivalent to a sample. Thus, a brain-driven sampling mechanism, to allow the specification of a cube-in-rotation, would have to be pre-adjusted to the symmetry period of the cube. This would require a form of pre-cognition. And what if there were two or more cubes rotating at different rates?

The sampling model also implies a set of static features within each sample – edges, vertices. But we have seen that these are only ephemeral constructs to the brain – sharp discontinuities in velocity fields, features which themselves, in their global specification of the form, are functions of Bayesian constraints. Destroy or change these constraints, the "features" disappear.

So let us discard sampling as an answer. The question may have arisen as to why bother to invoke sampling in the first place? We need only to imagine the continuous processes underlying the neural firing as the support for the ongoing perception. Taylor (2002), for example, notes:

> The features of an object, bound by various mechanisms to activity in working memory, thereby provide the content of consciousness of the associated object... In these [neural activity loops], neural activity "relaxes" to a temporally stable state, therefore providing the extended temporal duration of activity necessary for consciousness... (Taylor, 2002: 11)

Here we simply rely on the "temporal extension" of the neural processes to provide the support for the time-extended perception. But this is a gratuitous assumption. By what right do we grant this temporal extension to the material world, including the brain? If we can so easily grant it, how do we place a limit upon it? Why should the limit not extend for our entire lifetime? Or several lifetimes? Or to the entire history of the matter-field? And why would the limit, or lack thereof, apply only to the brain? On the other hand, science intently pursues the method whereby the brain *stores* experience. Why? Because our implicit model of matter is tied to the classical model of time. This model sees matter as existing only in the "present" instant.

Consider a buzzing fly, with its wings beating at approximately 200 cycles/second. For the sake of choosing a scale, assign each wing beat to a "present" instant. As each present instant arrives (with its wing beat), the previous moves into the past. The past, to us, is the symbol of *non-existence*. Therefore, to preserve the instant, it must be stored in the ever-"present" brain (matter), which is to say, in some brain-instantiated memory. The "buzzing" fly perception is comprised of a series of these "presents" that have long since come and gone. By this logic, each must be stored in the brain, i.e., in matter, else it is lost to non-existence.

But if we are not willing to grant infinite time-extension to the present instant, what is the time-extent? In fact, we view the classical "instant" as infinitely divisible. Being such, the best we can say is that the classical, "present" instant of time's evolution is the most infinitely minute amount of time imaginable. If the lifetime of the currently shortest lived micro-particle is, perhaps, 10^{-9} nanoseconds, then the present instant of the time-evolving matter-field is even less than this. This is the best we are allowed to say for the actual time-extent of the neurological processes.

I am insisting on a decision here. If we are storing experience in the brain because the brain is matter, and matter is always that which is present, therefore existent, as opposed to non-existent, then, for once, we must face the implications of this logic. Declare the actual time-extent of this present. If your model of time is a series of instants, what is the time-extent of an instant? If the answer is "infinitesimal," you must store each instant, instantaneously, in the brain. From a series of such stored, instantaneous snapshots of the rotating cube, you must reconstruct the cube's motion, with all the logical problems noted. If the answer is "infinitesimal," it goes without saying that the notion of "extended" neurological processes is a convenient, but invalid myth. And it goes without saying that the time-extension of these processes cannot then be simply invoked to support the perception of something even so simple as a "rotating" cube.

Memory as Non-Differentiable Motion

The very concept of time as a series of "instants" is founded within a framework of an *abstract* space and time. Bergson (1896/1912) argued that abstract space is derived from the world of separate "objects" gradually identified, ironically enough, by our perception. It is an elementary process, for perception must partition the continuous, dynamic field which surrounds the body into objects upon which the body can *act* - to throw a "rock," to hoist a "bottle of beer," to grasp a "cube" which is "rotating." This fundamental perceptual partition into "objects" and "motions" – at a particular scale of time we should note - is reified and extended in thought. The separate "objects" in the field are refined to the notion of the continuum of points or positions. As an object moves across this continuum, as for example, my hand moving across the desk from point A to point B, it is conceived to describe a *trajectory* - a line - consisting of the points or positions it traverses. Each point momentarily occupied is conceived to correspond to an "instant" of time. Thus arises the notion of abstract time - the series of instants - itself simply another dimension of the abstract space. This space, argued Bergson, is in essence a "principle of infinite divisibility." Having convinced ourselves that this motion is adequately described by the line/trajectory the object traversed, we can break up the line (space) into as many points as we please. But the concept of motion this implies is inherently an infinite regress. To account for the motion, we must - between each pair of static points/positions supposedly occupied by the object - re-introduce the motion, hence a new (smaller) trajectory of static points - ad infinitum.

Motion, Bergson argued, must be treated as *indivisible*. The paradoxes of Zeno, he held, had their origin in the logical implications of an abstract space and time; they were Zeno's attempts to force recognition of the invalidity of this treatment. When Achilles cannot catch the hare, it is because we view his indivisible steps through the lens of the abstract trajectory or line each step covers. We think of the abstract space traversed. We then propose that each such distance can be successively halved – infinitely divided in other words. Achilles never reaches the hare. But Achilles moves in an indivisible motion; he most definitely catches the hare.

I have argued, then, that neural processes have no intrinsic time-extent, that it is not possible to appeal to such a time-extent without implicitly violating the logic of the model by which we store experience in the brain in the first place. In effect, this argument is to force exactly the same recognition as that which Zeno intended. The classical abstraction – time as a series of instants – forces us to clarify our notion of matter. If matter is only that which is "present," else it is consigned to non-existence, then we are forced to ask, "what is the extent of the present instant?" Then, since we are committed to "instants," we are committed to abstract space with its principle of infinite divisibility. We end by taking any "instant" or extent of time, and dividing it unto its ultimate component – an abstract mathematical point. This is the inherent extent of the instant, the time-extent of matter, the time-extent of the brain and the time-extent of all neural processes. In truth, at the mathematical point, there is no time at all. If we accept abstract space and time, then it is on this logical and metaphysical basis that we must explain the perception of rotating cubes, buzzing flies, and singing notes of violins, that is, all qualia.

In this abstract continuum of positions, an "object" can move across the continuum, or the continuum may move beneath the object. All motion is relative. All *real* motion or change is lost. Depending purely on perspective, the object is at rest, or in motion. But there must be real motion, dynamic change or evolution of the matter-field.

> Though we are free to attribute rest or motion to any material point taken by itself, it is nonetheless true that the aspect of the material universe changes, that the internal configuration of every real system varies, and that here we have no longer the choice between mobility and rest. Movement, whatever its inner nature, becomes an indisputable reality. We may not be able to say what parts of the whole are in motion, motion there is in the whole nonetheless. (1896/1912, p. 255)

The alternative then is to view the "motions" of "objects" as *changes or transference state* within a globally, indivisibly transforming whole. The conception that colors, or as we have seen, somewhat absurdly, even forms must be "secondary," merely subjective properties, not intrinsic to the abstract motions of abstract objects, resolves here to a fiction of the abstract space. The matter-field is, must be, intrinsically qualitative.

Abstract space/time is a projection frame for our thought, derived from the necessity for practical action. Imported into the problem of consciousness, it is a barrier. For physics, the effort to break from this projection frame has been very real. If for physics itself it is true that,

"*...a theory of matter is an attempt to find the reality hidden beneath...customary images which are entirely relative to our needs...*" (Bergson, 1896/1912, 254), the abstraction has been the ultimate barrier.

Physics and the Abstraction

First to go was the concept of a trajectory of a moving object. This no longer exists in quantum mechanics. One can determine through a series of measurements only a series of instantaneous positions, while simultaneously renouncing all grasp of the object's state of motion, i.e., Heisenberg's famous principle of uncertainty. As de Broglie (1947) would note, writing his comparison of Bergson to current concepts of physics, the measurement is attempting to project the motion to a point in our continuum, but in doing so, we have lost the motion. Thus Bergson noted, over forty years before Heisenberg, "In space, there are only parts of space and at whatever point one considers the moving object, one will obtain only a position" (Bergson 1889, p. 111).

Nottale (1996) simply notes Feynman and Hibb's (1965) proof that the motion of a particle is continuous but not differentiable. Hence, he argues, we should reject the long held notion that space-time is differentiable. He opts for a fractal approach – indivisible elements which build patterns. The essence of differentiation is to divide (say, a motion from A to B, or the slope of a triangle) into small parts. This operation is carried out with smaller and smaller parts or divisions. It is understood that the divisions can be infinite in number, infinitely small. When the parts or divisions have become so minute, we envision "taking the limit" of the operation - obtaining the measure of say, "instantaneous" velocity, or slope, etc. To speak of non-differentiability is to say - "non-infinite divisibility." We have something - indivisible. To state that space-time is non-differentiable another way, we may say the global evolution of the matter-field over time is seen as non-differentiable; it cannot be treated as an infinitely divisible series of states.

Lynds (*Foundations of Physics Letters*, 2003) now argues that there is no precise static instant in time underlying a dynamical physical process. If there were such, motion and variation in all physical magnitudes would not be possible, as they would be frozen static at that precise instant, and remain that way. In effect, such an instant would imply a momentarily static universe. Such a universe is incapable of change, for the universe itself could not change to assume another static instant. Consequently, at no time is the position of a body (or edge, vertex, feature, etc.) or a physical magnitude precisely determined in an interval, no matter how small, as at no time is it not constantly changing and undetermined. It is by this very fact - that there is not a precise static instant of time underlying a dynamical physical process or motion - that variation in magnitudes is possible; it is a necessary tradeoff – precisely determined values for continuity through time. It is only the human observer, Lynds notes, who imposes a precise instant in time upon a physical process. Thus, there is no equation of physics, no wave equation, no equation of motion, no matter how complex, that is not subject to this indeterminacy.

With this view, there can be no static form at any instant, precisely because this static instant does not exist. The brain cannot base its computations on something that, to it, does not exist. The brain is equally embedded in the transforming matter-field, i.e., it is equally a part of this indeterminacy. It can only be responding to invariance over change.

The Origin of the External Image

Consider the picture thus far. On the one side, we have the transforming image of the cube. It is an image defining a scale on the matter-field. On the other side, we have the transforming neural patterns of the brain, supporting, we can posit, an attractor. It is a transformation, which we know, must determine the time scale of the image; it is structurally (via an invariance structure) related, it is even proportionally related. This dynamics, this proportionality, is a function of the energy state of the system. Gibson would have termed all this "resonance." But we come then to the critical problem. We see nothing in the brain that can possibly explain the experienced image of the cube. We see only attractors, neural patterns transforming. We stand before the famous explanatory gap.

Bergson explored beyond the gap. The dynamically changing field which carries the cube transforming, the fly buzzing, the neural patterns dynamically changing, Bergson, as Bohm (1980), saw as in essence a holographic field. In explaining the perception of events in this field, we have tended to take a photographic view of things, Bergson argued (and Gibson would echo), asking as it were how the brain develops a picture of the external world, or in current terms, how a representation (or code) is developed and interpreted as the external world. But, he argued, in holographic terms:

> "But is it not obvious that the photograph, if photograph there be, is already taken, already developed in the very heart of things and at all points in space. No metaphysics, no physics can escape this conclusion. Build up the universe with atoms: Each of them is subject to the action, variable in quantity and quality according to the distance, exerted on it by all material atoms. Bring in Faraday's centers of force: The lines of force emitted in every direction from every center bring to bear upon each the influence of the whole material world. Call up the Leibnizian monads: Each is the mirror of the universe." (1896/1912, p. 31)

Individual perception, he argued, is *virtual action*. An organism is a system of field elements organized for action. Embedded in the vast (holographic) field of real actions, those influences to which its action systems can respond are reflected as it were as virtual action, the rest simply pass through.

> "Only if when we consider any other given place in the universe we can regard the action of all matter as passing through it without resistance and without loss, and the photograph of the whole as translucent: Here there is wanting behind the plate the black screen on which the image could be shown. Our "zones of indetermination" [organisms] play in some sort the part of that screen. They add nothing to what is there; they effect merely this: That the real action passes through, the virtual action remains." (1896/1912, pp. 31-32)

While Bohm (1980) first introduced the notion of the holographic matter-field to physics, I think it safe to say that physics has routinely come to view this field as indeed a vast, dynamic interference pattern (cf. Beckenstein, 2003), where again the information for the whole is found at every point. If we take this as a postulate, the conjecture, then, is this: let us suppose the neural-dynamics with its re-entrant, resonant feedback, or if you will, the global wave of synchronous oscillations, is all conceived, very concretely, as supporting a wave, and more precisely, a modulated reconstructive wave "passing through" this holographic field. Now the dynamical, brain-supported pattern-wave "specifies" a virtual image of the matter-field. The modulation pattern is driven by the invariance structure or invariance laws defining the external event, while the energy-dynamics of the brain supporting this wave, with its underlying chemical velocities, in essence defines a ratio of proportion relative to the field's events at the micro-scale of time. Dependent on its energy-state (i.e., chemical velocities), it naturally defines the time-scale of the specified image of the field – a "buzzing" fly, or a "heron-like" fly, or a motionless, molecularly vibrating fly; a rotating cube or, as optimally as the available (invariance) information provided and constraints invoked - a wobbly, plastic-like object.

How can the image be specific to a past motion of the field? As in Figure 1, the initial rotation of the cube or the first wing-beat of the buzzing fly is long gone before the brain has begun its processing. It is the indivisibility or non-differentiability of the motion of the external field that allows the wave to be specific to the past. We need not hold that each "instant" of the cube's rotation ceases to exist unless stored within the (present) brain. This very property of the motion of the field provides the fundamental or "primary" memory supporting the time-extent of perceived events – a "rotating" cube, a "buzzing" fly.

This would be a concrete realization of Gibson's abstract "direct specification" of events or of dynamic forms. It is a direct realism that is not simply a naïve realism. The image is always an optimal function of the invariance information available in the field in conjunction with invariance laws (constraints) built into the brain's design. It is a specification of the past motion of the field given the best available information within the field and given the intrinsic uncertainty of "measuring" this field due to its temporal motion. Being a specification of the past, it is always, already a memory, a memory based in the primary memory supported by the non-differentiable time-evolution of the matter-field itself.

The Brain as Wave

A key element in this model is conceiving of the brain as a wave. This is certainly not unprecedented. Yasue, Jibu and Pribram (1991), see the evolving brain states in terms of complex valued wave flows, where constraints on the brain's (state) evolution are elegantly represented by Fourier coefficients of the wave spectrum of this formulation. Glassman (1999), for example, attempts to account for the limited capacity of working memory by viewing the brain, globally, as a set of waves whose frequencies are confined to a single octave. It has become common (Singer, 1998) to view the brain as a set of local and perhaps synchronous, oscillations, though we must be careful here of a category error in some of these cases, as an abstract oscillation is not equivalent to the concrete waves required by holographic reconstruction.

I will give no development of the physics and neuroscience required to model the brain as a very concrete reconstructive wave. There is sufficient work involved to unfold the model at the level of event invariance laws. It is a necessary endeavor to build a correspondent memory model at this level if only for the fact that the solution framework to the problem of perception described here may be the only one that handles the origin of the external image and the form of memory required for its ongoing extent in time. While even holographically oriented neuroscientists such as Pribram (1991; Yasue et. al., 1999) have tended to work within the storage metaphor, I am attempting to demonstrate that another framework is available in which to develop the neuroscience. And when the physics and neuroscience is all said and done, it will have the requirement in any case to support a description of memory retrieval operations at the event invariance law level of the sort that will be laid out in the following sections.

The brain-as-wave holds some fundamental implications. Given the inherent uncertainties of the information with which it deals and the fact that an optimal percept is being computed, on this basis alone, the brain's specification of events in the matter-field is based on probabilities. To construe direct realism as implying that we simply see "what is there" is in fact simply an expression of naïve realism. Given the inherent uncertainty of measurement, nothing is simply "there." This specification is nevertheless a specification, based upon information in the field, of a past form of motion of the field. In this sense it is a direct specification of events.

Yarrow et al. (2001) experimented with viewing a silently ticking clock, where, during rapid saccadic eye movements, the second hand appears to take longer than normal to move to its next position (as though the hand briefly stopped). Several experimental findings that appear to support indirect realism center around saccades. When we first look at a room, the eye darts from point to point over the area, in zigzag fashion, taking in information. During the movement itself, between the points, the eye is apparently blind, picking up no information. Under such conditions, objects presented during a saccade are actually invisible. The visual system appears to be shut down for an instant, but the brain computes what we would have seen during the saccade. Smythies (2002) notes that it would be most implausible to suggest, per direct realism, that we see directly only when our eyes are not in saccadic movement. The answer is that the perception is as direct as ever. During the clock hand's motion relative to a receptive eye, the always dynamic information from the field is taken in, the optimal percept computed, and the reconstructive wave/specification is still to the past. During the saccade, the brain-supported reconstructive wave does not cease – it continues to specify a state of the field based on the information available and the probabilistic algorithm employed by the architecture.

O'Regan (1992) is similar in this respect. He noted that an entire page of surrounding text can be changed without notice during a saccade while someone is reading as long as the 17-18 character window the eye is focused upon is undisturbed. This observation would lead to his treatment of "change blindness" (O'Regan and Noë, 2001). He opted to conceive of the environment as an "external memory store" to explain the persistence of the perceived world during saccades. He is one of the few that hold that perception is not "within," in some strange internal mini-world. But what is the time-scale of this external store (cf. Robbins, 2004b)? The "buzzing" fly? The molecular "fly?" We can better say that the reconstructive wave and/or the pattern supporting it within the brain is not affected by a substitution of the surrounding text during a saccade with its minute information gathering capacity (one estimate has this at 44 bits of information), the brain's specification yet being to the same states of the past.

There could be a long discussion here of many illusions, "filling in," etc., but this must suffice to give an indication of the potential of specification as a concept. As we shall see, the reconstructive wave can equally serve to retrieve memory experiences. These too can become part of the perceptual-illusory picture – for example the "bear" we suddenly see while walking through the woods, which on closer approach is seen to be merely a tree stump.

Direct Memory

The model of the conscious perception of time-extended events just described implies that experience is not occurring solely within the brain. It is truly a specification of past-motions of an already qualitative external field at a certain scale of time. As such, experience cannot be exclusively stored within the brain. There is a way, however, of conceiving the retrieval of experience as direct. Bergson (1896/1912) visualized the brain, embedded in the 4-D matter-field, as a form of "valve" which allows experiences from the past into consciousness depending on the array of action systems activated. In updated terms, we can say that the brain, embedded in the 4-D holographic field, again acts as a modulated reconstructive wave. Loss of memories – amnesias, aphasias, etc. – would be due, as Bergson (1896/1912) in essence argued, to damage that causes inability to assume the complex modulation patterns required. This might assume the form of damage to the complex connections between the pre-frontal areas and the temporal lobe, where the pre-frontal areas are charged with controlling the strategies and dynamics of *explicit* retrieval of past events, or as Piaget (1954) termed it, the "localization of events in time."

This does not mean that no form of memory is stored in the brain. Sherry and Schacter (1987) described two general forms of memory, labeled "System I" and "System II." The two systems correspond exactly to the distinction Bergson made in *Matter and Memory*. "System I" can also be termed the "procedural" – stored mechanisms or procedures for unrolling an action at will. It is amenable, at least partially, to the connectionist net, and is obviously brain-based. "System II" holds experiences. It corresponds to the memory Tulving (1972) termed "episodic." In Bergson's example, everyday I sit down at the piano, let us say, and practice Chopin's Waltz in C# minor. I do this day after day. Each experience is different. I have a head cold one day, the sun is bright the next and the room brilliant, the next day is dreary, I am depressed over exams in another. The resultant of all the practices is a nice motor program that unrolls effortlessly as the C# minor Waltz. This is clearly a neural modification in the brain. There are other neural storage effects. The layout of the piano keyboard, with its five black and seven white alternating keys, is experienced daily over and over. The particular black-white pattern is always the same, it is an *invariant* over these experiences. The spatial neural firing patterns in the visual cortex which respond to the layout of the keyboard must eventually be registered at some level of the neural structure or hierarchy as an invariant pattern. Hawkins (2004), for example, proposes a model for the formation of these all-important neural "invariants." The auditory patterns of the C# minor Waltz must similarly be registered. But these resultants, or invariant patterns, are not the same as each *experience* of practicing. These experiences are not "stored" as such in the brain, Bergson argued, but neither are they lost, and each experience is in principle retrievable.

System I includes the sensorimotor "schemas" of Piaget, where, for example, an object such as a cup becomes embedded as it were in a matrix of possible actions – lifting, drinking, pouring – which are initially overtly acted out when a cup is perceived and with age, ultimately inhibited. These become a basis for triggering wave-modulation patterns. The relation between these two forms of memory – that based in the brain and that which is not - is a complex one and a subject for much further theory.

The essential operation of direct memory is redintegration. The concept of redintegration can trace its genes back to the very origins of psychology. Thus it was Christian Wolff, a contemporary and disciple of Leibniz and a mathematics professor, who first introduced the "law of redintegration" in his *Psychologica Empirica* of 1732. In effect, Wolff's law stated that "when a present perception forms a part of a past perception, the whole past perception tends to reinstate itself." A 1912 formulation of this by Dessoir stated: "Every idea tends to recall to the mind the total idea of which it is a part."

Examples of this phenomenon abound in everyday experience. Thus the sound of thunder may serve to redintegrate a childhood memory of the day one's house was struck by lightning. Perhaps, for example, we are walking down a road in the summertime and suddenly notice a slight rustling or motion in the grass along the embankment. Immediately, an experience returns in which a snake was encountered in a similar situation. Klein (1970) notes that these remembered experiences are "structured or organized events or clusters of patterned, integrated impressions," and that Wolff had in effect noted that subsequent to the establishment of such patterns, the pattern might be recalled by reinstatement of a constituent part of the original pattern.

The Redintegrative Model

It is precisely the mathematical description of these "event patterns" that we have seen in Gibson's theory. Suppose then, "stirring coffee," and to appreciate the full dynamics that might be involved, let the cup be slowly rotating, successively presenting its flow field sides and simultaneously moving towards us across the table's gradient surface. When stirring this cup of coffee, we are involving multiple areas of the brain – visual areas, motor areas, auditory areas, haptic areas. Even the action-goal of "stirring" must be supported by the pre-frontal areas. Over these, we have a resonant feedback from the multiple re-entrant projections between all areas which supports a dynamical pattern occurring over time. For practical purposes, we have a near-global, time-extended pattern supported over the brain. The dynamical pattern itself, in some form, must support the ongoing, dynamic invariance structure of the coffee-stirring event being specified in perception.

The redintegration principle I am about to propose assumes a fundamental symmetry between perception and memory: the same invariance laws which determine the perception of an event also drive remembering. This implies a basic law of the fundamental operation of redintegration or direct retrieval:

> (1) An event E' will reconstruct a previous event E when E' is defined by the same invariance structure or by a sufficient subset of the same invariance structure.

In essence, when the same dynamic pattern, supporting the same invariance structure, is evoked over the global state of the brain, the correspondent *experience* is reconstructed. We are essentially relying upon the same mechanism Gibson argued supported the direct specification of an event, and this is why I term this a model of direct retrieval or *direct memory*.

Let us put this into our event context. Imagine a drive up a mountain road. The road curves back and forth, sinusoidal, rising at a particular grade. We have then a certain gradient of velocity vectors lawfully transforming as a function of the radius of the curves and the velocity of the vehicle. Over this flow field the tau (τ) ratio is defined, discussed above, which specifies time to impending contact and severity of impact, and has a critical value in controlling action. Our driver can rely directly on the τ value to modulate his velocity to avoid possible impacts with structures along the road. There are other components such as the contour and texture density gradients peculiar to a mountain terrain. An integral part of this transforming field (E) is the organism (O). The transformation specifying the flow field is also that defining the values of tuning parameters for the action systems. The velocity of field expansion/directional change is specific to the velocity of the car and to the muscular adjustments necessary to hold it on the road. Therefore the state of the body/brain with respect to future possible (virtual) action as well as that actually being carried out constitutes an integral component of the E-O event pattern.

I believe it is quite common for people to have past experiences redintegrated by this form of flowing, road-driving, invariance structure. My wife tells me that every time we drive along a certain curving section of the freeway near Milwaukee, she swears she is driving on a segment of a freeway in California where she once lived. Due to the indivisible time-evolution of the matter-field, neither the original transformation of the field nor its subsequent specification by the brain as an image (of its then-past motion) have moved into non-existence. The reason that the experience is reconstructed is that the brain is thrown by the invariance structure of the present event into the same reconstructive wave pattern as that which defined the original event. This is the essence of the principle of redintegration.

The more unique this invariance structure, the easier it is to reconstruct the specific event. It is exactly as if a series of wave fronts were recorded upon a hologram, each with a unique frequency of reference wave, as when we imagined storing the wave fronts of a pyramid/ball, chalice, toy truck and candle. Each wave front (or image) can then be reconstructed uniquely by modulating the reconstructive wave to each differing frequency. This implies a second law for *sets* of events:

> (2) For a set of events, $E_1, E_2, \ldots E_n$, the more unique the invariance structure defining each event, the greater the probability that they will be reconstructed by E' events with the same invariance structure.

Imagine a series of perceived events, for example, a man stirring coffee, a baseball hurtling by one's head, a boot crushing a can. Each has a unique invariance structure. To create the reconstructive wave for these, i.e., to evoke over the brain the needed modulation or dynamic wave pattern, I might use as a "cue" respectively - a stirring spoon, an abstract rendering of an approaching object capturing the composite tau value of the baseball event (cf. Craig and Bootsma, 2000), and an abstract rendering of one form descending upon and obscuring another (Verbrugge, 1977). But these events are multi-sensory (multi-modal) and the four-dimensional extent of experience is multi-modal. There are auditory invariants as well defined over the events. Our cues could become respectively – the swishing or clinking sound of stirring, while the steady "looming" of the approaching baseball, with its radial, expanding flow field, is proportional over a range of frequency values to the change of sound inherent in the Doppler effect, and finally, we would have the crinkling sound of collapse of a tin structure. Even the dynamics of the muscular (or haptic) component of the event has a mathematical structure we could employ to re-cue the event, namely Turvey's "inertia tensor," consisting of the mathematical specification of the forces and moments of inertia in three dimensions that describe the motion. We could cue our stirring event by wielding a "tensor object." that captures this inertia tensor (invariant) specific to spoon-stirring. Were we trying to catch the onrushing baseball, the grasping adjustment of the hand is precisely specified by the tau value (Savelsburgh et al., 1991), and conversely then, a specific grasping adjustment is an integral, and potentially redintegrating component of this event.

Note that the invariance laws above are *amodal*. The information cuts across modalities, allowing an event specified in one modality (for example, sound), to be redintegrative of the same event in another modality (e.g., the optical).

I would like to progress now from the abstract to the concrete, as research did historically, situating these principles first and briefly in the context of the much studied verbal tasks. I will move from there to imagery, then to Subject Performed Tasks (SPTs), and then view priming in the SPT context.

Verbal Tasks and Redintegration

Consider an experiment in the verbal learning tradition, in this case the A-B, A-C paired-associate list paradigm.

List 1 (A-B)	List 2 (A-C)
SPOON-COFFEE	SPOON-BATTER
KNIFE-SOAP	KNIFE-DOUGH
BOTTLE-THIMBLE	BOTTLE-PAN
	And so on......

After list 1 is learned, then the process begins again with list 2, and we must now keep the responses for list 1 (COFFEE for SPOON) separate from list 2 (BATTER for SPOON). Here, theory focuses on "inter-item" relations (or relational information) as critical to help us (e.g., Marschark et al., 1987). For example, we might notice that List 2 is mostly about baking/cooking-related response words. This helps us "delineate a search set," as the memory literature terms things. We know at least, when we are dealing with list 2, that baking/cooking response words are the targets. The ecological case is far simpler and it is primary.

Let us assume these are concrete events, enacted or perceived. The subject stirs the coffee with the spoon, or stirs the batter with the spoon. He cuts the soap with the knife, or cuts the dough. He pours water from the bottle into the pan, or into the thimble. Now in the verbal case, after learning the lists, we would simply present the word "SPOON" as a cue. But this is a very vague event; it has no *specificity*. Which object, or which event will it redintegrate? Even a concrete but static spoon, placed on the table before us, would have a questionable cueing power. We have at best the classic "response competition" model which McGeoch (1942) introduced early on. In the behaviorist terminology of the day, the "stimulus," SPOON, activates both BATTER and COFFEE as possible "responses." In modern terminology, we would say both words are "primed." In essence, we could say, we have sent a highly *unconstrained* wave though our holographic memory, as though we had a non-coherent wave containing frequencies f_1 and f_2, the frequencies of the original reference waves for recording two different wave fronts (or objects).

We can improve this by modulating the wave to a precise or coherent frequency, correspondent with the original reference wave, e.g., f_1, of the desired stored wave front. And concretely, in terms of events, we must put greater *constraints* on the cue event. For starters, a dynamism must be placed on the static spoon – the circular motion of stirring. But yet more precise constraint is needed to cue the proper event and object – batter or coffee. We can choose to create the greater resistance provided by the batter medium, or the larger amplitude of circular motion in the batter case assuming it was in a bowl, or both. The cue-event must force this precise modulatory pattern over the brain. Had one of the pairs been SPOON-OATMEAL, where the spoon was being used to shovel-in the oatmeal, a quite different transformation, involving scooping and lifting, and with the weight, mass and consistency constraints implied by oatmeal, would be placed on the cue-event with its spoon.

With this in mind, one can imagine an absurdly difficult paired-associate paradigm as far as verbal learning experiments are concerned. We'll call it the "A-B_i" paradigm. A list would look as follows:

SPOON-COFFEE
SPOON-BATTER
SPOON-OATMEAL
SPOON-BUTTER
SPOON-CORNFLAKES
SPOON-PEASOUP
SPOON-CATAPULT
SPOON-CHEESE
SPOON-TEETER TOTTER
And so on…

It is absurd since the stimulus words are exactly the same, the subject could have no clue what the appropriate response word is. But assume that the subject concretely acts out each event of the "absurd" list – stirring the coffee, stirring the batter, scooping/lifting the oatmeal, the cornflakes, cutting the cheese. To effectively cue the remembering, I have argued, the dynamics of each cue-event must be unique, and the invariance structure of an event in effect implies a structure of constraints. These constraints may be "parametrically" varied, where increasing fidelity to the original structure of constraints of a given event corresponds to a finer tuning of the reconstructive wave. Vicente and Wang (1998) alluded to this process in a different, more advanced memory context such as chess or baseball, as "constraint attunement." The (for example, blindfolded) subject may wield a Turvey type "tensor-object" in a circular motion within a liquid. The resistance of the liquid (a parameter value) may be appropriate to a thin liquid such as coffee or to a thicker medium such as the batter. The circular motion (a parameter value) may be appropriate to the spatial constraint defined by a cup or to the larger amplitude allowed by a bowl. The periodic motion may conform to the original adiabatic invariance (frequency/energy) within the event, or may diverge. We can predict that with sufficiently precise transformations and constraints on the motion of the spoon (either visual, or auditory or kinesthetic or combined), the entire list can be reconstructed, i.e., each event and associated response word. Each appropriately constrained cue-event corresponds to a precise modulation (or constraint) of the reconstructive wave defined over the brain.

The obvious inverse is that, as the parameter values diverge from the original event, cueing/recall performance and/or recognition performance will increasingly degrade.

Recognition tests are one method of testing these manipulations, employing familiarity ratings. In this case, we would present events transformed on various dimensions. The familiarity value should steadily decrease as the parameters are varied.

Parametric Variation of Cues in Concrete Events

These kinds of experiments are implicit in the literature. An example is found in a demonstration by Jenkins, Wald and Pittenger (1978). Capitalizing on the notion of the optical flow field, they showed subjects a series of slides that had been taken at fixed intervals as a cameraman walked across the university campus mall. Some slides, however, were purposely left out. Later, when subjects were shown various slides again and asked if they had seen the slide shown, they rejected easily any slide taken from a different perspective and which therefore did not share the same flow field invariant defined across the series. Slides not originally seen, but which fit the series were accepted as "having been seen" with high probability. But Jenkins et al. had created a "gap" in the original set shown to the subjects by leaving out a series of six continuous slides. Thus a portion of the transformation of the flow field was not specified. Subjects were quite easily able to identify these slides as "not seen." In this case, we are in effect varying parametric values defining a flow field. Other manipulations are possible, for example the slant of the gradient, the smoothness of the flow, the velocity of the flow, etc.

The many experiments of Freyd on “representational momentum” can be seen in this light (Freyd and Finke, 1984; Finke, Freyd and Shyi, 1986; Finke and Freyd, 1985; Freyd, 1987; Freyd et al., 1990). A subject may be shown three slides of a rotating rectangle. Each slide shows the rectangle rotated a little bit more. When subjects are given a recall test, they are likely to remember what would have been the fourth slide – the next rotated position or angle. A “probe” slide or memory cue of the never-seen fourth slide is rated the most likely to have been seen. The memory seems to represent the “momentum” of the moving rectangle. This however can be seen as a form of parametric manipulation of the cue-event. More straightforwardly, we could simply initially present the rectangle rotating at a certain velocity, then later attempt to cue the event, or ask for familiarity judgments, with rotations of different velocities.

On the visual side, consider, for example, presenting a simple static event of a field with a schematic tree (Figure 13). The trees in the figure have been grown with the precise mathematics defining real tree growth (Bingham, 1993).

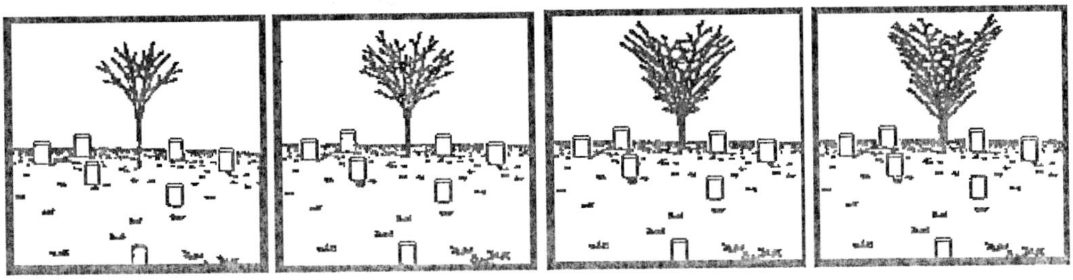

Figure 13. A generated, aging tree. (Adopted from Bingham, 1993).

The number of terminal branches (N) is a set function of height (H), $N=k(H)^2$, while the diameter (D) of trunk or branches at any point is a function of remaining length to the tip, $D=k(H)$. Suppose that one of the recognition items in our experiment is the leftmost or youngish tree in Figure 13. In the recognition test phase, the parametric values defining the structure of the trees can be varied increasingly from the original value. For example, we could re-represent the second tree, or third, or fourth tree and ask if this is recognized as part of the original set of items.

Familiarity ratings should drop the further we move along the age dimension. More dynamically, a time-accelerated view of the tree's growth under certain parametric values can be used as the stimulus. For a dynamic event such as an approaching rugby ball, the time to contact value (cf. Gray and Regan, 1999) can be varied increasingly from the original value.

Even the original experiments of Pittenger and Shaw (1978), with their aging facial profiles generated via strain transformations on a cardioid (Figure 11), could be re-cast in this redintegration test framework. Originally the subjects looked at many pairs of faces, judging each time which of the pair was the older. Changing this to a memory task, a face of a certain age can be included in a set of various items successively presented to a subject. On the recognition task, a face transformed by a certain parametric aging value is now presented. Familiarity values will be a function of the transformation. The aging transformation works for animal faces too, even for Volkswagons – it can generate increasingly aging "Beetles!" So we can have many different kinds of items in this test that eventually get aged (or un-aged) in a recognition phase.

It is good here to keep in mind the implications of virtual action relative to the previous rectangle example. We could have various possible rotation events of a rotating cube at various velocities and therefore various transitional forms - from slowly rotating, to multiple serrated edges, to fuzzy cylinder – with each transitional form conforming to a 4n-fold symmetry constraint. Each of these, by virtual action, would imply, for example, a possible modulation of the hand required to grasp either a cube, a serrated-edged object, or a cylinder. Therefore the implied muscular or haptic component of a perceived event, or parametric variation on grasping, is an equally possible cue-event manipulation.

Imagery and Concreteness

The introduction of imagery was perhaps one of the early things to show that there is far more going on than the laws of verbal learning, complex as they were becoming, were revealing. In introducing imagery as a variable in paired associate learning experiments, Paivio (1971) simultaneously moved to another *level of specificity*, yet closer to the concrete, ecological world of events. Research more clearly delineated the "facilitative" effect of images upon memory performance. Some important aspects noted by Paivio (1971) were the following:

1) Given a pair of objects, designated by words, or pictures, or simply the objects themselves, the more *dynamic* the image formed involving the two objects, the greater the probability of correct recall (given one object as the cue). As an example, Rowher et al. (1967) did a study in which subjects saw either (a) two objects simply appearing side by side, (b) two objects oriented towards each other spatially in a

manner corresponding to a prepositional phrase, e.g., a HAND *in* a BOWL, or a CUP *on* a TABLE, (c) two objects depicted in an action sequence corresponding to a verb phrase, e.g., the DOG *opening* the GATE. Different subjects were assigned to each type of case. After the sets of pairs were presented to each subject, there followed a test in which the experimenter named each stimulus object, e.g., HAND or DOG, and the subject was asked to recall the object paired with it. Performance was best in case (c) where the objects were in motion, followed by (b) where they were at least spatially related, and then by (a) or simple juxtaposition.

2) What forms in effect a corollary to the above is the finding that *interactive* images are more effective than non-interactive images. Again it was found (Wollen, 1969) that subjects produced better performance when told to create interactive images, rather than simply being told to image. To visualize a "jar *on* a table" was better than simply a "jar *and* a table."
3) The *concreteness* effect. Given a pair of words, it is the *specificity* of the *stimulus* (cue word) that is most crucial for recall. Paivio referred this "specificity" to the *concreteness* of the cue word. Paivio (1971) tested four conditions involving stimulus-response word-pairs which varied in abstractness-concreteness:

    a) Concrete stimulus, concrete response (house-shoe)
    b) Concrete stimulus, abstract response (house-truth)
    c) Abstract stimulus, concrete response (furniture-carrot)
    d) Abstract stimulus, abstract response (furniture-vegetable)

Learning was best in (a) where both members of the pair were concrete, followed by (b), then (c), and lastly (d) where both members of the pair were abstract. Ultimately this finding was dubbed the "concreteness effect" and has been considered one of the strongest or most "robust" effects in memory research (Marschark et al., 1987). Only the most special conditions seem able to destroy it.

Given the preceding discussion of redintegration, the reason for the effectiveness of imagery in paired-associate learning, particularly dynamic imagery entailing some event, should be quite clear. The creation of a mental image of an event firstly comes a step closer to the level of specificity of a concrete, perceived event. It inherently will possess some degree of invariance structure. Suppose for a moment our word-pairs were:

SPOON-WATER
KNIFE-SOAP
TURTLE-BOARD
HAMMER-ROCK
BOAT-CUP
And so on….

For these we envision the spoon stirring the water, the knife cutting flakes from the soap, the hammer crushing the rock, etc. These imaged events are a series of unique event structures along the time dimension. Uniqueness could also be termed "distinctiveness," but this term, used very vaguely in the literature (cf. Schmidt, 1991, for a critical review), now carries a very "distinctive" and precise meaning in this model – *it is the dynamic structure of transformations, invariants, and constraints defining each event.* Again, when we present simply the word SPOON as a cue, we are not using a very powerful cue. The relation of the cue to these event structures is clearly critical as we have seen. The cue-event gains its power by establishing the structure of constraints that are specific to the precise event. Simultaneously, the invariance structure of each cue (event) should be unique, for this corresponds to the unique reconstructive wave. This is why the "specificity of the stimulus" (cue) is so important. But at least, in these imagery experiments, we have the uniqueness of event structure.

To dig down a little deeper, we can ask why "prepositional" type imagery is less effective than the "actional" type. Consider "the hand in the bowl" versus "the hand stirring in the bowl." Here the "hand in the bowl" is but a snapshot of several possible events - a stirring hand, a hand moving up and down, a hand grabbing a goldfish, etc. The perceptual relations or mathematical structure supported over such a static scene are not as specific and therefore the resonance states not so sharply differentiated from states appropriate to a hand in relationship to some other object, e.g., a can, a cup, a briefcase. Given this it can be said that the dynamic image-cue by nature creates a more specific modulatory pattern such that the possible scenes that can be reconstructed are intrinsically constrained. To specify an event of a spoon-in-motion is already to constrain the scenes that can be reconstructed, while to restrict it to a spoon-in-a-circular-motion involving a force of a given strength is to constrain the (to-be-stirred) object – relative to the event invariance structure - to an equivalence class of objects, each stage, as we have seen, corresponding to a finer tuning of the reconstructive wave.

Therefore, a legitimate line of experimentation in imagery experiments is the introduction of dynamic cues. This could be in the form of images ("Imagine a spoon moving in a circle"), or more concrete events where the subject actually takes a real spoon and moves it in a stirring motion. The more powerful variants of this have been noted in the context of parametric variation of cues, but in general, performance will improve increasingly from verbal-static (SPOON), to image-dynamic (image of circling spoon) to concrete dynamic (concrete moving spoon).

Craik and Tulving (1975), in interpreting such results, would have been led to say that the more dynamic image leads to a "richer, more elaborate encoding," and the achievement by target and cue thereby of a greater "compatibility" with the structure and rules of "semantic" memory. But now we have insight into what "compatibility" means - the precise sharing of mathematical invariance defined over cue and target - and of what the rules of "semantic memory" actually consist, i.e., invariance laws, and how "richness" of encoding is actually to be described via the mathematics of events.

We must consider briefly the source of the concreteness effect itself. In essence, the abstractness of a word represents an increasing order of invariance (cf. Robbins, 2002). Intuitively we understand that the higher the order of invariance a phrase specifies, the more difficult it is to instantiate that structure as an image of a particular event. When we start from the specification, "A utensil is interacting with a piece of furniture," rather than "A knife is cutting the wooden top of the table," we have complicated the modulatory task. From this perspective, the concreteness effect is very real, but it is in one sense an artifact, created by the intrinsic difficulty of transducing these stimuli to something nearer the concrete, ecological events with invariance structures allowing redintegrative laws to operate effectively.

Subject-Performed Tasks

There is a line of memory research, reviewed in detail and summarized in Engelkamp and Zimmer (1994) and Engelkamp (1998), on subject-performed tasks (SPTs). The research has generally shown that simple action phrases (such as "break the toothpick") are better recalled when participants perform the actions themselves as opposed to simply hearing or reading the action description (Cohen, 1981; Engelkamp, 1998, and Nilsson, 2000 for reviews). The large memory effect of the SPT relative to the largely predominant verbal tasks (VTs) has been called the SPT effect. Tasks performed by the experimenter and simply observed by the subject, i.e., experimenter performed tasks (EPTs), have virtually the same effect as the SPT in between- subjects designs with relatively short (18-20 item) lists. The SPT gains an advantage over the EPT for lists employed in a within-subjects design, or for very long (e.g., 48 items) lists (cf. Engelkamp, 1998, pp. 55-59).

SPTs are also impervious to the "generation effects" of VTs. In a verbal task, if the subject is given the word BALL and asked to generate an event, e.g., imagining a bouncing ball, he tends to do better in later recall than a subject who was simply presented the phrase, "The ball is bouncing." In an SPT, it makes no difference in later recall if the subject thought up the act of bouncing the ball and performed it, or merely performed it upon the supplied command, "Bounce the ball." Similarly, in verbal tasks, it can make a difference if the subject is told to check a word for spelling, or imagine its use in a sentence. The spelling check is a "shallow encoding" of the word, the sentence is a "deeper encoding." These types of instructions are virtually meaningless and have no effect in an SPT.

Two views have competed for the explanation of the effect. The multi-modal view (Backman and Nilsson, 1985; Backman, Nilsson, and Kormi-Nouri, 1993) has emphasized the multi-modal nature of enacted events, arguing SPTs activate the verbal-semantic content of the action as well as information from perceptual cues. This combination, it is felt, accounts for the improved retention. Engelkamp (1998; Engelkamp and Zimmer, 1985, 1997) focused on the motor component. Central to the encoding of actions is the fact that they must be planned and initiated. Rather than all sensory and motor features contributing to the effect, only the motor features contribute to the enactment advantage.

For the holographic redintegration model, these findings are fully expected (cf. Robbins, 1976). Purely from the ecological perspective, a subject performed task, e.g., "break the match," or "stir the coffee," is a completely specified multi-modal invariance structure. It sits at the highest level of an order of *completeness of specification*, which is to say completeness of specified event constraints. Whether the event is self-generated or performed on command, there is little difference in the invariance structure defining the event, or in the "modulated wave" required to reconstruct the event. The event carries none of the baggage of variability that abounds in purely verbally based experiments where subjects' mental operations are generally uncontrolled. In the purely verbal case of the presentation of the event (a sentence), we have very little idea what the "event" actually is. It may involve a visual image, it may not; the sentence may have been comprehended, it may not. Therefore the actual structure of event constraints is unknown. The use of imagery instructions comes closer, attempting to create an imaged, concrete event. But we are unsure of the veridicality of the image with respect to the concrete event; we are unsure that the complete structure of transformations and invariants was produced or to what extent.

Let us note the implications of the model for several specific aspects of the SPT research.

1) The Transitve-Intransitve Pattern

In the SPT experiments, there has been some controversy over the role of objects (cf. Zimmer and Cohen, 2001). The Swedish group used real objects in their experiments, while the Saarbrücken group had the subjects perform actions with imaginary objects. The latter group still found an effect from acting out the event, but found the effect got a boost when real objects were used. While action was clearly seen as important, the question became, why? Zimmer (2001) considered the concept of brain-embedded programs for action or "action schema." For example, the action schema for "lifting" has a "slot" for *something to lift*, and in this sense action programs might be the units that "bind" events together. In this respect, he noted an experiment by Ratner and Hill (1991) using actions with transitive vs. intransitive verbs (push the refrigerator vs. sit by the desk). Only the actions were re-performed in recall, with care taken to constrain the specifics of the action. If the original action involved pushing a refrigerator, then as a recall cue, the subject pretended to push something difficult to move. The cueing effect was stronger for transitive verbs. The subject was much more likely to remember that the action involved pushing a refrigerator. But just "sitting by" something, even if sitting in exactly the same way, was less likely to retrieve the fact that it was a desk one was sitting by.

We have seen now that the "transitive-intransitive" effect holds for SPTs, EPTs, VTs and imagery. This indicates that there is a memory mechanism or law that cuts across all modes of experiencing an event. It cannot be a purely motor effect; it is a more general effect than the SPT, yet applies to the SPT. The principle acting must be more general and deeper than "action as the glue of events." The concept of a reconstructive wave faithful to, or supportive of, the invariance structure of events, to include their virtual motor component, is such a general principle.

2) The Role of Objects

The role of actual objects in the events, noted above, indexes how the SPT research efforts have exposed the concept that there are obvious levels of specificity. From worst to best:

- Verbally specified events
- Imagined events
- Observed events (as in EPTs)
- Imitated, concretely acted events (as in SPTs)
- Concretely acted events (as in SPTs).

The presence of objects - their actual usage in the event - can only aid more precise specification of the invariance structure and its constraints, and therefore the differentiation of events. This is because "specificity" *corresponds precisely to the degree of instantiation of the full dynamics supporting the perception of an event.* In cued recall, as we have reviewed, this becomes increasingly important. The discussion of the fine tuning of memory performance that is possible via the parametric manipulation of invariance structures highlights this. With respect to the role of action, *enactment guarantees the specificity.* The precise action constraint, used as a cue, again is a precise constraint on the reconstructive wave. Based on the invariance structure in which the cue is normally embedded it specifies, if not the actual event, an equivalence class of objects. Perhaps we should say, just as in McGeoch's model, that a set of past events has been "primed." In a reconstructive wave, we are dealing with something more dynamic and concrete than an abstract "slot" or argument for an object in an action schema.

3) Verb to Verb Failure

In this context, it can also be seen why one should not have expected the attempts of SPT researchers to associate verbs to verbs (actions to arbitrary actions) in SPTs to be particularly successful (they were not), e.g., "lifting the book" as a cue for "tapping the wall," (cf. Engelkamp, 1998). There is nothing in the invariance structure of E' capable of redintegrating E. This was in effect a nonsense syllable PA task imported into the context of SPTs.

4) EPT vs. SPT Performance

Why is the performance on EPTs so nearly equal to that of the SPT? If action or motor encoding is the primary principle operating in the SPT effect, why is there not a greater difference? The virtually equal performance of the EPT in between-subjects designs with lists of 18-20 items is ascribed to the episodic-relational capabilities of EPTs. Buttressing this is the observation that in within-subjects designs, the EPT performance degrades (somewhat), apparently because in the switch from observing the tasks to acting the tasks, the relation-formation and its advantage is disrupted. Engelkamp (1998, p.95) argues that carrying out an action forces focusing onto the information relevant to the action in such a way that the planning of the action is screened off from other information, ensuring that the action is carried out without interference. This is not the case in other modalities. While watching someone pick apples, he notes, it doesn't hurt if I widen my range of vision and include the context, but if picking the apple ourselves and our attention wanders, we can miss the apple. This may certainly be true, yet we can ask, if the experimental context, as is usual, is relatively invariant across items, what good could context information for each item/action actually do?

In truth, there is no truly principled reason within the curent SPT/motor action framework of theory for the supposed EPT episodic-relational advantage, nor especially for the larger question as to why the EPT is within a hair of SPT performance. The redintegrative model makes perfect sense of the virtual equality of EPT performance. We have seen that the EPT, as a concrete, ecological event, is highly specific of the invariance structure of events, and especially when coupled with the principle of perception as virtual action, the redintegrative model described would fully predict very strong memory performance in this very concrete, ecological context. The SPT, at the greatest level of specificity, would be expected to eventually prove superior. This model does not answer why the performance break-point is 18-20, but no theory does.

5) EPT vs. SPT and Reenactment

The SPT effect occurred when participants were blindfolded at study, therefore being denied visual information (Engelkamp et al., 1993). Engelkamp et al. (1994) found that for items enacted at study, enacting during test produced greater recognition accuracy (known as the *reenactment effect*). Both studies support a pure motoric explanation of the SPT effect. Mulligan and Hornstein (2003) replicated the reenactment effect, showing that it existed for both SPTs and EPTs. However, they were able to show that the SPT effect existed even when the subjects were blindfolded at test, indicating, they argued, that visual information is not critical for reenactment recognition in the case of SPTs, and that the basis for the reenactment effect differs across SPTs and EPTs. Mulligan and Hornstein did not test the EPT case with blindfolds, but we can predict that the EPT condition will also show a reenactment effect, for the basis of the effect is the same for both: reenactment, in respecting the motor invariance laws defining the event, creates a reconstructive wave redintegrative of the event. Further, in the earlier discussion of parametric variation of cues, e.g., varying the periodicity, or diameter, or resistance in stirring, I have already indicated that both EPT and SPT recall will be affected by these manipulations. There is, further, the (apparently) anomalous fact that visual interference, relative to motor task interference, equally reduces enacted task memory. The reason proposed is that enactment may also activate visual-sensory processes (Engelkamp, 1998, p.31), but this is coordinate with the position that invariance laws are amodal, cutting across modalities, and again pointing to the commonality of the redintegrative mechanism for EPT and SPT.

Priming

Priming is considered to have major implications for the structure of memory. In one experimental paradigm a word is presented briefly, e.g., "spoon" followed quickly by another word or non-word, e.g., in the word case, "coffee." The subject's task is usually a simple one like indicating whether "coffee" is a word or a non-word. In the SPOON-COFFEE pair, there would be an expected priming effect since SPOON is a close “associate” of COFFEE and has prepared the way in some sense for the response. In a pair like SPOON-BOOK we might expect little or no priming effect as BOOK is not a close associate of SPOON.

A major theoretical explanation for the priming effect has been the spreading activation model (Anderson, 1983). Here memory is conceived as a network of "nodes" consisting of concepts related by semantic links or associative links. Consider the concept of SLEEP with its semantic network (Figure 14). Roediger et al. (2001) describe the classic, spreading activation-explained phenomenon, where the subjects hear fifteen of the surrounding concepts/words (bed, rest, awake, tired, etc.). Though "sleep" is not presented, on a later recognition test, the subjects are extremely likely to recognize it as having been part of the original list they heard (Roediger and McDermott, 1995).

“Stirring" is no less a dynamic invariance structure than “sleep.” On seeing SPOON, activation would be conceived to spread through the network of nodes related to SPOON, ultimately reaching COFFEE and facilitating response time to COFFEE. But what is stored at these nodes? If our node is STIR, is it the dynamic, time-extended, multi-modal invariance structure we have described for a coffee stirring event, or a yet higher order invariance defined across many forms of stirring? But how is this invariance, which has no reality other than as an invariant defined across concrete *experience*, stored "at a node?"

Another competing model is the compound cue theory. Here the SPOON (prime) – COFFEE (target) pair is viewed as forming a compound cue in short-term memory which is used to create a match to information in long-term memory. This joint-cue is a more powerful cue, providing the basis for a familiarity or parallel matching process to all items in memory. Facilitation of a response then is considered a function of “familiarity.” A pair like

MOTHER-CHILD is more familiar than MOTHER-HOSPITAL (Shelton and Martin, 1992). The familiarity value is conceived to relate directly to the response time required to categorize CHILD or HOSPITAL (as a word or non-word).

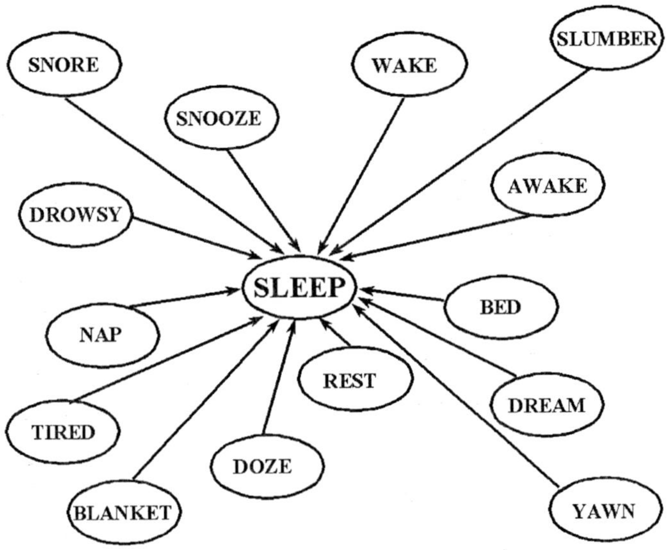

Figure 14. A semantic activation network for the concept "sleep." The words shown are the 15 highest associates to sleep. (After Roediger et al., 2001).

The SPOON-COFFEE pair is really but a compacted version of an experimental paradigm where sentences are presented such as:

(1) The spoon stirred the [COFFEE].
or
(2) The spoon stirred the [BOOK].

There is again a quicker response time in (word/non-word) categorizing COFFEE in (1) than BOOK in (2). Again, (1) is presumed to have greater "familiarity" than (2), enhancing the response process. Mckoon and Ratcliff (1992) however rejected the usefulness of this type of experimental material because they saw no way to get "familiarity" values from the sentences, whereas as with single words they could use associative frequency norms, e.g., the frequency that MOTHER appears as an associate to CHILD as opposed to HOSPITAL, or SPOON with COFFEE as opposed to BOOK.

Yet, with the sentence paradigm, we begin to approach the ecological case - real, specified events. Again we have extremely little control over the events in the subject's mind when we present word pairs like SPOON-COFFEE or DEER-GRAIN. Suppose we had this set of sentences:

(3) He stirred the coffee with the [spoon].
(4) He stirred the coffee with the [knife].
(5) He stirred the coffee with the [orange peel].
(6) He stirred the coffee with the [truck].

Here we are clearly in the case of an event invariance structure. "Coffee stirring" specifies an equivalence class of objects that can participate in the event, and that can fill in the blank. We have sent, in effect, a reconstructive wave through memory defined by the constraints of the invariance structure. Sentence (3) is the level of invariance defining normal (global) context. It is most "familiar." Sentences (4), and (5) begin defining a dimension of possible substances and structures which can participate in the event given they support certain structural invariances. Sentence (6) sits way at the end of this dimension, if at all. Nevertheless, with proper (global) context, for example a pre-discussion of childhood play, I could likely bring up the response time on (6). "Familiarity" or networks of "associates" are only a poor approximation to describing the effect of the dynamic patterns of activity and invariance structures involved here.

Priming - An Hypothesis

Priming is another case of redintegration with its inherent reliance on event invariance structures. This means that priming is also subject to the parametric variation of these structures. This can then be kept in the very ecological dimension where it must be initially understood. Therefore we might have the equivalent of a "priming sentence" such as:

(7) The spoon stirred the __________.

But let the event be concretely acted out, e.g., the (blindfolded) subject actually stirs with the spoon within standard spatial constraints, where the substance stirred has liquid properties, thus resistance, similar to coffee. Now we present words/non-words (or better, concrete objects/events?) for recognition reaction time. Again in this case, we must reckon with normal context, i.e., coffee as normally stirred, as providing the shortest time. But there should eventually be some equivalence class of liquids which have been primed. As we vary the parameters of the substance, for example, now moving to a thick, batter-like substance, this effect should become more pronounced. Now something like "batter" should be primed more quickly, or "dough," etc. Conversely, as parameters diverge from the coffee stirring event, for example, the diameter of the circular motion grows too large, or the periodicity too different, etc., categorization times to associate words such as "coffee" will increase.

There are cross-modal invariants that may be manipulated. Let the event be pouring water into a glass, an event normally accompanied by a increasing rise of pitch (Cabe and Pittenger, 2000). In this case the pitch may be manipulated to actually fall, or rise in a manner not coordinate with the invariance law. This, we can propose, should disrupt or lower categorization response time of words, e.g., POUR.

Admittedly, we must be careful. "Martini" may be in the equivalence class of substances when taken relative to the resistance of the liquid to the stirring-spoon, but not when viewed from a larger perspective - relative to the complete experience of the wielding of the object. The martini-stirring event is characterized by a different stirrer (a stirring stick), a different container (a martini glass), and therefore a different dynamics. This is a context law for this kind of event and priming "martini" may then require this event structure. In fact, then, it is the complete dynamics of the event, i.e., the full invariance structure that is determining what is being primed. Again we are visualizing a brain-supported wave through our "holographic memory," the dynamical pattern supporting this being determined by the invariance structure of the (stirring) event. To complete the hypothesis then, we would say that, firstly, all the normal components ("associates") of the invariance structure are primed, to include visual, auditory, haptic invariants, etc. Secondly, as in the stirring case, objects or substances within an equivalence class are primed.

This direct retrieval model of priming will support the non-word inhibition effect (Ratcliff and McKoon, 1995) where, for example, "duty" still facilitates the response to spoon compared to a nonword such as "glant," a problem for the spreading activation model, though not for the compound-cue model. It is also amenable to the mediated priming effect (McNamara and Altarriba, 1988) where, for example, "diameter" primes coffee even though indirectly related through "circle" and "stirring," an effect problematic for the compound cue theory though not for spreading activation (cf. Beer and Diehl, 2001).

The model has affinities to a response competition model of priming (cf. Klinger and Burton, 2000) already precursed, as noted, by McGeoch (1942), though obviously extended here beyond the S-R formulation. Interference is intrinsic in such a model, but theory has for some time held that priming is not subject to interference. Lustig and Hasher (2001), in a recent review, have effectively shown that priming is indeed subject to interference – in consonance with this model. Neither spreading activation nor compound cues have anything inherently within their theoretical structure that supports or predicts the parametric manipulation of invariance structures proposed here.

General Discussion

I would like to consider now certain aspects of this model that might appear very similar to current models, but which in fact are greatly different. It will also be helpful to at least sketch the beginnings of how such a model would support cognition.

Encoding Specificity - Not

This retrieval model is not simply encoding specificity (Tulving and Thomson, 1973) in other terms. Encoding specificity states that the more similar the situation is in retrieval to that of encoding, the more successful the search for the event. Tulving and Thomson showed that "context" words, when presented during learning together with items to be memorized, could be helpful later as retrieval cues. These experimenters gave subjects a list of paired words such as "ground-COLD" and asked them to remember the capitalized word while also noting the accompanying word which might be of some later use. Later subjects were asked to freely associate to words such as "hot." They might produce a list of words in which "cold" was included, e.g., "potato, soup, summer, cold, swimming, pot-handler." But when asked if any of the associates they had produced were also part of the list learned previously, they were likely to say no. However, if they had been asked to associate to "ground" and they produced "cold" as one of the associates, they were highly likely to recognize it as part of the earlier list of pairs. Tulving and Thomson interpreted this to mean that the "specific encoding" at the time of learning determines the accessibility to retrieval. Yet this is but a more subtle restatement of Wolff's law.

The question is, as always, what was the actual event, and what was its invariance structure? Did the subject vaguely remember an experience of walking or laying on the cold ground? The "cold" stated as mere opposite to "hot" (in our free associate list to "hot") can hardly be considered a "part" of the pattern-event of "laying on the cold ground," and simply can't redintegrate it. The whole point is to describe the patterns (invariance laws) that define events. Since Tulving and Thomson and their successors have not done this, the concept of context is itself left unexplicated. If memory theory is satisfied with description of events at the level of Tulving and Thomson, then indeed the principles being described here are useless to memory theory.

A criticism may be made that I have not given a simple recipe for memory theorists and experimenters for describing the invariance structure of events. There is no simple recipe. Discovering invariance laws is the name of the game in science (cf. Kugler and Turvey, 1987: Wigner, 1970; Woodward, 2000, 2001). The Gibson school has been working on this endeavor for years. I have given as many examples as I am able; more can be culled from the literature.

Distinctiveness - Not

Another critique may be leveled at this model for its use of uniqueness or distinctiveness as employed in law (2), saying that the role of uniqueness or distinctiveness of events is common knowledge in the literature. But again, the question is what makes an event unique? This comes down to the structure of the event, and this is a matter of its invariance structure. When we can manipulate the form of the event, e.g., by changing the value of the strain transformation applied to the cardioid defining the growth of the facial profile, we control the similarity (uniqueness) of events, and therefore redintegration. Current memory theory contains no statement on this beyond the intuitive notion that events can be different, and as noted, Schmidt (1991) gave an extensive critique of the vague use of distinctiveness in current theory. Vargas, Cuevas and Marsharck (1996), referencing Jacoby and Craik (1979) could give distinctiveness no more definition than that of "being enhanced by more complete descriptions, more meaningful processing of relational information, or the emphasis of distinguishing features (p. 49)."

Storage - Not

What has been described is clearly a retrieval theory, not a theory of brain-storage. This is because, in this model, *events* cannot be stored. Consider the rotating cube mentioned earlier, where the form of the cube is specified by velocity (flow) fields in conjunction with Bayesian constraints. A general tendency in current memory theory is to view the rotating cube residing in memory as a set of stored features and stored (static) states. The tendency is expressed in Barsalou (1993), where a 'biting' transformation would be stored in discrete, schematic states – "a mouth closed next to the object, followed by a mouth open, and then the mouth around the object" (p. 53). The cube, then, would be stored as samples or slices of its motion. Connectionism would envision vectors, or a series of such vectors, containing elements representing the presence of various such features. But these static features are simply invariants defined over velocity fields. It is the velocity fields or flows that would have to be stored. Other than taking samples of such a flow, which leads to the earlier discussion on the infinite regress concerning motion, I am aware of no workable model of storage of such flows. Recall that out-of-phase strobing (sampling) destroyed the information specifying the cube. To which strobe rate would Barsalou-like samples of the cube's rotation transformation correspond? The sampler would have to be precognizantly adjusted to the cube's symmetry period. What if there were two cubes rotating at different rates?

But, for the sake of argument, suppose three "states" were indeed stored of a rotating cube event. Then assume on a subsequent event, the cube is bulging in and out. For a standard observer, comparing against the two whole events, the difference between the two events is immediate. But the discrete sample method observer could in principle sample three states of the "bulging" cube and in fact "match" his three stored states of the previous, normal rotating cube, detecting no difference. Sampling begs the description of change.

The perceived event, I think we should hold, a) because it is occurring externally and not solely within the brain, and, b) because it is inherently four-dimensional or time-extended, must be "*stored*" in the holographic matter-field with its non-differentiable time-motion.

Current memory theory has little conception or worry as to how the elements it stores are reconstructed as *events*, i.e., experiences. Given a connectionist vector of elements [-1, -1, 0, +1, 0, -1] representing the features of a cup/coffee-stirring event, there is no theory as to how these features represent the invariance structure of the event, or ever were the image of the cup-being-stirred, or ever again become so as a memory image. If we are stirring coffee with a spoon, we have the swirling surface, the mixing cream and brown color, the clinking sound, the feel and forces of the motion, the resistance of the liquid, and more. We have in this event an extremely rich, dynamic structure. We do not know how such events are mapped or decoded or unfolded from vectors of features. As Murdock (1982) said some time ago, speaking in the context of TODAM:

> Although one can make memory performance as good as desired by increasing N - the number of elements in the memory vector - what are these elements? If it takes 50, 100, 1000, or 10,000 elements to produce the necessary results, they are certainly not the cognitive features others have in mind. (p. 625)

The problem is increased by orders of magnitude when making this cup part of a dynamic coffee-stirring event, or considering a rotating cube. That this is the essence of the dilemma presented by the SPT is attested to by Zimmer et al. (2000). We ask how an action, in and of itself, redintegrates a specific object within a past event – a pen, a wire, a refrigerator, a coffee cup – or even the whole experience? Motor action, by itself, is not the full experience. Speculating on the mechanism behind the free recall of such acted events in SPTs, Zimmer et al. use the notion of "popping into mind," as in cued recall, where "sets of features," "bound together by actions," can pop out from the noise if their "conjunctions" are sufficiently unique (p. 669). These "spontaneously reconstitute" the former episode. This is little improvement, however, albeit with a greater appreciation of action, beyond Klein's reformulation of Wolff's statement of 1732, and it has no theory as to how these static features are assembled to become an event or event-image.

Cognition and Compositionality

Can this model support cognition? This is partly to ask, "How does our concrete experience become abstract?" How does experience become *symbolized* in words or images such that these become elements we can employ in thought? Perceptions are "modal" or multi-modal. Symbols are considered amodal. How does the modal become amodal? Barsalou (1999) dealt at length with the problem of how perceptual symbols can exist such that they are subject to operations that *compositionally* combine them. Consider a phrase, the SAD CLOWN. To understand the phrase, we are relying here on experiences of sadness and our experiences of clowns. The meaning of SAD CLOWN is derived by composing or combining the two compositional elements, SAD and CLOWN. The BITING MOUTH is similarly composed of BITING and MOUTH, two compositional elements. Clearly this compositionality underlies the operation of language. Fodor and Pylyshyn (1995) argued that compositionality is one of two utterly basic features, or required capacities, of intelligence. The other is *systematicity* – the capacity to combine these compositional elements in lawful ways.

Barsalou is in some respects an "abstractionist" (Crowder, 1993). Perceptions inherently must be *reduced* and stored as schematizations. Concrete transformations such as the "buzzing" of the fly, the "stirring" of a spoon, or "biting" a cookie become snapshots. When perception is treated as information reduction, as Goldinger (1998) notes, with processing "stages" generating progressively more abstract representations, the *recoding* of perceived events into canonical representations becomes a basic tenet. For words, or better word-events, the models of spoken-word perception generally assume a collection of canonical representations that are somehow accessible by noisy symbols. For events, these become sets of features, schemas, or as Barsalou argued, schematic representations somehow reduced from the full concrete event via the operation of attention, and capable of supporting compositionality. But there is another and opposite direction from which to support abstraction and the resulting compositionality for which Fodor and Pylyshyn argue so effectively. This direction, Goldinger noted, was already developed by Semon (1909/1923). Semon had assumed that every experience, such as perceiving a spoken word, leaves a unique memory trace. On hearing a new word, all stored traces are activated, each according to its similarity to the stimulus. The most activated traces connect the new word to stored knowledge, in effect - recognition. How, from this implicit mass of stored knowledge, to derive abstractions? Semon would borrow Galton's (1883) observation that blending faces in a photographic composite creates a *generic* face. Thus abstraction occurs over retrieval as countless partially redundant traces respond to an input.

Goldinger notes the large number of research findings indicating outstanding memory for the "surface" details of experience, to include pictures, musical tempo, faces, social interactions, physical dynamics, and more. Due to the bias for normalization or storing only abstract elements, this detailed memory is not generally thought true of linguistic processes (its general manifestation being ignored theoretically in any case), but in fact there are numerous studies showing the same memory for detail in the linguistic realm. Not only has there never been any evidence of actual reduction, he argued, but theory and data show, he felt, that *detailed* episodes, to include all the particulars of voice, inflection, pronunciation, tone, etc., for the presented words, constitute the basic substrate of the mental lexicon. But the elements of the lexicon, Goldinger pointed out, are artificially delimited events. The words are embedded in whole sentences and conversations; the boundaries of these events are in fact flexible. The episodic lexicon becomes, then, more than a collection of multiply experienced words, but rather "a rich linguistic history of words in various contexts, nuances, fonts, voices" (p. 268). By experiencing a word in many contexts, we come to appreciate its frequency status, syntactic roles, "associative links" to other words. If words are indeed stored as such, he argued, as elements or phases in the larger context of their sentences with full accompanying particulars, then any *context free* retrieval of a word will seem abstract, just as Semon foresaw. "SPOON," presented for processing on a computer screen, will be functionally abstract.

Goldinger stops here. But we have already visited the next step on this path. The acoustical wave flows in which we identify states termed "words," are simply part of the overall flow of the matter-field, a flow in which we identify portions termed "events." There is, in other words, the flowing, concrete world where we stir our coffee with a spoon, lift the cup to our mouth, put out the fire, get in the canoe, plunge the paddle in the water, paddle across the lake with the wind in our face. Language is simply part of this flow. The concrete events of SPTs were in fact extensively prefigured in the 1960's in second language learning experiments based on action performed by Asher and his associates (Asher, 1965, 1966, 1972; Asher and Price, 1967). If Goldinger is led by his logic to the storage of the entire set of flowing, experienced sentences in their full contextual and experiential fabric, then we are equally led to the storage of *the entire multi-modal flow of concrete events* in which the language is embedded. By the same logic, this flow of experience is individuated, just as separate "words," into abstract events - spoon stirrings, coffee drinkings, etc. Thus a present event, confronting this vast memory, activates this entire set of "traces," and all similar events "respond."

Abstraction and Redintegration

This concept of abstraction, where abstraction is achieved by activating a large number of similar events or memory "traces," has significant support in memory theory, and is often termed *exemplar* theory. Smolensky (1995), a connectionist theorist, in essence comes at least close to this as well, speaking of a "coffee cup" as a family resemblance across activation patterns in his neural nets. Rovee-Collier et al. (2000) wonder if the memory for experiences Tulving termed "episodic" memory becomes Tulving's "semantic" memory as the *context* of individual events fades. In other words, again, is abstraction (the semantic) now a context free retrieval across all these events? But note that this requires a device that can store the totality of experienced events in all modalities, in *complete* detail. We have noted that perception, i.e., experience, in the holographic model being described, is not solely occurring in the brain. The concept of "traces" itself denotes only a vague idea of the storage of events, events that have never truly been found in the brain. We have, however, already previewed the mechanism for abstraction in the holographic model.

We have seen that the modulatory pattern defined over the brain and supporting invariance structures can be conceived as a continuously modulated reconstructive wave traversing 4-D extended and multi-modal experience. The computer theorist, Gelernter, visualized an operation of taking a "stack" of events across which the invariants stand out. One may conceive of the basis for a "concept" as a wave of less than perfect coherence supported by the dynamics of the brain (e.g., a composite of f_1, f_2, in Figure 3) reconstructing a composite of images or wave fronts (stirring-events) across 4-D memory, over which the invariants across the images/events stand out. “STIRRING” itself, as a *concept*, is an invariant across multiple stirring events in 4-D memory as defined by this operation. In this sense, the operation of redintegration or direct recall is the basis of abstraction. It is equally then the basis for “compositionality.”

The Piagetian Base of Systematicity

Though I have argued here that this form of abstraction provides a basis for compositional elements, compositionality and systematicity go hand in hand. The two are Fodor’s fundamental criteria for an intelligent device. How do we learn to use these compositional elements in structured patterns, to “put them together” is a systematic, rule-governed way? The systematic rules for composition also seem to be carved out of dynamic flows, which is to say that these too are invariance laws.

This dynamical approach to compositionality was the essence of Piaget's approach. Consider his simple experiment on children aged 3-7 (*The Child's Conception of Movement and Speed*, 1946). Here three beads are strung on a wire which in turn can be fitted into a small cylindrical "tunnel." The beads are of different colors, but we'll call them A, B, and C (Figure 15). The beads are run into the tunnel and the tunnel semi-rotated from 1 to N times.

A series of questions are asked, ranging from a simple, "What order will they come out?" after one semi-rotation (or half-turn), to the ultimate question on their order after any (n) number of half-turns. The child comes to a point of development where he can imagine the consequences of a 180^0 rotation which moves ABC to CBA and another 180^0 rotation which moves things back again to ABC, i.e., an invariance of order under a 360^0 rotation. When now asked in which order would the beads come out when the tunnel is semi-rotated 5 (or 4, or 6, or 7, etc) times, he evidences great difficulty.

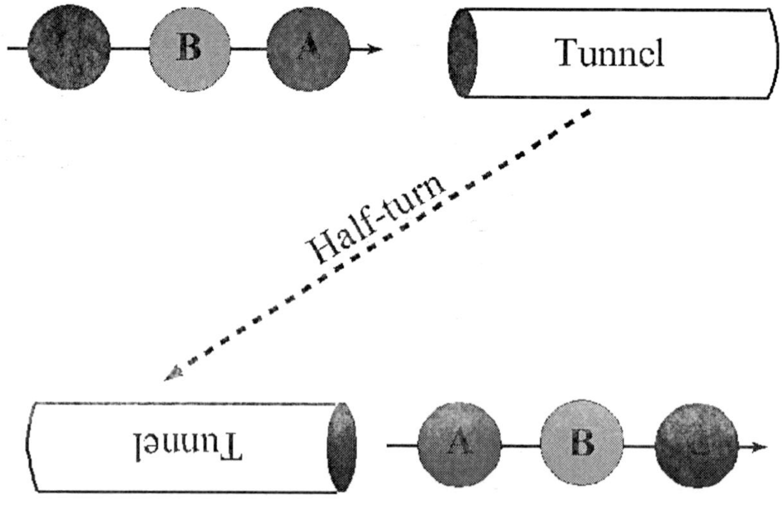

Figure 15. The Tunnel-Bead Experiment.

Some children appear to be exhausted after imagining three or possibly four semi-rotations, and they become lost when jumps are made from one number to another. As Piaget notes:

> But since the child, upon each half turn, endeavors to follow the inversion in every detail in his thoughts, he only gradually manages accurately to forecast the result of three, four, five half turns. Once this game of visualizing the objects in alternation is set in train, he finally discovers ...that upon each half-turn the order changes once more. Only the fact that up to this upper limit the subject continues to rely on visualizing intuitively and therefore needs to image one by one the half-turn, is proved because he is lost when a jump is made from one number of half-turns to any other. (1946, p. 30)

After this gradual perception of a higher order invariant (the "oscillation of order") defined over events of semi-rotations, there comes a point then when the child can easily answer the ultimate question for the resultant order for any n-turns. Piaget's explanation, describing the "operational" character of thought, is foundational to his theory and its "group" operations:

> Operations, one might say, are nothing other than articulated intuitions rendered adaptable and completely reversible since they are emptied of their visual content and survive as pure intention... In other words, *operations come into being in their pure state when there is sufficient schematization.* Thus, instead of demanding actual representation, each inversion will be conceived as a potential representation, like the outline for an experiment to be performed, but which is not useful to follow to the letter, even in the form of performing it mentally. (1946, p. 30, emphasis added.)

Thus, according to Piaget, operations, freed of their imaginable content, become infinitely compositional. This becomes the basis for forecasting the result of n-turns, and it takes the child to about the age of seven. The operations become the generalization of actions performed through mental experiment. This is not simply abstract rules and symbols. It is not simple "rule learning." As we have seen, these "schematic" operations are built upon and do not exist without the dynamic figural transformations over which invariance emerges. They are the result of a dynamical developmental trajectory incorporating these figural transformations which requires on average seven years.

Clearly the theory of this form of dynamically embedded compositionality and systematicity has a long way to go, but at least the "device" being described here provides a beginning basis for the dynamical imagery supporting invariance involved and its "modulation." It is in the context of this form of a device, I believe, that Piaget and his compositionality must be understood.

Imagery and Thought

Let us note that when the wave supported by the brain is functioning as a reconstructive wave within the 4-D field, an essential symmetry assumption has been made. It implies a very specific dynamical structure supported over the brain and its action tuning parameters which is reflective of the invariance structure of an event. This structure will provide constraints on the characteristics of this wave when described at the neuro-dynamical level, or the quantum level, or whatever level of the brain's hierarchical scales one chooses. We should view the *global* dynamics of the brain as comprising this wave. We do not see retrieval processes fetching stored elements – object "features" or "schematized" objects or events – and re-assembling them as an "image" or experience, viewed somehow by an homunculus in the brain. We are not then "inspecting" images. We are not using visual mechanisms to "see" or look around at images. The images are a natural adjunct of a definite, concept-driven (and/or motor-driven) modulatory pattern, perhaps an attempt to fix a precise event for thought to proceed, e.g., the spatial relation of the beads ABC, or now the turning or rotating of this structure according to an invariance law, in this case rigidity of the wire and therefore the fixed position of the beads upon it.

Neither do we imagine waves coursing through the brain, reconstructing images/wave fronts *within* the brain, or re-projecting images/wave fronts outside the brain, again for an homunculus to view. Body/brain and 4-D universal field comprise a coherent system. The changing dynamical pattern of the brain modulates virtual objects in time. If the modulatory pattern is sufficiently precise, these may be experienced as images (for example "a knife cutting a tabletop"), or depending on the order of invariance (level of abstraction), may be increasingly image-less (as in, "the utensil interacting with the furniture"). The debated representational status of the brain's dynamical patterns – the attractors, bifurcations, etc. - supporting these invariance structures is given clear place in this model. If we must still call them "representations," (and I would not) they are clearly in the relation of the part to the whole. They cannot be equated with the whole of thought. Thought is comprised of the simultaneous relation of dynamical patterns with virtual objects of the four-dimensional mind.

This picture is quite different from the concept of storing things under imaginal or verbal "codes" (e.g., Paivio, 1971). In accordance with our symmetry assumption, an event E with a given structure evokes a structurally related dynamic pattern over the brain. If E is a "concrete" word-pair and thus a structure that moves the brain into a dynamical pattern normally supporting some concrete event, e.g., coffee stirring, this may indeed evoke an image, but the dynamical pattern cannot be reduced to a set of imaginal "codes" that can be stored, no more than we could reduce the pattern or attractor supporting the rotating cube to a discrete set of code values. We are taking a non-differentiable motion, both in the environment and in the brain, and attempting to reduce it, as a "code" implies, to a discrete set of "symbols" or objects which represent the event. This was the essence of Pylyshyn's (1973) early reduction of the experienced image to propositions in a data structure:

> In other words, the image has lost all its picture-like qualities and has become a data-structure meeting all the requirements of the form of representation set forth in earlier sections. In fact, it can be put directly into one-to-one correspondence with a finite set of propositions... Similarly, "seeing the image" has been replaced by a set of common elementary and completely mechanical operations, such as testing the identity of two symbols. (Pylyshyn, 1973)

Though he asserted that the experience of the image "is not to be questioned," one would ask why not? Clearly we have worked to the point where, with a great sigh of relief, we can throw the pesky things away. They are indeed difficult to account for or justify in a computer. Even if the machine were to generate one, would it then "look" at it? A useless effort surely, especially given that it can't obtain any knowledge from it - it generated it in the first place from its data structures.

Imagery theorists, Kosslyn and Koenig, are, I think, less logically consistent about what is essentially the same concept:

> We use imagery to access stored information about an object by generating an image and then inspecting the imaged object for the sought information. This is accomplished by first looking up a description of the object in associative memory, and then using the code corresponding to the object to activate the appropriate visual memory of the object. This will produce a spatial pattern of activation in the visual buffer, which is the image proper. (Kosslyn and Koenig, 1992, pp. 144-145)

Questions on this passage that immediately come to mind are: (1) What is in the image that is not already in the "description of the object in associative memory?" If all the information is there to generate the object, what more information is there in the image. (2) The spatial pattern of activation in the visual buffer *is the image proper*? The visual buffer here is literally a screen on which a picture/pattern can be displayed, connected either to a camera (the eyes) or a tape recorder (memory). But this is typical current theoretical sleight of hand. This picture/pattern is again a pattern of *neural activity*. How can it be a pattern of neural activity *and* the phenomenal experience of the image as well? If it is a neural activity pattern what is the experience of the image? And who sees it? The visual buffer is only a handy theater screen for viewing by the theoretician's friend – the homuncular eye.

Kosslyn would argue that the homunculus regress indicated above is "easily" avoided. The "mind's eye" is simply a set of "tests" after the computer analogy. A matrix of values defining line patterns can undergo certain tests to see, for example, if two lines meet at a point or diverge. These tests, they say, constitute "seeing" the image. But this is simply the coding problem revisited. A set of values in a matrix can "stand for" anything. Three dots (...) in a cell of the matrix, as I have pointed out, can stand for the letter S, the number 3, a cloudy day, or the three blind mice. Something must again understand the "image" to use the code (or an encoding) just as something needs to understand the external world to know what a (perceptual) code would "stand for." Tests can be run on the code at great length, but running tests does not solve this problem. The test processes no more know what the image (or the external world in the case of perception) looks like than does the homunculus, for which "tests" are a subtle substitution. In reality, the debate on the nature and origin of mental images is simply symptomatic of the complete theoretical gap in current memory theory as to the means by which supposed abstracted, stored elements of events are reassembled to form a complete, event-image.

Pylyshyn (2002) later offered a more powerful challenge and critique of imagery theories. He particularly focused on Kosslyn with arguments similar to those expressed above and in more depth. The challenge he issued is in the form of a "null hypothesis." Though admitting that his abstract symbol manipulations are likely insufficient to account for the form our representations take when experienced as imagery, he asks any future theory to explain, why not? Formal language and symbolic calculi, he notes, at least meet the dual requirements of compositionality and systematicity essential for reasoning. Further, he is able to show that a large degree of imagery phenomena, particularly in reasoning and thought, could be handled in this limited, null hypothesis-like way.

I have addressed the origin of compositional (symbolic) elements above. In this, the very nature of Pylyshyn's "symbolic" medium itself is redefined. The first answer to why there is imagery is simply this: the redintegrative process, i.e., the reconstructive wave through 4-D memory over which even compositional elements are defined, inherently has the ability to reconstruct specific events or schematic events defined over composites of events. Not even the most abstract of "symbols" or compositional elements is utterly abstract. Such a symbol is always defined over a set of concrete events. The "abstractness" or amodality that Pylyshyn assumes in his null hypothesis of "symbol manipulation," while true in the sense of amodal invariants, is already a fiction by the very method through which this abstraction is defined.

Pylyshyn further noted that the process of imagistic reasoning involves the same mechanisms and the same forms of representation as are involved in general reasoning, "though with different content or subject matter." This statement, I think we would amend, given our recent view of Piagetian operations in the tunnel-bead experiment. This was as much "general reasoning" as one gets, and yet involved dynamic transformations expressed in imagery. Only if "reasoning" is conceived as pure, abstract symbol manipulation, do we get "different processes" underlying thought. It is a common misconception of the computer metaphor that the *abstract can exist without the concrete*. But we have seen in Piaget that the abstract is defined upon the concrete (see also Wertheimer, 1945). In fact, it was the failure to realize this that has supported the illusion for many years that Piaget is amenable to the information processing model. But an entirely different form of "device" is required for Piaget.

But Pylyshyn's key question was this: "What does the real work in solving the problem by [mental] simulation - a special property of images... or tacit knowledge?" (p. 9) Thus, in contemplating the folding experiments of Shepard and Feng (1972), where subjects were required to mentally fold paper into objects of certain forms, he noted that the subjects had, by necessity, to proceed sequentially through a series of folds to attain the result. Why? "Because," he argued, "*we know what happens when we make a fold*" (p. 13, original emphasis). It has to do, he stated, with "how one's knowledge of the effects of folding is organized" (p. 13).

What is a "fold" other than an invariant defined over a transformation in concrete experience? We have seen folds made in sheets, folds made in paper, folds made in arms/elbows, folds made in sails, folds made by Penrose (1994) in three-faced hexagonal structures to make partial cubes (see below), and even folds made with poker hands. And we have made the folds with bodily action. *Something* is always being folded. There is no such thing as an abstract "folding." A folding is a dynamic transformation preserving an invariant in our concrete experience. It is defined by a transformational and a structural invariant. It is an event with an invariance structure, and an event E' with similar structure can effect a wave through 4-D memory defining an abstraction across all these events. This invariance is at least the beginning of the "knowledge of the effects of folding" and the "organization" of this knowledge, and the form of device we have been reviewing thus far is what is required, I have been arguing, to support this form of knowledge.

Supporting and initiating the modulation pattern underlying the reconstructive wave for "folding" is in all probability a *motor attitude* as Bergson (1896/1912) termed it. Yes, we know how to make a fold - we know *bodily* as well. We know then how to move the body, overtly or covertly, into such an action. These "action syntagms" are likely ubiquitous. An object such as a cup is used to hold liquids; we pour liquid into it, pour out of it, pour from the cup into mouths, etc. This begins early. At 9-15 months infants often act out an action syntagm (such as the actions of drinking) when they encounter or perceive an object such as a cup. This overt tie to action (or assimilation to a sensorimotor scheme in Piaget's terms) disappears with age, and can be (strongly) supposed to have been internalized as the "core" of an object-action-word invariance which ties the functional-motor and perceptual information in terms of their formal packaging under a "word" or concept – what has been termed their "canonical correlation" (Sinha, 1982). Curiously, this compulsive acting out can return in patients with certain prefrontal lesions, presumably because the tracts that carry inhibitory signals that prevent this behavior (that the child must have eventually formed) have been destroyed (cf. Jeannerod, 1994). But clearly, this gives a glimpse of the complexity of the neural involvement and its relation to action systems or mechanisms triggering a reconstructive modulation pattern and which is supporting an image.

Ultimately, as Piaget attempts to chronicle, this bodily action, for example, folding, becomes an "operation," it is capable of being carried out in the mental or imaginary plane. Piaget is well aware that the figural aspect and the operative aspect of thought are complimentary (1974, pp. 74-75). He is at some pains to distinguish the two, concerned as he is to emphasize the foundational role of action (becoming then "transformations") in thought, but compliments they are. There is no folding without something being folded. The implicit actions or operations are simultaneously the basis for a modulated wave through memory. But the road to raise bodily action to this representative or *symbolic* level is a long developmental dynamic, as discussed in detail by Piaget.

Thought, Consciousness and the Non-Computational

Finally, on this subject of thought, we inevitably come back to the point that our model of memory is key to the theory thought and of consciousness. It has been little remarked that the "non-computational" thought of Penrose (1994), which he felt demanded conscious awareness, rests upon time-extended transformations defining invariance. Consider the proof that successive sums of hexagonal numbers are always a cubical number (hence a computation that does not stop). He has us imagine building up any cube by successively stacking three-faced arrangements that comprise hexagons - a back, a side, and a ceiling – giving each time an ever larger cube (Figure 16).

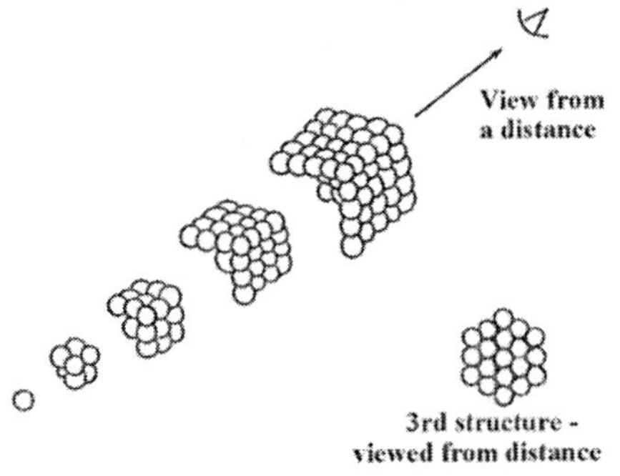

Figure 16. Successive cubes built from side, wall, and ceiling. Each side, wall, and ceiling structure make a hexagonal number. (Adapted from Penrose, 1994).

This is a dynamic transformation over time, in fact multiple transformations defining invariance. We can expand the hexagonal structures successively, from 1, to 7, to 19, etc., each time preserving the visual hexagonal invariant. Then, each is folded successively, each time preserving the 3-faced structural invariant. Then imagine them successively stacking, one upon the other, each operation preserving the cubical invariance. Over this event, the features (or transformational invariance) of the transformation are defined.

As another example, he notes (1994) that if we consider an elementary fact of arithmetic, namely that given any two natural numbers a and b (i.e., non-negative whole numbers 0, 1, 2, 3,...), we have the property that a x b = b x a.

Consider the case where a=3, b=5. Each side of the equation is different, and the two different groupings expressed can be displayed visually as:

axb (●●●●●) (●●●●●) (●●●●●)
bxa (●●●) (●●●) (●●●) (●●●) (●●●).

A computational procedure to ascertain the equality of axb and bxa would now involve counting the elements in each group to see that we have 15 in each. But we can see this equality must be true by visualizing the array:

●●●●●
●●●●●
●●●●●

If we rotate this through a right angle in our mind's eye, we can see that nothing has changed - the new 5x3 array we see has the same number of elements as the 3x5 array pictured. We see here, as in the case of the cubes, that the thing to which Penrose gravitates as a natural exemplar of non-computational thought is the perception of invariance. These perceived invariants form his "obvious understandings" that become the building blocks for mathematical proofs. As we have seen of invariants, these obvious understandings, Penrose felt, are inexhaustible. From this he argued in effect, will arise the elements of an object language employed in a proof. But in this he was well preceded by the likes of Wertheimer (*Productive Thinking*, 1945), Arnheim (*Visual Thinking*, 1969), Bruner (*Beyond the Information Given*, 1973), Montessori (e.g., her mathematical program), Hanson (1958; 1970), and if one looks closely, Piaget (1946), and others.

Wertheimer (1945) described a visit to a classroom of children learning how to compute the area of a parallelogram. The teaching followed the traditional method of dropping perpendiculars and extending the baseline, and the teacher gave the students several problems to work involving different sizes of parallelograms. Wertheimer then got up before the class, drew a rotated figure on the board, and asked the class to work out the area. Only a small minority of the class was able to solve the problem, some of the rest responding that, "they had not had that yet." Implicit in Wertheimer's discussion of the incident was the purely mechanical, "human computer-like" knowledge the children had obtained. It went without saying that this was a degenerate form of knowledge in his opinion. It did not compare to the five year-old he observed who looked at a cardboard cutout of a parallelogram, then asked for a scissors so she could cut the (triangular) end off and move it to the other side to make a rectangle. Nor did it compare to the dynamic transformation exhibited by a five year-old child who formed the cardboard parallelogram into a cylinder, then asked for a scissors to cut it in half, announcing it would now make a rectangle.

Yet, as Copeland (2000) has emphasized, Turing specifically defined the form of computation that he would formalize in terms of *mechanical* operations. He was thinking of the ubiquitous types of computation then found everywhere – the calculations of a bank officer balancing the ledger or of a clerk computing a total cost of purchase. "Computation" consisted of the steps a human computer could carry out, a human acting mechanically *without intelligence,* i.e., *without semantics.* It was this form of computation that he would formalize in terms of the Turing machine.

As we have viewed the form and nature of the understanding underlying that which we can term a *semantic* "computation," it is clear that the Turing concept of computation is purely derivative. By this I mean that computation, in the Turing sense, is a simply a residue, a spatialized husk of far more powerful operations of mind supporting representative thought, in turn based in the non-differentiable motion of the matter-field. In a word, Turing computation is again a limiting case, fundamentally based in the "projection frame" of the ever underlying abstract space and abstract time in which we tend to think (and theorize), itself a derivative concept from perception and its "objects." As with physics, this frame is what must be peeled away.

Free Recall and the Explicit

Can this retrieval theory support free recall? The short answer is, yes. A theory of redintegration is primary – the base. Note that Zimmer et al's (2000) statement on events "popping into mind" via "conjunctions of features" was made in the context of the free recall operation for SPTs. At a minimum, one can see that the interference effects in such experiments must take into account the invariance structure of the events being recalled. The usage and effectiveness of internal cues will ultimately rely on these laws. Simple free-recall memory techniques such as the "method of loci" and "one-bun, two-shoe…" rely on a learned, automated mechanism which ultimately employs event invariance structures to retrieve the target events. The case can also be made that language is itself a form of mediating device, via its lexicon and syntax, to move the brain into the appropriate modulation patterns for the reconstruction of events.

But free recall also takes us to the realm of explicit memory. This relies on a far more complex dynamical state, the developmental trajectory of which was described extensively by Piaget (1954) as the "localization of events in time," and includes the simultaneous development of the symbolic function such that events can become *symbols* of the past. This integrally relates to the development of the prefrontal cortex and the simultaneous development of the concepts of causality, object, space and time (what I like to term the "COST" of explicit memory). Disruption to this complex dynamic would be hypothesized to underlie amnesia, not damage to experiences stored within the brain.

The essence of the four-dimensional memory argued for here is, as Bergson argued, "to have a date." Each event or experience, just as each note of a melody, is the reflection of the preceding series. Such a property is an intrinsic basis for the order of events in time. This is far from the ad hoc "date tagging" schemes for events one can find in computer simulation models. Nevertheless, Piaget's (1927/1967) explorations of COST show that the ability to order events in time is a complex one, and follows a dynamic developmental trajectory. The past is seen through this dynamical lens.

This is a subject that would require far more space – some further aspects of it are touched upon below. The model of direct memory described here provides the fundamental basis for retrieval of events which in turn become symbolic of the past, i.e., *explicit* recall.

Is Everything Stored?

Is everything stored? This model would say, yes, all experience is "stored" in the sense that we are inherently four-dimensional beings, that the holographic field is four-dimensional. In principle, given the right precision of modulation, i.e., the precise reconstructive wave, any event in the past should be capable of reconstruction. In addition to Goldinger's discussion of the large evidence for the retention of surface details of events, we could add examples like those provided by Oliver Sacks (1987), for example his "Martin A.," suffering from a form of brain damage, who could nevertheless quote verbatim *Grove's Dictionary of Music and Musicians* - any of its six thousand pages. He heard these quotes in his father's voice - memories from the long hours his father devoted to reading and sharing the history of music with his beloved, though handicapped son. Sack's retardate "Twins" could, given a date in their lives anywhere after roughly the age of four, give its details in total - the weather, the political events of which they might have heard, personally related events - as though they were simply reviewing a vast panorama unfolding before their inward eye. Kotre (1994) reports the feats of some Jewish scholars, discovered in Poland around the turn of the century, who had memorized the entire contents of the Talmud, twelve volumes of thousands of pages. In demonstrating their ability, they would ask a volunteer to open the Talmud to any page. The volunteer would then take a pin and touch it to one of the words on the page, any word at all. The scholar would then ask the people in the room to call out other pages. Without looking he would tell them what words were in the same position as the pin on those other pages. The people could check out his accuracy by pushing the pin through the pages. Cases were documented in which the scholar never failed.

Such phenomena are troublesome for the prevailing trend in memory theory, but more experimentation is needed to prove the concept of complete recording of experience. Hitherto, however, I think it can be said that it has not been taken seriously. The prevailing trend has at least partial origins in the "constructivist" tradition of Neisser (1967). This conception shares the abstractionist image of more general (abstracted) elements of experience stored in the brain from which specific experiences are reconstructed. Say Mayes and Roberts (2001), "Only a tiny fraction of experienced episodes are put into long term storage, and, even with those that are, only a small proportion of the experienced episode is later retrievable" (p. 91). This ubiquitous view is intended to alleviate the burden on the brain of storing the vast volume of our experience, as well as eliminate the burden of how images could be stored. One only needs to get up and walk outside for five minutes, observing the vastness of visual detail presented in experience to feel sympathetic for this position. However there are only vague notions on how the brain makes this selection of elements or events, or given any event, which elements these would be, or how dynamic and multi-modal events are then reconstructed from fragmented pieces or "features" of an event stored in different spots in the brain.

Nevertheless, the problem of obtaining the right precision of modulation to reconstruct any given event, and exactly what this might mean, is a real one in this holographic theory. Further, it is doubtful that the concept of simply moving the brain into the right modulation pattern is a real basis to explain *all* these phenomena. It is reported for example (Tart, 1975) that Aldous Huxley, author of *Brave New World* and *1984*, could enter a meditative state in which he could view any page from any book he had ever read. Bergson made it quite clear that we are dealing with a four-dimensional being and aspects of consciousness that modern science has not yet addressed. In a case like Huxley's, the mind is abstracting from the present as far as possible, moving away from the perception-action state of the brain and deeply into the past. Glenberg (1997) would later term this ability to ignore the call of the present perceptual array "suppression." Bergson expressed this "movement of the mind" in terms of the diagram of Figure 17. The point of the cone is the most "focused" or concentrated point of the mind in the physical plane, completely concentrated on action. At the most spread-out plane of the cone, we have the realm of dream, of reverie, of the pure memory of experience. Between are various degrees of "focus," and indeed the computer scientist Gelernter used just this term to express the phenomenon as he observed it in *The Muse and the Machine* (1994). Near the highly "focused" end or point, observed Gelernter, thought is abstract, conceptual. The operation (abstraction) of taking an entire "stack" of memories to examine one aspect of all them (an invariant) is one of high focus, and the complex process of working with the results of these operations, e.g., via symbols, is yet higher in terms of focus. The full understanding of this process of modulating degrees of focus is far from us, yet we are better off accepting the need for a four-dimensional model of mind and working to understand it, or to put it differently, working within a model of the non-differentiable motion of the matter-field.

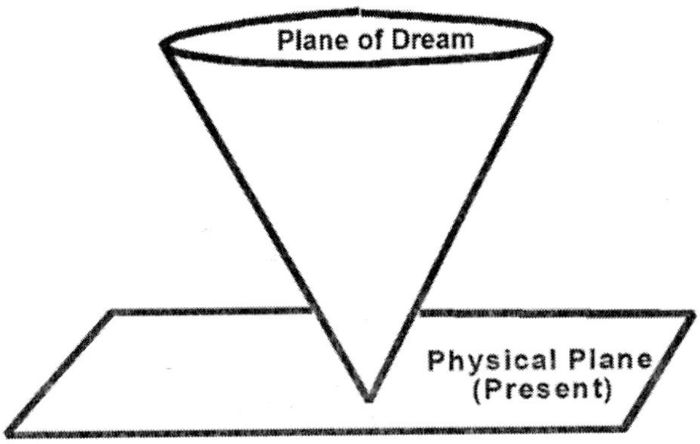

Figure 17. Bergson's Planes of Memory.

Interference Theory and Eye-Witness Phenomena

Forgetting (normal type - not due to brain damage) has generally been assumed in memory theory to arise from "interference." As we place "items" into memory, they tend to interfere with one another and cause difficulties in memory retrieval. As noted earlier,

McGeoch (1942) first proposed that interference occurred at the time of retrieval, i.e., at the time we actually try to recall an item. Thus, for example in cued recall, a cue word such as BOY, seeking its appropriate paired word, e.g., PLAY, may in fact arouse several interfering responses - BALL, SON, MOTHER, PARK, SMALL, etc., from which we must "choose" the correct response. In the then current stimulus-response framework inherited from behaviorism, this was termed "response competition."

All of this relates to "Retroactive Interference" (RI). RI can be created in the paired associate learning paradigm as follows: We give the subject a set of A-B pairs, e.g., BOY-PLAY, KNIFE-STRING, etc., then follow this with a set of "A-D" pairs, e.g., BOY-RUN, KNIFE-MEAT, etc. In this A-B, A-D format, we have the same stimulus portion "A" in each case. A control group of subjects gets an A-B, C-D set, i.e., different stimulus portions, different response portions.

Typically the group with the A-B, A-D set suffer the greatest RI, i.e., they remember less of the A-B's - due to the "retroactive" effect of A-D's. In McGeoch's original interference hypothesis, this was a natural. The "A" portion (e.g., KNIFE) was conceived to activate both the B (STRING) and the D portion (MEAT). This causes "interference," and makes it problematic which response, if any, the subject will give. Thus far, all this is in complete accord with the holographic model. In the A-B, A-D case we have the same reconstructive wave, due to its imprecision (i.e., lack of coherence) redintegrating two events, B+D, a composite wave front, so to speak. Note again the natural relation to "priming" of multiple events. (Cf. Hintzman, 1984, re Semon's highly related "homophony.") But from this point of clarity, the theoretical development became very tangled. The response competition metaphor was the focus of competing explanations, some arguing that the subject suffers a "bias" to respond to the interpolated items (A-D), some that the D response occurs because B was never learned, or vice versa. The storage metaphor also became a point of controversy. In the "memory trace" terminology now current, there are theoretical positions for *independent* memory traces (where events are stored separately), *altered* traces (where the trace for A-B has been "changed" to A-D), and *mingled* (A-B, A-D are meshed together in some form). Chandler (1989), in experiments which appeared to eliminate the response "bias" positions and defend the independent trace idea, posited a "convergence" hypothesis for the A-B, A-D case, arguing that the A portion activates both B and D, the features of each mingling, and making it difficult for the subject to disentangle the information. This is of course the same as McGeoch, and it is exactly the holographic model, where an imprecise wave or cue (A) reconstructs both wave fronts (B+D).

We create such a circular deja vu due to inattention to a theory of the information defining events, and therefore of redintegrative laws. Chandler (1989), for example, notes an experiment by Zaragoga et al. (1987) where all RI is eliminated by "category" cues, (in an attempt to destroy the "altered trace" position). Subjects were shown, for example, a Pepsi can. Later, in a narrative story it was implied that they had seen a peanut butter jar (i.e., a different category - "jar" rather than "can"). A control group was not given this category switch. Subjects were then given the cue, "can." Subjects in the experimental group remembered the Pepsi can as easily as those in the control group. Chandler felt that since "can" is a category, it may be masking other effects that might have resulted in RI. It is unfortunate that things have become so confused. The invariance structure of the cue event – the constraint of the reconstructive wave - is critical for the reconstruction of events. This is a simple principle. If we wish to reconstruct B or D uniquely, we must have a cue with an invariance structure defining/specifying the event B or D. If our pairs are SPOON-COFFEE and SPOON-ICE CREAM, then if we want to destroy RI, let the cue be an event - a spoon in a stirring motion in one case, a spoon in a scooping motion in another. With SPOON-CEREAL we might still have interference, the visual scooping motions being too similar, so now we further constrain the reconstructive wave, specifying the forces and kinesthetics involved - which are quite different for ice cream vs. cereal. But clearly, experimental control is in an ecologically well-specified event in the first place.

As the "altered trace" theories mentioned above already imply, alternative models were proposed later where the source of interference occurs as the items are stored. The damage has already been done in other words *before* the operation of attempting to recall a given item. This model has, by a form of default, held sway for the last several years due to the fact that most of the associative mathematical models developed recently, including neural nets, virtually assume it. Eich's CHARM (1985) throws all the items in mathematically jumbled form into its single memory vector M. Anderson et al. (1977) distributed every item over a matrix where they all coexist, and so on for several others. Neural nets store an "item" across every neuron, and thus multiple items are jumbled over the same neurons as synaptic weight adjustments.

A simple phenomenon has put this interference-at-storage model in jeopardy. It has long been a respected law that the longer a list of items to be remembered, the more the interference. We will remember a lower percentage of words from a list of 30 words for example than from a list of 10 words. This holds for free recall, recognition tasks, and for cued recall. But "length" of a list is one factor. "Strength" of items in a list is another. I can "strengthen" some items on the list by giving them more practice repetitions or a longer time to be looked at. This too has an effect on the other items, lowering the ability to recall items in general just like length. Except for one thing. Unlike length, strengthening some items really only has its effect on free recall type situations, and little if any on recognition tasks or cued recall.

This has been pointed out as a real dilemma for interference-at-storage models. Interference at storage should be interference at storage. A mess in the memory vector M, matrix A, or your neural net, is still a mess. Every retrieval operation should then be affected. Why, when "strength" is manipulated, is only free recall affected? At present there are only unsatisfying ways to save these mathematical models. The authors of the dilemma (Ratcliff, Clark, and Shiffrin, 1991), in their attempt to explain the phenomenon, rely on the critical point that it appears necessary that "items" (events) be stored separately. But this leads us back to interference-at-retrieval type of models.

The physical process of holography, to which I feel we should cling, can in effect have interference at either point. With a unique reference wave and a unique reconstructive wave, even though all the information in the hologram is distributed, there is no "interference" in reconstructing a wave front. A unique reference wave in effect provides independent storage of events. However, when the reconstructive wave is not modulated precisely, we have interference in the recall process - multiple superimposed wave fronts can be reconstructed - though in principle, with precise modulation, each wave front *could* be uniquely recalled. The reference wave associated with each object-wave could also be non-unique and this could be construed as "interference" at storage. I have assumed here though that by the very nature of time, where each state is the reflection of previous states (read previous experiences), there is always a unique referencing aspect in each event, but in practice, it is obviously possible for events to be so similar as to be in effect interfering at storage. The holographic model, in fact though, allows for "separate storage," i.e., reconstruction, of each wave front (or event).

The list "length" effect, we should note, where memory performance decreases as the length of lists to be remembered increases, indeed has a reality, but yet appears somewhat of an artifact. It seems somewhat a legacy of Ebbinghaus. It has a reality when we drive the machine to perform at a particular low level, but what is the ecological case? I have already, in effect, speculated that the length effect can be defeated, at least in recognition and cued recall, if we respect ecological laws, i.e., if we are careful to create events defined by unique invariance structures. The SPT experiments are already close to showing this (c.f. Zimmer et al., 2000.). A set of 10 uniquely defined events that can be reconstructed by unique cues is no different than a set of 20 of the same.

In effect, it is for this reason that manipulating "strength" in a list has so little effect on recognition or cued recall. A unique invariance structure, i.e., reference/reconstructive wave, is a unique structure no matter how many times we repeat the item or item-pair. If all 10 word-pairs in the list have a unique structure, it should matter little to the laws of redintegration how many times a selected subset of these words has been favored by increased repetition.

The interference-at-storage argument has its relation to the subject of "eye-witness" type phenomena. As in the Pepsi can vs. peanut butter jar of Zaragoga et al. just discussed, one study (Loftus et al., 1978) had subjects view a video showing a car accident in which a *stop* sign appeared. Subjects were later *told* it was a *yield* sign, and proceeded to remember it this way. Similarly, in another study (Loftus, 1977), subjects saw a sequence involving a *blue* car. Later they were informed it was a *green* car. In later judgments, matching color samples to the witnessed car, they tended to choose a color near the green. This has been interpreted by some (Hintzman et al., 1992) as interference at storage, as though the yield sign replaced the stop sign, and the green replaced the blue, in memory.

The original perception of the “car as blue” was an event. The announcement that “car as green” was simply another event. In general, I feel that the holographic model described here allows us best to keep clear of these difficulties, letting us hold to the concept that each event is recorded and in principle able to be reconstructed. In practice, this may indeed be virtually impossible – the confused or new event (e.g., yield sign) being always reconstructed. But this framework would predict that it can be done, i.e., experiments can be arranged where analogously, the yield sign appears to be winning, yet a cue can be introduced which reconstructs the original (stop sign) event.

Brain Storage: No Contrary Proof

It could well be argued that the model described here is entirely unnecessary, that it is completely unneeded until there is some definitive experiment or proof that experience is not stored in the brain. We must be careful over the narrowness of this stance. It assumes that what is in fact only an hypothesis, has, by virtue of historical precedent, a superior right to assume the need for disproof. Yet it remains just that – an hypothesis. Current theory does not explain how time-scaled, time-extended *events* are stored and retrieved. Nor does current theory attempt to align itself with any form of solution to the problem of conscious perception. It simply assumes there will be one and that it will have little effect on the model of storage. As far as the model of time in which current theory operates, it can be argued that it is aligned with an outmoded physics. Further, we can note, given the model just presented, how easily the situation is reversed. This new model could equally say, "This (brain as reconstructive wave) hypothesis will never need to change until there is proof that experience is indeed stored in the brain. The fact, for example, that damage to the brain causes failures to retrieve experience is absolutely no proof that experience is stored there." The fact is, each position can demand, legitimately, the definitive disproof.

Is there a deciding experiment? From what might be termed a phenomenal level, even Bergson (1896/1912) thought the answer to be, "no." Both models can support the same memory storage/loss phenomena. I have not dwelt here in any detail on how this theory would deal with amnesia (memory loss), but have done enough theoretical explorations to see that it can. From a scientific theory level, I have searched for a deciding experiment, but have found none. One difficulty with this search, I have discovered, concerns the nature of the theories that are contesting. In a quest for the decisive theoretical experiment, we imply that we have a theory A (current) of the storage/retrieval of experience and a theory B (new). But I would submit that the current theory, A, is somewhat a phantom. There are multiple theories, most ambivalent over what is truly stored, most holding for a selected subset of the event or events. None actually deal with the storage and retrieval of *events* as discussed here. In what we are learning today about the true nature of the perception of form as invariance over velocity flows, there is no corresponding theory of memory storage of such events, and the difficulties for a storage theory loom large. The theory must account for the scale of time of events, factor in virtual action, deal with what I have termed parametric variation of cues or event structures, and ultimately be compatible with a theory of conscious perception. So when we ask for a decisive experiment to prove theory B against theory A, I find myself asking, decisive relative to what? What is current theory A (storage of experience in the brain) offering that begins to deal with actually storing experience, let alone making some counter-prediction? This does not mean a decisive experiment does not exist, simply that none is clear at this point of time.

PROBLEMS/DIFFICULTIES

I have focused the discussion on the invariance law-guided retrieval aspect of memory, which I think the model liberates us to explore. I would be the first to acknowledge that there are difficult and problematic dimensions in this general framework that require further theoretical work. The subject of the deciding experiment broached above raises an extremely difficult area.

The holographic matter-field is imageless in the root sense of the word: it is unimaginable. The state of each "point-event" is the reflection of all other point-events. As such, the field is perspective-less; it looks nothing like the world we see from a given spatial perspective. In essence, an ensemble of such point-events is Kant's "thing-in-itself." The brain's specification process, as an ongoing reconstructive wave, is an integral part of the time-flow of the matter-field. This wave is specifying the field's past motion from a spatial, action-relative perspective at a scale of time. This is "experience." Experience is not the (perspective-less, null-scaled, holographic) matter-field per se. It is, the best we can say, of a different, perhaps we can say, supervenient, order. The experience is not simply *in* the matter-field in its perspective-less state at the null scale at some past position/extent along the fourth dimension. It is the interactive, perspective-based, scaled specification of the past. It is, however, simultaneously and equally part of the field's non-differentiable motion. It is an aspect of the four-dimensionality of our being. Therefore, when we again pass a reconstructive wave through the matter-field to reconstruct this experiential image, it is not as though we are simply passing the wave through a holographic interference pattern to reconstruct a wave front. How then, when the brain assumes the same modulated wave pattern, do we truly conceive this experience-reconstruction process?

As noted earlier, Bergson visualized the brain as a "valve," where the proper configuration of the brain's action systems allows the experiential dimension of the field to actualize as an image. The past experience is virtual – only becoming an image as it "fits" the action-state configuration. In this sense, Bergson saw the modulation pattern, which is supportive of a specific invariance structure, as allowing the similar experiential dimension to become enfolded in the ongoing state. A deeper understanding is needed here.

How are past, present and future experience differentiated in such a model? The distinguishing factor, in Bergson's theory, is action. The present is the display of virtual action, of how we can indeed act upon the world. Past experiences, as indicated above, no longer hold such a relation to the present action state. It is in this very real sense, that present and past are distinguishable.

Conclusion

The theory of consciousness and the theory of memory are intimately related. Their union begins with the problem of the perception of time-extended, external events. It continues through the very mechanism and nature of the retrieval of past experience and its explicit recall. And in the wings, unmentioned here, is the even greater problem of voluntary action and how the image of past actions guides the present act. The problem of consciousness has recently emerged with such force and difficulty as to make it extremely dangerous to simply assume that conscious experiences "are stored in the brain." There are profound consequences to such an assumption. I believe we have seen that the holographic, direct memory model described here can at least hold its own with current theorization on several areas of memory. If such is the case, the concept that storage (and retrieval) of experience does not demand storage within the brain is made available to enter the ongoing debate on the brain's role in consciousness.

References

Anderson, J. A., Silverstein, J. W., Ritz, S. A., and Jones, R. S. (1977). Distinctive features, categorical perception, and probability learning: Some applications of a neural model. *Psychological Review*, 84, 413-451.

Arnheim, R. (1969). *Visual Thinking.* London: Faber and Faber Ltd.

Asher, J. J. (1965). The strategy of total physical response: An application to learning Russian. *International Review of Applied Linguistics*, 3, 291-300.

Asher, J. J. (1966). The learning strategy of total physical response: a review. *The Modern Language Journal*, 50, 79-84.

Asher, J. J. (1972). The child's first language as a model for second language learning. *Modern Language Journal,* 56, 135-150.

Asher, J. J., and Price, B. (1967). The learning strategy of total physical response. *Child Development*, 38, 125-137.

Backman, L., and Nilsson, L.G. (1985). Prerequisites for lack of age differences in memory performance. *Experimental Aging Research*, 11, 67-73.

Backman, L., Nilsson, L.G., and Kourmi-Nouri, R. (1993). Attentional demands and recall of verbal and color information in action events. *Scandinavian Journal of Psychology*, 34, 246-254.

Barsalou, L. W. (1993). Flexibility, structure and linguistic vagary in concepts: Manifestations of a compositional system of perceptual symbols. In A Collins, S. Gathercole, M. Conway, and P. Morris (Eds.), *Theories of Memory,* New Jersey: Erlbaum.

Barsalou, L. (1999). Perceptual symbol systems. *Behavioral and Brain Sciences*, 22, 577-660.

Beckenstein, J. (2003). Information in the holographic universe. *Scientific American*, 289(2), 58-66.

Beer, A. L., and Diehl, V. A. (2001). The role of short-term memory in semantic priming. *Journal of General Psychology.*

Bergson, H. (1889). *Time and Free Will: An Essay on the Immediate Data of Consciousness.* London: George Allen and Unwin Ltd.

Bergson, H. (1896/1912). *Matter and Memory.* New York: Macmillan.

Bickhard, M. H. (2000). Dynamic representing and representational dynamics. In E. Dietrich and A. B. Markman (Eds.), *Cognitive Dynamics: Conceptual and Representational Change in Humans and Machines*, New Jersey: Erlbaum.

Bickhard, M. H. and Richie, D. M. (1983). *On the Nature of Representation*. New York: Praeger.

Bingham, G. P. (1993). Perceiving the size of trees: Form as information about scale. *Journal of Experimental Psychology: Human Perception and Performance*, 19, 1139-1161.

Bohm, David (1980), *Wholeness and the Implicate Order (*London: Routledge and Kegan-Paul).

Bruner, J. S. (1973). *Beyond the Information Given.* New York: W. W. Norton Co.

Byrne, A., and Hilbert, D. (2004). Color realism and color science. *Behavioral and Brain Sciences* 26 (1): 3-21.

Cabe, P. A. and Pittenger, J. B. (2000). Human sensitivity to acoustic information from vessel filling. *Journal of Experimental Psychology: Human Perception and Performance*, 26, 313-324.

Chalmers, D. (1995). Facing up to the problem of consciousness. *Journal of Consciousness Studies*, 2(3), 200-219.

Chandler, C.C. (1989). Specific retroactive interference in modified recognition tests: Evidence for a new cause of interference. *Journal of Experimental Psychology: Learning, Memory, and Cognition*, 15, 256-271.

Churchland, P. S., Ramachandran, V. S., and Sejnowski, T. J. (1994). A critique of pure vision. In C. Koch and J. Davis (Eds.), *Large-scale Neuronal Theories of the Brain*, Cambridge: MIT Press.

Cisek, P. (2001). Embodiment is all in the head. *Behavioral and Brain Sciences*. 24(1): 36-38.

Cisek, P. and Kalaska, J. F. (2002). Simultaneous encoding of multiple potential reach directions in dorsal premotor cortex. *J. Neurophysiol.* 87, 1149–1154.

Clark, A. (1997). *Being There: Putting Brain, Body and World Together Again.* Cambridge: MIT Press.

Clark, A. (1999). Where brain, body and world collide. *Cognitive Systems Research*, *1*, 5-17.

Cohen, R. L. (1981). On the generality of some memory laws. *Scandinavian Journal of Psychology*, 22 267-281.

Copeland, B. J. (2000). Narrow versus wide mechanism: including a re-examination of Turing's views on the mind-machine issue. *Journal of Philosophy*, XCVI, 1, 5-32.

Craig, C. M. and Bootsma, R. J., (2000). Judging time to passage. In M. A. Grealy and J. A. Thomson (Eds.), *Studies in Perception and Action V.* New Jersey: Erlbaum.

Craik, F.I.M., and Lockhart, R. S. (1972). Levels of processing: A framework for memory research. *Journal of Verbal Learning and Verbal Behavior*, 11, 671-684.

Craik, F., and Tulving, E. (1975). Depth of processing and the retention of words in episodic memory. *Journal of Experimental Psychology: General*, *104*, 268-294.

Crooks, M. (2002). Intertheoretic identification and mind-brain reductionism. *Journal of Mind and Behavior*, 23, 193-222.

Crowder, R. G. (1993). Systems and principles in memory theory: another critique of pure memory, in A Collins, S. Gathercole, M. Conway, P. Morris (Eds.), *Theories of Memory*, New Jersey: Erlbaum.

De Broglie, L. 1947/1969. The concepts of contemporary physics and Bergson's ideas on time and motion. In P.A.Y. Gunter (ed.), *Bergson and the Evolution of Physics,* University of Tennessee Press.

Dennett, D. C. (1995). What RoboMary knows. *Sweet Dreams: Philosophical Obstacles to a Science of Consciousness.* : New York: Oxford University Press.

Dessoir, M. (1912), *Outlines of the history of psychology.* New York: MacMillan Co.

Domini, F., Vuong, Q. C., and Caudek, C. (2002). Temporal integration in structure from motion. *Journal of Experimental Psychology: Human Perception and Performance, 28* (4), 816-838.

Eich, J. (1985). Levels of processing, encoding specificity, elaboration, and CHARM. *Psychological Review. 92* (1), 1-38.

Engelkamp, J. (1998). *Memory for Actions.* East Sussex: Psychology Press.

Engelkamp, J., and Zimmer, H. D. (1985). Motor programs and their relation to semantic memory. *German Journal of Psychology*, 9, 239-254.

Engelkamp, J., and Zimmer, H. D. (1994). *The Human Memory: A Multi-Modal Approach*, (Seattle: Hogrefe and Huber).

Engelkamp, J., and Zimmer, H. D. (1997). Sensory factors in memory for subject performed tasks. *Acta Psychologica*, 96, 43-60.

Engelkamp, J., Zimmer, H. D., and Biegelmann, U. E. (1993). Bizarreness effects in verbal tasks and subject performed tasks. *European Journal of Cognitive Psychology*, 5, 393-415.

Engelkamp, J., Zimmer, H. D., Morh, G. and Sellen, O. (1994). Memory of self-perforned tasks: Self-performing during recognition. *Memory and Cognition*, 22, 34-39.

Feynman, R. (1965). *The Character of Physical Law*. Cambridge, M.A.: MIT Press.

Feynman, R. P. and Hibbs, A. R. (1965). *Quantum Mechanics and Path Integrals.* New York: MacGraw-Hill.

Finke, R. A., and Freyd, J.J. (1985). Transformations of visual memory induced by implied motions of pattern elements. *Journal of Experimental Psychology: Learning, Memory and Cognition*, 11, 780-794.

Finke, R. A., Freyd, J. J., and Shyi, G. C. (1986). Implied velocity and acceleration induce trasnformation of visual imagery. *Journal of Experimental Psychology: General*, 115, 175-188.

Fodor, J. and Pylyshyn, Z. (1995). Connectionism and cognitive architecture. In C. Mac Donald and G. Mac Donald (Eds.), *Connectionism: Debates on Psychological Explanation.* Oxford: Basil Blackwell.

Freyd, J.J. (1987). Dynamic mental representations. *Psychological Review*, 94, 427-438.

Freyd, J.J., and Finke, R. A. (1984). Representational momentum. *Journal of Experimental Psychology: Learning, Memory and Cognition*, 10, 126-132.

Freyd, J. J., Kelly, M. H., and DeKay, M. L. (1990). Representational momentum in memory for pitch. *Journal of Experimental Psychology: Learning, Memory and Cognition*, 16, 1107-1117.

Fuster, J. M. (1994). In search of the engrammer. *Behavioral and Brain Sciences. 17*, 476.

Galton, F. (1883). *Inquiries into Human Faculty and its Development.* London: Macmillan.

Gelernter, D. (1994). *The Muse in the Machine: Computerizing the Poetry of Human Thought.* New York: Free Press.

Gennaro, R. J. (2005). The HOT Theory of consciousness. *Journal of Consciousness Studies*, 12(2), 3-21.

Glassman, R. B. (1999). Hypothesized neural dynamics of working memory: Several chunks might be marked simultaneously by harmonic frequencies within an octave bank of brain waves. *Brain Research Bulletin*, 30(2), pp. 77-93.

Glenberg, A. M. (1997). What memory is for. *Behavioral and Brain Sciences*, 20:1-55.

Gibson, J. J. (1950). *The Perception of the Visual World.* Boston: Houghton-Mifflin.

Gibson, J. J. (1966). *The Senses Considered as Visual Systems.* Boston: Houghton-Mifflin.

Gibson, J. J. (1979). *The Ecological Approach to Visual Perception.* Boston: Houghton-Mifflin.

Goguen, J.A. (2004). Musical qualia, context, time and emotion. *Journal of Consciousness Studies*, 11, 117-147.

Goldinger, S. (1998). Echoes of echoes? An episodic theory of lexical access. *Psychological Review*, *105*(2), 251-279.

Gray, R. and Regan, D. (1999). Estimating time to collision with a rotating nonspherical object. In M. A. Grealy and J. A. Thomson (Eds.), *Studies in Perception and Action V.* New Jersey: Erlbaum.

Hanson, N. R. (1958). *Patterns of Discovery.* Cambridge: University Press.

Hanson, N. R. (1970). A picture theory of theory meaning. In M. Radnur and S. Winokur (Eds.), *Analyses of Theories and Methods of Physics and Psychology,* Minneapolis: University of Minnesota Press.

Hawkins, J. (2004). *On Intelligence*. New York: Henry Holt.

Hintzman, D. L. (1986). Schema abstraction in a multiple-trace memory model. *Psychological Review, 93*, 411-428.

Hintzman, D. L. (1984). Episodic versus semantic memory. A distinction whose time has come - and gone?, *The behavioral and brain sciences,* **7**, 223-268.

Hintzman, D.L., Curran, T., Oppy, B. (1992). Effects of similarity and repetition on memory: Registration without learning, *Journal of Experimental Psychology: Learning, Memory and Cognition*, 18 (4), 667-680.

Hoaglund, H. (1966), Some bio-chemical considerations of time. In J.T. Fraser (Ed.), *The Voices of Time*, New York: Braziller.

Jacoby, L. L., and Craik, F.I.M. (1979). Effects of elaboration of processing at encoding and retrieval: Trace distinctiveness and recovery of initial context. In L. S. Cermack and F. I. M. Craik (Eds.), *Levels of Processing in Human Memory.* New Jersey: Erlbaum.

James, W. (1890). *Principles of Psychology.* New York: Holt and Co.

Jeannerod, M. (1994). The representing brain: Neural correlates of motor intention and imagery. *Behavioral and Brain Sciences*, *17*, 187-245.

Jenkins, J. J., Wald, J., and Pittenger, J. B. (1978). Apprehending pictorial events: An instance of psychological cohesion. *Minnesota Studies of the philosophy of science*, Vol. 9, 1978.

Kelly, M. H., and Freyd, J. J. (1987). Explorations of representational momentum. *Cognitive Psychology*, 19, 369-401.

Kim, N., Turvey, M., Carrelo, C. (1993), Optimal information about the severity of upcoming contacts. *Journal of Experimental Psychology: Human Perception and Performance,* 19(1), 179-193.

Kingma, I., van de Langenberg, R., and Beek, P. (2004). Which mechanical invariants are associated with the perception of length and heaviness on a nonvisible handheld rod? Testing the inertia tensor hypothesis. *Journal of Experimental Psychology: Human Perception and Performance*, 30, 346-354.

Klein, D. B. (1970), *A history of scientific psychology.* New York: Basic Books.

Klinger, M. R. and Burton, P. R. (2000). Mechanisms of unconscious priming I: Response competition, not spreading activation. *Journal of Experimental Psychology: Learniing, Memory and Cognition*, 26(2), 441-456.

Kock, W. E. (1969). *Lasers and Holography*. New York: Doubleday-Anchor.

Kosslyn, S., and Koenig, O. (1992). *Wet Mind: The New Cognitive Neural Science.* New York: The Free Press.

Kotre, J. (1994). *White Gloves.* New York: Free Press.

Kugler, P. and Turvey, M. (1987). *Information, Natural Law, and the Self-assembly of Rhythmic Movement*. Hillsdale, NJ: Erlbaum.

Loftus, E. F. (1977). Shifting Human Color Memory, *Memory and Cognition*, **5**, 595-599.

Loftus, E. F., Miller, D. G and Burns, H. J. (1978). Semantic Integration of Verbal Information Into a Visual Memory, *Journal of Experimental Psychology: Human Learning and Memory*, 4, 19-31.

Lombardo, T. (1987). *The Reciprocity of Perceiver and Environment: The Evolution of James J. Gibson's Ecological Psychology*. Hillsdale, NJ: Erlbaum.

Lustig, C., and Hasher, L. (2001). Implicit memory is not immune to interference. *Psychological Bulletin, 127*, 618-628.

Lynds, P. (2003). Time and Classical and Quantum mechanics: Indeterminacy versus discontinuity. *Foundations of Physics Letters* 16(4): 343-355.

Marschark, M., Richman, C., Yuille, J., and Hunt, R. (1987). The role of imagery in memory: On shared and distinctive information. *Psychological Bulletin, 102*, 28-41.

Marsharck, M., and Hunt, R. (1989). A re-examination of the role of imagery in learning and memory. *Journal of Experimental Psychology: Learning, Memory and Cognition*, 15, 710-720.

Mayes, A.R., and Roberts, N. (2001). Theories of episodic memory. In A. Baddeley, M. Conway and J. Appleton (Eds.), *Episodic Memory*. New York: Oxford.

McFadden, J. (2002). Synchronous Firing and its influence on the brain's electromagnetic field: Evidence for an electromagnetic field theory of consciousness. *Journal of Consciousness Studies*, 9(4), 23-50.

McGeoch, J. A. (1942), *The psychology of human learning*. New York: Longmans, Greene.

McKoon, G. and Ratcliff, R. (1992). Spreading activation versus compound cue accounts of priming: Mediated priming revisited. *Journal of Experimental Psychology: Learning, Memory, and Cognition,* 18, 1155-1172.

McNamara, T. P., and Altarriba, S. (1988). Depth of spreading activation revisited: Semantic mediated priming occurs in lexical decisions. *Journal of Memory and Language*, 27, 545-559.

Mulligan, N. W., and Hornstein, S. L. (2003). Memory for actions: Self-perforned tasks and the reenactment effect. *Memory and Cognition*, 31, 412-421.

Murdock, B.B. (1982). A theory for the storage and retrieval of item and associative information. *Psychological Review*, *89* (6), 609-626.

Murname, K., Shiffrin, R.M. (1991). Interference and the representation of events in memory. *Journal of Experimental Psychology: Learning, Memory, and Cognition*, 1991, 17, 855-874.

Mussati, C. L. (1924). Sui fenomeni stereocinetici. *Archivo Italiano di Psycologia,* 3, 105-120.

Nakamura, R.K. and Mishkin, M. (1980). Blindness in monkeys following non-visual cortical lesions. *Brain Research, 188*, 572-577.

Nakamura, R. K. and Mishkin, M. (1982). Chronic blindness following non-visual lesions in monkeys: Partial lesions and disconnection effects. *Society of Neuroscience Abstracts, 8*, 812.

Neisser, U. (1967). *Cognitive Psychology.* New York: Appleton-Century-Crofts.

Nilsson, L. G. (2000). Remembering actions and words. In F.I.M. Craik and E. Tulving (Eds.), *Oxford Handbook of Memory* (pp. 137-148), Oxford: Oxford University Press.

Nottale, L. (1996). Scale relativity and fractal space-time: applications to quantum physics, cosmology and chaotic systems. *Chaos, Solitons and Fractals* 7: 877-938.

O'Regan, J. K. (1992). Solving the real mysteries of perception: The world as an outside memory. *Canadian Journal of Psychology* 46(3): 461-488.

O'Regan, J. K. and Noë, A. (2001). A sensori-motor account of vision and visual consciousness. *Behavioral and Brain Sciences*, 24(5), 939-973.

Paivio, A. (1971) *Imagery and verbal processes.* New York: Holt, Rinehart, and Winston.

Paivio, A., Walsh, M., and Bons, T. (1994). Concreteness effects on memory: when and why? *Journal of Experimental Psychology: Learning, Memory and Cognition*, *20* (5), 1196-1204.

Penrose, R. (1994). *Shadows of the Mind.* Oxford: Oxford University Press.

Piaget, J. (1927/1969). *The Child's Conception of Time*. New York: Basic Books.

Piaget, J. (1946). *The Child's Conception of Movement and Speed.* New York: Ballentine.

Piaget, J. (1954). *The Construction of Reality in the Child.* New York: Ballentine.

Piaget, J. (1974). *The Child and Reality*. New York: Viking Press.

Pittenger, J. B. and Shaw, R. E. (1975). Aging faces as viscal elastic events: Implications for a theory of non rigid shape perception. J*ournal of Experimental Psychology: Human Perception and Performance,* 1, 374-382.

Pribram, K. 1971. *Languages of the Brain.* New Jersey: Prentice-Hall.

Pribram, K. 1991. *Brain and Perception.* New Jersey: Erlbaum.

Pylyshyn, Z. (1973). What the mind's eye tells the mind's brain: a critique of mental imagery. *Psychological Bulletin*, *80*, 1-22.

Pylyshyn, Z. (2002). Mental imagery: In search of a theory. *Behavioral and Brain Sciences,* 25, 157-238.

Raasmussen, J. (1986), *Information processing and human-machine interaction: An approach to cognitive engineering*, (Amsterdam: North-Holland).

Ratcliff, R., Clark, S. E., Shiffrin, R. M. (1991). List-Strength Effect I. Data and discussion, *Journal of Experimental Psychology: Learning, Memory, and Cognition*, 16, 163-178.

Ratcliff, R., and McKoon, G. (1995). Sequential effects in lexical decision: Tests of compound-cue retrieval theory. *Journal of Experimental Psychology: Learning, Memory and Cognition*, 21, 1380-1388.

Ratner, H. H., and Hill, L. (1991). The development of children's action memory: When do actions speak louder than words? *Psychological Research*, 53, 195-202.

Reichardt W, (1959). Autocorrelation and the central nervous system. In W. A. Rosenblith (Ed.) Sensory Communication MIT Press Cambridge 303-318.

Robbins, S. E. (1976), *Time and memory: the basis for a semantic-directed processor and its meaning for education*, Doctoral dissertation, University of Minnesota.

Robbins, S. E. (2000). Bergson, perception and Gibson. *Journal of Consciousness Studies*. 7(5), 24-46.

Robbins, S. E. (2001). Bergson's virtual action. In A. Riegler, M. Peschl, K. Edlinger, and G. Fleck (Eds.), *Virtual Reality: Philosophical Issues, Cognitive Foundations, Technological Implications.* Frankfurt: Peter Lang Verlag.

Robbins, S. E. (2002). Semantics, experience and time. *Cognitive Systems Research*, 301-335.

Robbins, S.E. (2004a). On time, memory and dynamic form. *Consciousness and Cognition*, 13, 762-788.

Robbins, S. E. (2004b). Virtual action: O'Regan and Noë meet Bergson. *Behavioral and Brain Sciences*, 24(7), 906-907.

Roediger, H. L., Balota, D., and Watson, J. (2001). Spreading Activation and Arousal of False Memories. In H. L. Roediger III, J. Nairne, I. Neath, A. Surprenant (Eds.), *The Nature of Remembering: Essays in Honor Robert G. Crowder*. Washington, D. C.: American Psychological Association.

Roediger, H. L, and McDermott, K. B. (1995). Creating false memories: Remembering words not presented in lists. *Journal of Experimental Psychology: Learning, Memory and Cognition*, *21*, 803-814.

Rosenthal, D. (2002). Explaining consciousness. In *Philosophy of Mind: Classical and Contemporary Readings*. ed. David Chalmers (New York: Oxford University Press).

Rovee-Collier, C., Hayne, H., Colombo, M. (2000). *The Development of Implicit and Explicit Memory*. Amsterdam: John Benjamins.

Rowher, W. D. Jr. (1967). Pictorial and verbal factors in the efficient learning of paired-associates. *Journal of Educational Psychology*, 58(5), 278-284.

Ruiz-Vargas, J. M., Cuevas, I. and Marschark, M. (1996). The effects of concreteness on memory: dual codes or dual processing? *European Journal of Cognitive Psychology*, 8(1), 45-72.

Sacks, O. (1987). *The Man Who Mistook His Wife for a Hat.* New York: Harper and Row.

Savelsbergh, G. J. P., Whiting, H.T., and Bootsma, R. J. (1991). Grasping tau. *Journal of Experimental Psychology: Human Perception and Performance*, 17, 315-322.

Schmidt, S. R. (1991). Can we have a distinctive theory of memory? *Memory and Cognition*, 19(6), 523-542.

Searle, J. R. (2000), Consciousness, Free Action and the Brain. *Journal of Consciousness Studies*. 7 (10), pp. 3-22.

Semon, R. (1909/1923), *Mnemic Psychology* (B. Duffy, Trans.). Concord, MA: George Allen and Unwin.

Shaw, R.E., and McIntyre, M. (1974). The algoristic foundations of cognitive psychology. In D. Palermo and W. Weimer (Eds.), *Cognition and the Symbolic Processes,* New Jersey: Lawrence Erlbaum Associates.

Shelton, J.R. and Martin, R.C. (1992). How semantic is automatic semantic priming? *Journal of Experimental Psychology: Learning, Memory, and Cognition*, 18(6), 1191-1210.

Shepard, R. N., and Feng, C. (1972). A Chronometric Study of Mental Paper Folding. *Cognitive Psychology*, *3*, 228-243.

Sherry D., and Schacter, D. (1987). The Evolution of Multiple Memory Systems. *Pscyhological Review*, 94(4): 439-454.

Singer, W. (1998). Consciousness and the structure of neural representations. *Philos Trans R Soc Lond B Biol Sci*, *353*, 1829-40.

Sinha, C. (1982) Representational development and the structure of action. In G. Butterworth and P. Light (Eds.), *Social Cognition: Studies in the Development of Understanding*. New York: Harvester.

Smythies, J. (2002). Comment on Crook's "Intertheoretic Identification and Mind-Brain Reductionism." *Journal of Mind and Behavior*, 23: 245-248.

Smolensky, P. (1995). Connectionism, Constituency and the Language of Thought. In C. MacDonald and G. MacDonald (Eds.), *Connectionism*, Cambridge: Blackwell.

Tart, C. (1975). *Altered States of Consciousness*. New York: Dutton.

Taylor, J. G. (2002). From matter to mind. *Journal of Consciousness Studies*. *9* (4), 3-22.

Thelen, E., Schoner, G., Scheler, C., and Smith, L. (2001). The dynamics of embodiment: A field theory of infant preseverative reaching. *Behavioral and Brain Sciences, 24*, 1-86.

Tulving, E. (1972). Episodic and Semantic Memory. In Tulving, E. and Donaldson, W. (Eds.). *Organization of Memory*. Academic Press.

Tulving, E. and Thomson, D. (1973). Encoding specificity and retrieval processes in episodic memory. *Psychological Review*, 80, 352-373.

Turvey, M. (1977) Preliminaries to a theory of action with references to vision. In: R.E. Shaw and J. Bransford (Eds.), *Perceiving, Acting and Knowing.* New Jersey: Erlbaum.

Turvey, M. and Carello, C. (1995). Dynamic Touch. In W. Epstein and S. Rogers, (Eds.), *Perception of Space and Motion.* San Diego: Academic Press.

Verbrugge, R. (1977). Resemblances in language and perception. In R.E. Shaw and J. D. Bransford (Eds.), *Perceiving, Acting and Knowing*. New Jersey: Lawrence Erlbaum Associates.

Vicente, K. J., and Wang, J. H. (1998). An ecological theory of expertise effects in memory recall. *Psychological Review*, 105 (1), 33-57.

Viviani, P. and Stucchi, N. (1992). Biological movements look uniform: Evidence of motor-perceptual interactions. *Journal of Experimental Psychology: Human Perception and Performance*, *18*, 603-623.

Viviani, P. and Mounoud, P. (1990). Perceptuo-motor compatibility in pursuit tracking of two-dimensional movements. *Journal of Motor Behavior*, 22, 407-443.

Weiss, Y., and Adelson, E. (1998). Slow and smooth: a Bayesian theory for the combination of local motion signals in human vision. MIT A. I. Memo No. 1624.

Weiss, Y., Simoncelli, E., and Adelson, E. (2002). Motion illusions as optimal percepts. *Nature Neuroscience* 5: 598-604.

Weiskrantz, L. (1997). *Consciousness Lost and Found.* New York: Oxford.

Wertheimer, M. (1945). *Productive Thinking*. New York: Harper and Row.

Wollen, K. A. (1969). Variables that determine the effectiveness of picture mediators in paired-associate learning. Paper presented at the Meeting of the Psychonomic Society, St. Louis (cited in Paivio, 1971).

Woodward, J. (2000). Explanation and invariance in the special sciences. *British Journal for the Philosophy of Science*, 51, 197-214.

Woodward, J. (2001). Law and explanation in biology: Invariance is the kind of stability that matters. *Philosophy of Science*, 68, 1-20.

Yarrow, K., Haggard, P., Heal,, R., Brown, P., and Rothwell, J. C. (2001). Illusory perceptions of space and time preserve cross-saccadic perceptual continuity. *Nature* 414: 302-304.

Yasue, K., Jibu, M., and Pribram, K. H. (1991). A theory of non-local cortical processing in the brain, in *Brain and Perception*, ed. K. H. Pribram, (New Jersey: Erlbaum)

Zaragoga, M. S., McCloskey, M., and Janis, M. (1987), 'Misleading post-event information and recall of the original event: Further evidence against the memory impairment hypothesis', *Journal of Experimental Psychology: Learning, Memory, and Cognition*, 13, 36-44.

Zimmer, H. D., Helstrup, T., and Engelkamp, J. (2000). Pop-Out into Memory: A Retrieval Mechanism That is Enhanced with the Recall of Subject-Performed Tasks. *Journal of Experimental Psychology: Learning, Memory and Cognition*, 26, 3, 658-670.

Zimmer, H. D., and Cohen, R.L. (2001). Remembering actions: A specific type of memory? In H. D. Zimmer and R. L. Cohen (Eds.), *Memory for Actions: A Distinct Form of Episodic Memory?* Oxford: Oxford University Press, pp. 3-24.

Zimmer, H. D. (2001). Why do actions speak louder than words?: Action memory as a variant of encoding manipulations or the result of a specific memory system? In H. D. Zimmer and R. L. Cohen (Eds.), *Memory for Actions: A Distinct Form of Episodic Memory?* Oxford: Oxford University Press, pp. 151-198.

In: Perspectives in Psychiatry Research
Editors: Nicole M. Levine and Donna J. Campbell
ISBN: 978-1-61209-236-2

Chapter 5

THE MONTREAL ADOLESCENT DEPRESSION DEVELOPMENT PROJECT (MADDP): SCHOOL LIFE AND DEPRESSION FOLLOWING HIGH SCHOOL TRANSITION

Alexandre J.S. Morin[1*], Michel Janosz[2] and Serge Larivée[2]
[1]Department of Psychology, University of Sherbrooke
[2]School of Psycho-Education, University of Montreal

ABSTRACT

The present study was designed to evaluate the relationship between school life and depression development in adolescents. More precisely, this study sought to determine which specific aspects of school life (in-school psychological characteristics, school-related socialization experiences, perceived school environment) could be considered as risk factors for depression development once students' background characteristics are taken into account. The possibility that these relationships could be moderated by gender and by students' previous levels of depression was also evaluated. These exploratory questions were evaluated with data from the transitional component of the Montreal Adolescent Depression Development Project (MADDP), a one-year follow-up study of 1167 seventh grade students having just experienced high school transition. The results clearly suggested that various aspects of students' school life represent significant predictors of depression development, particularly among girls. One of the main conclusions from this study is that school-based prevention programs, would be likely to diminish students' risk of developing depression following high school transition.

Keywords: depression, adolescence, risk factors, school life, transition.

[*]Corresponding author: University of Sherbrooke, F.L.S.H., Department of Psychology, 2500 boulevard de l'Université, Sherbrooke, Qc, Canada, J1K 2R1, E-mail: alexandre.morin@usherbrooke.ca

INTRODUCTION

Depression, through its lifelong chronic, recurrent, comorbid, and disabling nature, clearly represents a preeminent challenge for mental health researchers and preventionists (Angold, Costello, & Erkanli, 1999; Lewinsohn & Essau, 2002; Murray & Lopez, 1996). Developing efficient depression prevention programs was therefore identified as a key priority for developmental research by national and international health organizations (Dawson & Tylee, 2001; Mrazek & Haggerty, 1994). Developing such programs requires a precise and integrated understanding of the many risk and protective factors involved (Coie *et al.*, 1993; Mrazek & Haggerty, 1994). Moreover, as depression usually develops during adolescence and shows great continuity across the lifespan, the impact of these factors would have to be studied in child and adolescent populations (Newman, Moffitt, Caspi, Magdol, Silva, & Stanton, 1996).

Children and adolescents spend a significant part of their life at school. It is thus not surprising that studying the relationships between school life and mental health has often been identified as a priority for developmental research (Rutter, 1999; Zaslow & Takanishi, 1993). Schools represent some of youths' central life settings as well as a key socialization area. School life also encompasses many non-academic aspects of youths' social existence, such as the beginning of friendships, romance, and autonomy from parents. Consequently, school life may play a vital part in the fulfillment of youths' basic developmental needs for affiliation, security, autonomy, bonding, and achievement (Eccles, Lord, & Midgley, 1991; Mortimore, 1995).

Depression prevalence rates were found to increase in recent adolescent birth cohorts (Lewinsohn, Rohde, Seeley, & Fisher, 1993), and current hypotheses indirectly suggest that school life may be implicated in this phenomenon. For instance, Eccles (Eccles *et al.*, 1991, 1993) argued that whereas adolescents' basic developmental needs imply autonomy, intimacy, identity formation, and abstract thinking, modern middle schools (versus elementary ones) are often characterized by increased discipline, academic and social competition, social network disruptions, and lower cognitive demands. The resulting mismatch may create an increased risk for the development of psychosocial problems, especially in already vulnerable students (Eccles *et al.*, 1991, 1993; Janosz, Georges, & Parent, 1998). More precisely, adolescents whose school life is characterized by a mismatch between developmental needs and socialization experiences may come to internalize the idea that their needs are unworthy of attention and develop chronic feelings of helplessness, which in turn may lead to depression (Haaga, Dyck, &Ernst, 1991). The fact that depression often develops in early to mid-adolescence, following high school transition (Cyranowski, Frank, Young, & Shear, 2000; Nolen-Hoeksema, 2002), provides further support to Eccles *et al.*'s (1991, 1993) hypothesis.

Additionally, Diekstra (1995) and Robins (1995) indicated that the lives of modern adolescents are characterized by an earlier onset of puberty, by lengthier academic training and by the breakdown of traditional sources of social support (e.g., families, community cohesion, churches, etc.). In this context, modern adolescents have to deal earlier with adult bodies and physiological functions without being able to assume adult roles. Diekstra (1995) and Robins (1995) hypothesized that these new challenges represent one potential explanation for the increased rates of depression observed among modern adolescents. In addition to these challenges, schools may themselves contribute to adolescents' exposure to various forms of stressful experiences (e.g., being bullied at school, having a conflictual relationship with one's teachers, etc.): the relationship between stress exposure and depression is a well-documented phenomenon (Ge, Lorenz, Conger, Elder, & Simons, 1994; Lewinsohn, Allen, Seeley, & Gotlib, 1999). Moreover, due to the breakdown of traditional institutions, modern adolescents often must face alone the identity crisis that may result from these new challenges and stressful experiences (Diekstra; 1995; Robins, 1995). Schools occupy a privileged position to provide modern youths with alternate sources of social support to help them build up an integrated sense of identity. Once again, social support represents a known protective factor against depression development (Kiesner, 2002; Stein, Newcomb, & Bentler, 1996). Unfortunately, as Eccles *et al.* (1991, 1993) indicated, modern schools may not be equipped to deal with these new challenges.

Surprisingly, although many risk and protective factors were studied in relation to depression development in children and adolescents (for a review, see Morin, Janosz, & Larivée, submitted), very few studies attempted to understand the precise role of various dimensions of school life in depression development. This is the objective of the present exploratory study.

School Life and Depression Development

Schools are highly complex social systems. In schools, multiple sources of influence converge to influence students' development. Accordingly, students' school life quality will be determined by a combination of various factors related to their psychological characteristics, socialization experiences, and by the specific characteristics of their schools (Janosz, Georges *et al.*, 1998). Reaching a complete understanding of school life's effects on depression requires the simultaneous consideration of these multiple sources of influence.

Psychological Characteristics

Because individuals may choose and modify environments, it is unlikely that students with different psychological characteristics will be exposed to similar school experiences (Mortimore, 1995; Rutter, 1999). Studies should thus attempt to evaluate whether the effects of school life on depression are real or an artifact of students' psychological characteristics (body image, neuroticism, anxiety, self-esteem, behavioral disorders), themselves related to depression (Jaffe *et al.*, 2002; Krueger, 1999; Lewinsohn *et al.*, 1994; Siegel, 2002). However, specific psychological characteristics (school adaptation, achievement, motivation, etc.) are more direct determinants of school life and their effects on depression should be more directly evaluated.

Many studies showed significant negative relations between depression development and various dimensions of students' motivation at school, such as academic self-efficacy, perceived academic competencies, and involvement in school extracurricular activities (Bandura, Pastorelli, Barbaranelli, & Caprara, 1999; Gore, Farell, & Gordon, 2001; Hilsman & Garber, 1995; Lewinsohn *et al.*, 1994; Mahoney, Schweder, & Stattin, 2002). Nevertheless, studies usually failed to demonstrate a relationship between academic achievement and depression development (Bandura *et al.*, 1999; Cole, Martin, Powers, & Truglio, 1996;

Lewinsohn *et al.*, 1994; Reinherz *et al.*, 1993). This last result should be considered cautiously, as Chase-Lansdale, Cherlin, and Kiernan (1995) reported an association between academic achievement at age 7 and depression development in young adulthood. Fergusson and Woodward (2000) also noted a long-term relation between academic achievement at age 12 and depression at age 18.

For their part, Lewinsohn *et al.* (1994) concluded that students who were dissatisfied with their academic achievement and/or who did not regularly complete their homework presented an increased risk of developing depression. Yet, they obtained no significant relationship between depression and school failures, truancy, and lateness, suggesting that only some facets of school-based motivation and misbehaviors are related to depression. Further studies also reported a relation between depression and bullying, another specific form of school misbehavior (Austin & Joseph, 1996; Kaltiala-Heino, Rimpelä, Marttunen, Rimpelä, & Rantanen, 1999; Kaltiala-Heino, Rimpelä, Rantanen, & Rimpelä, 2000; Nansel *et al.*, 2001).

Socialization Experiences

Previous studies clearly showed that children's and adolescents' socialization experiences within families and peer groups influenced their risk of developing depression (Ge *et al.*, 1994; Jaffe *et al.*, 2002; Kiesner, 2002; Lewinsohn *et al.*, 1994, 1999; Stein *et al.*, 1996). Moreover, these experiences may also indirectly affect the quality of school life. For instance, parents may choose to send their children to schools that conform to their values and practices. Moreover, youths also tend to reproduce at school the various skills and interactional patterns that they learned with peers and parents (Cicchetti & Rogosch, 2002; Cicchetti & Toth, 1998). It is therefore important to evaluate whether the effects of school life on depression development represent an artifact of students' background socialization experiences or whether these effects are real and specific to school-based socialization experiences. Three kinds of socialization experiences may be more directly involved in the quality of students' school life: parental school-related educative practices, school-based interactions with peers, and interactions with school adults (teachers and other members of the school personnel).

Regarding the role of parental school-related educative practices, Hilsman and Garber (1995) indicated that parental dissatisfaction with children's grades was related to a small increase in children's depressive symptoms in the following days, but not a week later. Conversely, Lewinsohn *et al.* (1994) found no support for a relation between parental dissatisfaction with adolescents' grades and depression in a longer term follow-up study.

Second, preliminary evidence indicates that specific aspects of in-school peer relationships might be associated with depression development. For instance, Gazelle and Ladd (2003) suggested that peer exclusion at kindergarten entry could be particularly predictive of depression development for anxious-solitary children. Other studies noted similar relationships between depression development and peer rejection, conflict and victimization at school (Austin & Joseph, 1996; Brendgen, Vitaro, Bukowski, Doyle, & Markiewicz, 2001; Hodges & Perry, 1999; Jaffe *et al.*, 2002; Kaltiala-Heino *et al.*, 1999, 2000; Kiesner, 2002; Nansel *et al.*, 2001), and affiliation with deviant peers (Cantin, Wanner, Brendgen, & Vitaro, 2002).

Finally, some studies revealed a relationship between various aspects of students' socialization experiences with school adults and depression. Generally, those revealed that higher levels of teacher support and positive teacher regard were related to lower risk of subsequently developing depression (Kaltiala-Heino *et al.*, 1999; Roeser & Eccles, 1998; Roeser, Eccles, & Sameroff, 1998), although this effect may be more important for girls (Sim, 2002). Similarly, scholars were able to identify a significant relationship between school and teacher-related stress and depression development (Siddique & D'Arcy, 1984; Turner & Cole, 1994).

School Environment

In themselves, schools are social systems with their own rules and characteristics which are relatively independent from the specific socialization experiences and characteristics of their students (Janosz, Georges *et al.*, 1998). For example, whereas the school experience of a specific student might be characterized by repeated victimization, very few other students may be victimized in the school. Consequently, studying the effects of school life on depression implies that specific school characteristics should also be considered. Three methods have generally been used to evaluate school environment characteristics. First, some scholars relied on students' perceptions of their school environment. This approach is referred to as the evaluation of school *psychological environment* (Roeser & Eccles, 1998; Roeser, Eccles *et al.*, 1998). Second, students' perceptions could also be aggregated at the school level to obtain a less subjective estimate of school characteristics. Third, structural school characteristics could be more directly evaluated through observation and school records (i.e., architectural design, size, curricular diversity, demographic characteristics, state of the buildings, etc.). Both the second and third approaches represent attempts to evaluate more objectively school characteristics (Anderman, 2002). Unfortunately, we are aware of no studies in which aggregated or structural school characteristics effects on depression were directly evaluated.

Some studies reported a significant relationship between the overall quality of school climate and lower levels of depression among students (Garnefski, 2000; Kuperminc, Leadbeater, & Blatt, 2001; Way & Chen, 2000). Other studies, however, failed to replicate this result (Hadley-Ives, Stiffman, Elze, Johnson, & Dore, 2000) or found this effect to be limited to girls (Kuperminc, Leadbeater, Emmons, & Blatt, 1997). Measurement differences could explain this discrepancy, as the school climate scales used in these studies were generally idiosyncratic. Similarly, other studies used combined scales of students' academic motivation, in-school socialization experiences, and school climate perceptions and found that lower scores on these omnibus scales predicted higher levels of depression (Anderman, 2002; Aseltine & Gore, 1993; Eccles, Early, Frasier, Belansky, & McCarthy, 1997; Resnick *et al.*, 1997). In a more detailed cross-sectional analysis of the relationships between school climate and depression, Morin and Janosz (2002) noted a negative relationship between students' levels of depression and several dimensions of school climate quality (e.g., relational, security, educative and justice climate).

Among more specific aspects of school psychological environment, some studies discovered that school-based discrimination and injustice were related to higher levels of depression among students (Resnick *et al.*, 1997; Roeser, Eccles *et al.*, 1998), whereas school practices designed to facilitate proactive social relationships (Kasen, Johnson, & Cohens 1990) and efficient discipline (Eccles *et al.*, 1997) were related to lower levels of depression. However, scholars generally failed to find significant associations between students' levels of depression and their perceptions of their schools' curricular meaningfulness and valorization of learning (Kasen *et al.*, 1990; Roeser, Eccles *et al.*, 1998).

In the only prospective longitudinal study in which students' previous levels of depression were controlled, Roeser and Eccles (1998) verified the relationships between specific aspects of school environment and adolescents' depression development. In this study, no relationship was noted between depression and school facilitation of student autonomy – an aspect of school discipline. The authors also observed that students who perceived their schools as emphasizing learning over achievement presented less risk of developing depression, whereas those who perceived their schools as more competitive places presented a higher risk.

Remaining Questions

From the previous results, at least three limits of current knowledge are apparent. First, the impact of many facets of school life on depression development remains to be evaluated in an integrated, coherent and methodologically sound fashion. Indeed, current studies generally focused on very limited and idiosyncratic aspects of school life and seldom provided controls for students' personal and social background characteristics. Moreover, given that schools are highly complex environments, a complete and precise understanding of school life effects on depression development ideally requires the simultaneous consideration of the multiple facets of school life.

Second, some results pinpoint gender differences regarding school life effects on depression development. Consequently, as these studies are still few, the moderating role of gender should be more thoroughly examined. Given that gender differences in depression emerge during early adolescence, following high school transition (Cyranowski *et al.*, 2000; Nolen-Hoeksema, 2002), changes in school life from elementary to middle school may represent potentially important determinants of these differences. Indeed, some hypotheses posit that girls' increased rates of depression might be explained by the fact that they experience more often than boys the simultaneous occurrence of pubertal and school-related social changes (Bebbington, 1996). Moreover, Eccles and colleagues (Eccles *et al.*, 1991, 1993) indicate that middle schools are often characterized by academic and social competitiveness and by social network disruptions. Both of these characteristics are known predictors of depression, particularly amongst females (Bebbington, 1996; Nolen-Hoeksema, 2002).

Finally, although the previously cited studies often provided control for previous levels of depression, these controls were insufficient to disentangle the effects of school life on the *emergence* versus *aggravation* of depressive states. Briefly, controls of previous levels of depression are used to account for the bidirectionality of the relationships between depression and purported risk factors. For example, depression represents a known predictor of school adaptation problems (Kessler, Foster, Saunders, & Stang, 1995). Consequently, to clearly conclude that school adaptation problems predict depression development, one must demonstrate that the effects observed are not due to students' baseline levels of depression.

Although doing so allows depression antecedents to be identified more clearly, it remains insufficient for research in which the ultimate goal is to guide preventive efforts. Indeed, depression prevention programs usually target undepressed individuals and strive to help them to remain well (Mrazeck & Haggerty, 1994). Prevention programs should therefore be based on risk factors related to the *emergence* of depression rather than on factors related to its *aggravation*. For instance, if a risk factor predicts elevated levels of depression in already depressed individuals and shows no relationship with depression development in previously well individuals, this factor would be useless for preventionists, although very useful for clinicians. Kessler (1997) therefore urges scientists to systematically verify if the relationships between risk factors and depression development are moderated by subjects' baseline levels of depression.

Depending on how scholars define depression, two approaches can be used to this end. First, in a categorical conception of depression in which one defines depression as a diagnostic entity qualitatively distinct from subclinical symptomatology, a subject is seen as either depressed or non-depressed (APA, 1994). In such a view, scholars can either eliminate already depressed subjects from their analyses (Lewinsohn *et al.*, 1994) or verify interactions between predictors and previous levels of depression defined in a present/absent manner. Resulting interactions can then be decomposed to evaluate if the proposed risk factors differently predict onsets versus recurrences of depression (Lewinsohn *et al.*, 1999). Second, the dimensional view depicts depression as a "normative" phenomenon positioned on a continuum somewhere between a state of complete emotional well-being and of handicapping depression (Akiskal, 2001; Zuckerman, 1999). In such a view, interactions are more complex to interpret. Indeed, a significant interaction may mean that a risk factor exerts more significant effects at the lowest levels of the depressive spectrum or the reverse. However, risk factors may also be more or less potent at the midpoint of the spectrum.

THE PRESENT STUDY

The present exploratory study will attempt to provide preliminary answers to these remaining questions. More precisely, this study was designed to evaluate the specific nature of the relation between school life and depression development in adolescents. School life was defined in a global manner and encompasses three major dimensions: (a) *in-school psychological characteristics*, such as school motivation (academic self-efficacy, academic involvement, and extracurricular involvement) and school adaptation (school misbehaviors, academic delay, and academic achievement); (b) *school-related socialization experiences* involving parents (parental academic support and pressure), peers (loneliness at school, transitional difficulties, friends' school adaptation, and victimization at school), and school adults (school-related daily hassles, warm and supportive teacher-student relationships, conflictual teacher-students relations, and dissatisfaction with school discipline, academic control, help practices and encouragement); and (c) *students' perceptions of their schools'* climates (inter-students and teacher-student relational, bonding, justice, educational, and security climates), problems (minor violence, major violence, school-related problems), and practices (discipline, consultation, classroom management, extracurricular activities, support, school-family collaboration). More specifically, the present study will verify which specific aspects of school life predict depression development once adolescents' background characteristics are taken into account. Additionally, this study will verify whether: (a) these relationships are different for boys and girls (moderating role of gender), and (b) these aspects are equally relevant to the prediction of depressive symptoms' emergence among well students, aggravation among symptomatic students, and aggravation among clinically depressed students (moderating role of previous levels of depression).

METHODOLOGY OF THE MADDP

Sample and Procedure

The Montreal Adolescent Depression Development Project (MADDP) is an ongoing prospective longitudinal study of over 1000 adolescents. All seventh grade students from five Montreal-area high schools (two private and three public) were asked to participate in the project in September 2000, right after high school transition. Parents of the 1553 eligible participants were informed through a letter of the objective of the project and had the option to call the research team if they wished to withdraw their child from the study. The letter was accompanied by a consent form that described the initial transitional project, which comprised three measurement points across the school year: September/October 2000 (two classroom periods, Time 1), January/February 2001 (two classroom periods, Time 2), and May/June 2001 (one classroom period, Time 3). Only 10 parents decided to withdraw their children from the study.

The remaining 1543 students were asked sign a consent form similar to the parental one. Valid answers were provided by 1289 participants to both Time 1 questionnaires, which included most of the control variables: 66 participants refused to participate, 104 participants were absent, and 84 participants failed to provide valid answers to the questionnaires[3]. From these 1289 participants, 1167 (90.54%) provided valid answers to the Inventory to Diagnose Depression-Lifetime Version (IDD-L) administered at Time 3 (May/June 2001): 13 participants opted out of the study, 62 were absent, 41 failed to provide valid answers, and 6 were present but failed to complete the IDD-L. These 1167 subjects represent the sample used in the present analyses. This sample was predominantly of a French-speaking Caucasian background (78.2%) and almost equally split across gender (52.7% males). Of these students, 50.6% attended public schools, 29.5% attended private schools, and 19.9% attended a public school for gifted students. Regarding school curricula, 19.54% of the students followed a regular program, 32.13% an enriched program, 29.31% a program for gifted students, and 19.02% attended a special education program. At Time 1, the mean age of the participants was 12.75 years ($SD = 0.65$).

All eligible students were also offered the option to participate in the five testing sessions. Thus, students from the final sample could be compared with non-participants on most of the variables used in this study. Results from these attrition analyses revealed that non-participants generally differed in that they presented a more problematic profile of psychosocial adaptation on most variables. More precisely, non-participants generally presented lower levels of personal adaptation (lower self-esteem, more behavioral disorders, higher levels of anxiety, etc.), came from more dysfunctional families, had more problems

[3]More details regarding this last exclusion criterion are available upon request from first author.

with their peers, and described their in-school socialization experiences and school environments more negatively.

Instruments

Dependent Variable: Depressive Symptoms

Depressive symptoms were evaluated at Time 1 and Time 3 using the French translation (Pariente, Smith, & Guelfi, 1989) of Zimmerman and Coryell's (1987 b) Inventory to Diagnose Depression – Lifetime Version (IDD-L). This instrument was developed to specifically answer the main criticisms generally addressed to self-reported depression severity scales: (a) non-specificity, or the fact that severity scales often include items which are not related to diagnostic criteria; (b) incompleteness, or the fact that severity scales sometimes do not cover the entire range of diagnostic criteria; (c) diagnostic usefulness, or the fact that one can score high on a severity scale without meeting diagnostic criteria[4]; and (d) temporal specificity, or the fact that severity scales draw a time-specific portrait ignoring the possibility of recent remission. To answer the non-specificity and incompleteness criticisms, the authors chose items directly related to depression diagnostic criteria and covering their entire range (APA, 1994). The resulting instrument comprises 22 items scored on a five-point rating scale[5]. To answer the usefulness criticism, the authors developed three alternate scoring procedures for the IDD-L. Thus, a severity score highly similar to that of other self-reported depression scales can be obtained by adding participants' results on the different items (severity scoring). The authors also suggested cut-off scores for each symptom that allow for a more precise form of severity score based on the number of symptoms presented by participants (symptom scoring). Finally, once symptoms are scored, one can simply apply DSM-IV criteria to obtain a categorical diagnostic of depression. Finally, to address the time-specificity question, the IDD-L asks participants to answer by referring to the week of their life in which they felt the most depressed. Validation studies showed that both the present and lifetime versions of the IDD present strong cross-cultural psychometric properties and a very high level of diagnostic sensitivity and specificity (e.g., Ackerson, Dick, Manson, & Baron, 1990; Krause, Philipp, Maier, & Schlegel, 1989; Sakado, Sato, Uehara, Sato, & Kameda, 1996; Zimmerman, & Coryell, 1987 a, 1987 b, 1988). In this study, the alpha for the severity scoring was 0.87 at Time 1 and 0.91 at Time 3, and the KR-20 coefficient for the symptom scoring was 0.79 at Time 1 and 0.84 at Time 3.

In this study, a continuous measure of depression based on the number of symptoms (symptom scoring) presented by each participant was used. However, analyses were replicated using severity scoring, and few differences were observed. Additionally, two modifications were made. First, as this instrument was designed for a previous version of the DSM, three items referring to non-diagnostic symptoms (sexual drive and anxiety) were excluded from the final scoring. The final version thus comprises 19 items. Second, the Time

[4]For example, six items of the Beck Depression Inventory (Beck, Steer, & Brown, 1993) assess feelings of guilt and worthlessness. Thus, one can score up to 18 only by feeling guilty.

[5]As an example, the item evaluating insomnia is: (0) I was not sleeping less than normal; (1) I occasionally had slight difficulty sleeping; (2) I clearly didn't sleep as well as usual; (3) I slept about half my normal amount of time; (4) I slept less than two hours per night.

3 IDD-L was modified to refer to the week in which participants felt the most depressed during the school year.

Controlled Variables [6]

The MADDP was designed specifically to study the mechanisms implicated in depression development. Most available variables therefore represented potential risk factors for depression. Among those, every variable which was not used as a predictor and which represented a known predictor of depression development was used as a potential control. It should be noted that controlled variables were measured at Time 1. The source, number of items, sample items, answer choices and internal consistency of the questionnaires are reported in Table 1.

Demographic information. Gender and age (at October 1st, 2000) of the participants were obtained from school records.

Personal background characteristics. Measures of participants' personal background characteristics included their levels of *neuroticism* (or emotional instability), *anxiety*, *self-esteem*, and *body image satisfaction*, the frequency with which they exhibited socially deviant behaviors in the past year (*behavioral disorders*), and their levels of *pubertal development.* The behavioral disorder scale originally comprised 12 items, 2 of which referred to school misbehaviors. These 2 items were retrieved to be included in another subscale (see below).

Life event exposure. Youths' exposures to stressful life events during the past year and to *past personal difficulties* were evaluated. The *generic stressful life events* scale included 39 items from which five items had to be excluded for theoretical and methodological considerations.

Out-of-school socialization experiences. Measures of participants' out-of-school socialization experiences include *parental monitoring*, or parental knowledge of adolescents' activities; *legitimacy of familial rules*, or the perceived legitimacy of parental rules; *parental punishment*, or the use of punishment practices by parents; *familial attachment*, or the affective quality of parent-adolescent contacts; *familial instability*, or the amount of changes experienced within the participants' families;

Table 1. Description of the measurement instruments used in the present study.

Questionnaires	Authors	Items	Sample item	Answer choices	Consistency[1]
Controls: Personal background characteristics					
Neuroticism	Eysenk & Eysenk, (1963), LeBlanc (1998)	22	"Are your feelings easily hurt "	Yes/no	0.78
Self-esteem	Rosenberg (1965), Vallières & Vallerand (1990)	10	"I feel that I have a number of good qualities"	1- strongly disagree; 2- disagree; 3- agree; 4- strongly agree.	0.75 to 0.83
Body image	Marsh (1990), Ayotte et al. (2003)	8	"I am good looking"	1- false; 2- mostly false; 3- mostly true; 4- true	0.88 to 0.90

[6] Additional controls were tested (parental education, familial rules, time spent with family members and peers, trust in peers) and did not demonstrate linear relationships with depression.

Questionnaires	Authors	Items	Sample item	Answer choices	Consistency
Controls: Personal background characteristics					
Anxiety	Beck, & Steer (1993), Freeston et al. (1994)	21	"Terrified,""Difficulty breathing"	0- not at all; 1- mildly; 2 moderately; 3- severely	0.89 to 0.91
Behavioral disorders	LeBlanc (1998)	10	In the last 12 months, did you: "Use hashish or marijuana," "Refuse to obey your parents"	1- never; 2- one or two times; 3- many times; 4- very often	0.77 to 0.79
Pubertal development	Petersen, Crockett, Richards, & Boxer (1988), Héroux (1997)	7	Generic (3 items): height Girls (2 items): menarche Boys (2 items): voice change	1 to 4 rating scale with body change descriptors.	Girls: 0.70 to 0.73 (0.79 to 0.81) Boys: 0.73 to 0.75 (0.81 to 0.83)
Controls: Life event exposure					
Stressful life events	Newcomb, Huba, and Bentler (1981), Baron, Joubert, & Mercier (1991)	34	In the last 12 months, did the following things happen to you: "I had acne eruptions," "I fell deeply in love,"	Treated as yes/no	Not applicable (NA)
Past difficulties	MADDP	2	"Were you ever forced to participate in sexual acts without your consent," "Were you ever hospitalized for more than 20 days because you were very sick or had an accident"	Treated as yes/no	NA
Controls: Out-of school socialization experiences					
Parental monitoring	LeBlanc (1998)	2	"Your parents know where you are when you're not at home"	1- always; 2- often; 3- from time to time; 4- never	0.95*
Familial rules legitimacy	LeBlanc (1998)	1	"Do your parents create unfair rules?"	1-never; 2- from time to time; 3- many times; 4- often	NA
Parental punishment	LeBlanc (1998)	4	"Do your parents hit you when they want to punish you?"	1- never; 2- from time to time; 3- many times; 4- often	0.82*
Familial attachment	LeBlanc (1998)	10	"Do your parents let you know what they think and how they feel about things"	1- often, 2- many times, 3- from time to time, 4- never	0.83*
Familial instability	MADDP	5	"Did you move within the last year," "Are your parents still together?"	Treated as yes/no	NA
Familial daily hassles	MADDP	3	Do the following elements stress you: "your parents/ stepparents"	1- not at all; 2- a bit; 3- somewhat; 4- a lot	0.68 to 0.63 (0.82 to 0.85)
Communication with friends	LeBlanc (1998)	4	"Do you discuss the problems you have at home with your best friend"	1- often; 2- sometimes; 3- seldom; 4- never	0.83*
School-related psychological characteristics					
Academic self-efficacy	Skinner (1995), Janosz et al. (2001)	4	"I can get good grades at school when I want to"	1- false; 2- mostly false; 3- mostly true, 4- true	0.60 to 0.81 (0.86 to 0.94)

Table 1. (Continued).

Questionnaires	Authors	Items	Sample item	Answer choices	Consistency
School-related psychological characteristics					
Academic involvement	Skinner (1995), Janosz et al. (2001)	6	"I study or do my homework everyday"	1- false; 2- mostly false; 3- mostly true, 4- true	0.52 to 0.80 (0.81 to 0.94)
Extracurricular involvement	Skinner (1995), Janosz et al. (2001)	2	"I spent many hours a week in extracurricular activities"	1- false; 2- mostly false; 3- mostly true, 4- true	0.59 to 0.71 (0.85 to 0.91)
School misbehaviors	LeBlanc (1998)	6	"Did you intentionally disturb your class"	1- never; 2- one or two times; 3- many times; 4- often	0.79*
Academic delay	LeBlanc (1998)	1	"Since you began elementary school, did you ever have to repeat a grade?"	1- never; 2- one time; 3- two times; 4- three times; 5- four times	NA
Academic achievement	MADDP	2	"What are your actual grades in French?," "What are your actual grades in mathematics"	1- Less than 60%; 2- 60 to 69%; 3- 70 to 79%; 4- 80 to 89%; 5- 90% +	NA
Parental school-related educative practices					
Parental support	Janosz et al. (2001)	6	"I can count on my parents when I have school difficulties"	1- false; 2- mostly false; 3- mostly true, 4- true	0.61 to 0.66 (0.68 to 0.72)
Parental pressure	MADDP	4	"When I get low grades, my parents make me feel guilty,"	Idem	0.72 (0.84)
In-school peer relationships					
Loneliness at school	Asher, Hymel and Renshaw (1984), Vitaro, Pelletier, Gagnon, & Baron (1995)	5	"I feel lonely at school"	1- not true; 2- a little bit true; 3- somewhat true; 4- very true	0.82 to 0.85 (0.88 to 0.90)
Peer-related daily hassles	MADDP	2	Do the following elements stress you: "My friends," "My classmates"	1- not at all; 2- a bit; 3- somewhat; 4- a lot	0.54 to 0.61 (0.82 to 0.86)
Transitional difficulties	MADDP	2	1) "How easy is it to make new friends at school?" 2) "Are you satisfied with the number of friends you have?"	1) 1- very easy; 2- easy; 3- hard; 4- very hard 2) 1-very satisfied; 2- satisfied; 3- unsatisfied; 4- very unsatisfied	0.57 to 0.61 (0.84 to 0.86)
Friends' school adaptation	Janosz, Rondeau, and Lacroix (1998)	8	"My best friends often talk about dropping out of school"	1- false; 2- mostly false; 3- mostly true, 4- true	0.71 to 0.74
Minor victimization	Janosz (2000)	5	Since the beginning of the school year: "An adult insulted or humiliated you at school"	1- never; 2- one time; 3- two times; 4- three times; 5- four times and more	0.57 (0.68)
Major victimization	Janosz (2000)	6	Since the beginning of the school year: "Students physically attacked you"	1- never; 2- one time; 3- two times; 4- three times; 5- four times and more	0.69 (0.75)
Sexual victimization	Janosz (2000)	3	Since the beginning of the school year: "My boyfriend or girlfriend shook, hit, or squeezed me"	1- never; 2- one time; 3- two times; 4- three times; 5- four times and more	0.70 (0.86)

Questionnaires	Authors	Items	Sample item	Answer choices	Consistency
Socialization experiences involving school adults					
School-related daily hassles	MADDP	6	Do the following elements stress you: "Your teachers," "Homework"	1- not at all; 2- a bit; 3- somewhat; 4- a lot	0.80 (0.84)
Warm and supportive teacher-student relations	Pianta and Steinberg (1992), Larose, Bernier, Soucy, & Duchesne (1999)	6	"I share warm and friendly relationships with my teachers"	1- not at all; 2- not really; 3- neutral; 4- somewhat; 5- very much	0.76 (0.81)
Conflictual teacher-student relations	Pianta and Steinberg (1992), Larose et al. (1999)	7	"Sometimes, I feel that I am unfairly treated by my teachers"	1- not at all; 2- not really; 3- neutral; 4- somewhat; 5- very much	0.85 (0.87)
Dissatisfaction: discipline	MADDP	3	"severity of school rules"	The elements are: not enough (1), enough (0), or too much (1) present	0.69 (0.86)
Dissatisfaction: academic control	MADDP	2	"amount of homework and exams"	The elements are: not enough (1), enough (0), or too much (1) present.	0.57 (0.84)
Dissatisfaction: help	MADDP	3	"availability of help services for personal problems"	Should these elements be more present: yes/no	0.67 (0.84)
Dissatisfaction: encouragement	MADDP	2	"teachers' efforts to be motivating and interesting"	Should these elements be more present : yes/no	0.55 (0.83)
Perceived school climate					
Relational: inter-student	Janosz (2000)	6	"In this school, students can count on each other"	1- totally agree; 2- agree; 3- disagree; 4- totally disagree	0.76 (0.81)
Relational: teacher-student	Janosz (2000)	7	"In this school, teachers treat students with respect,"	1- totally agree; 2- agree; 3- disagree; 4- totally disagree	0.61 to 0.64 (0.83 to 0.86)
Bonding	Janosz (2000)	5	"Students feel at home in this school"	1- totally agree; 2- agree; 3- disagree; 4- totally disagree	0.78 (0.85)
Justice	Janosz (2000)	4	"The rules of this school are fair"	1- totally agree; 2- agree; 3- disagree; 4- totally disagree	0.75 (0.86)
Educational	Janosz (2000)	5	"What we learn in this school is important"	1- totally agree; 2- agree; 3- disagree; 4- totally disagree	0.75 (0.83)
Security	Janosz (2000)	5	"There are places in this school were students are afraid to go."	1- totally agree; 2- agree; 3- disagree; 4- totally disagree	0.67 to 0.73 (0.88 to 0.89)
Perceived school problems					
Minor violence	Janosz (2000)	6	Since the beginning of the school year, how often did you observe: "thefts," "insults," "vandalism."	1- never; 2- a few times during the school year; 3- a few times per months; 4- a few times per week; 5- nearly every day	0.79 (0.83)
Major violence	Janosz (2000)	4	Since the beginning of the school year, how often did you observe: "fights," "attacks of adults by students"	1- never; 2- a few times during the school year; 3- a few times per months; 4- a few times per week; 5- nearly every day	0.67 (0.80)

Table 1. (Continued).

Questionnaires	Authors	Items	Sample item	Answer choices	Consistency
Perceived school problems					
School-related	Janosz (2000)	5	Since the beginning of the school year, how often did you observe: "cheating," "truancy," "classroom disturbance"	1- never; 2- a few times during the school year; 3- a few times per months; 4- a few times per week; 5- nearly every day	0.79 (0.86)
Perceived school practices					
Disciplinary practices	Janosz (2000)	11	"School rules are easy to understand," "Teachers apply school rules as prescribed"	1- totally agree; 2- agree; 3- disagree; 4- totally disagree	0.61 to 0.64 (0.83 to 0.86)
Student consultation	Janosz (2000)	2	"Students' opinions regarding school operations are taken into consideration "	1- totally agree; 2- agree; 3- disagree; 4- totally disagree	0.64 (0.88)
Classroom management	Janosz (2000)	16	"We seldom see teachers yelling at students," "Teachers explain why new subject matters are important"	1- totally agree; 2- agree; 3- disagree; 4- totally disagree	0.64 to 0.80 (0.80 to 0.83)
Extracurricular activities	Janosz (2000)	3	"Extracurricular activities are interesting"	1- totally agree; 2- agree; 3- disagree; 4- totally disagree	0.64 (0.83)
Support mechanisms	Janosz (2000)	3	"In this school, the different help services/resources can really help students who encounter academic or personal problems"	1- totally agree; 2- agree; 3- disagree; 4- totally disagree	0.76 (0.89)
School-family collaboration	Janosz (2000)	5	"Parents often participate in school committees or activities"	1- totally agree; 2- agree; 3- disagree; 4- totally disagree	0.71 (0.80)

[1]For most scales, we report the internal consistency coefficients (α, KR-20) found in this study. However, for the scales included in LeBlanc (1998) SIQ (Social Inventory Questionnaire) and used integrally in this study, we report internal consistency coefficients taken from the SIQ manual (marked by*Table). Additionally, coefficients of shorter scales were adjusted (in parentheses) to eight equivalent items using the Spearman Brown prophecy formula.

familial daily hassles, or participants' perceptions of their families' stressfulness ; and *communication with friends*, or the degree to which participants feel free to discuss personal matters and problems with their peers.

Predictors

All the predictors used in the present study were measured at Time 2. Three dimensions of school life were tested as potential predictors of depression development: students' *school-related psychological characteristics*, *school-based socialization experiences*, and *perceptions of their school environment*. Students' *school-based socialization experiences* were further divided into three sub-dimensions: *parental school-related educative practices*, *in-school peer relationships*, and *socialization experiences involving school adults*. Finally, students' *perceptions of their school environment* were also divided into three sub-dimensions: *school climate*, or the generic atmosphere permeating the school environment; *school problems*, or aspects of students' behaviors that may negatively affect the overall quality of the school environment; and *school practices*, or school attempts to regulate and facilitate students' behaviors. These three sub-dimensions were evaluated with Janosz' (2000) SEQ (Socio Educational Questionnaire), a questionnaire validated in a large sample of Quebec adolescents.

School-related psychological characteristics. Measures of participants' school-related psychological characteristics included *academic self-efficacy*, or feelings of academic competency and of personal control; *academic involvement*, or levels of involvement in academic tasks, attitudes toward school, and academic aspirations; *extracurricular involvement*, or degree of participation in extracurricular activities; *school misbehaviors*, or the frequency with which students' exhibit school misbehaviors; *academic delay*, or the number of times students had to repeat a school year; and *academic achievement*, or participants' average grades in French (main language) and mathematics. It should be noted that whereas we had access only to students' self-reports of academic achievement at Time 2, the observed correlations between students' Time 2 self-reports and their Time 3 report cards varied between $r = 0.671$ ($p = 0.000$) and $r = 0.798$ ($p = 0.000$), which confirms the validity of students' self-reports at Time 2.

Parental school-related educative practices. Measures of parental school-related educative practices include *parental academic support*, or parental provision of academic help and support; and *parental pressure*, or the students' exposure to parental achievement pressure.

In-school peer relationships. Measures of in-school peer relationships include *loneliness*, or the degree to which students feel lonely at school; *peer-related daily hassles*, or participants' perceptions of the stressfulness of relationships with classmates; *transitional difficulties*, or participants' friendship difficulties due to school transition; *friends' school adaptation*, or participants' perceptions of the degree of school involvement, adjustment and valorization of their peers; and *minor, major and sexual victimization*, or the frequency with which participants were victims of minor, major or sexual acts of violence at school since the beginning of the year.

Socialization experiences involving school adults. Measures of participants' socialization experiences involving school adults include *school-related daily hassles*, participants' perceptions of the stressfulness of their school life; *warm and supportive teacher-student relationships*, or the degree to which participants' relationships with their teachers are characterized by warmth and support; *conflictual teacher-student relationships*, or the degree to which participants' relationships with their teachers are characterized by conflict. Four additional subscales assessed students' personal dissatisfaction with their school's *disciplinary control practices* (rules, punishments, etc.), *academic control practices* (amount of homework, exams, etc.), *help services* (academic/personal), and *encouragement practices* (offered by teachers).

Perceived school climate. Measures of perceived school climate include *inter-student relational climate*, or the degree to which interactions between students are characterized by warmth, trust, and respect; *teacher-student relational climate*, or students' respect for their teachers, and teachers' respect, warmth and support toward students; *bonding climate*, or the general feeling of school belongingness; *justice climate*, or the degree to which students perceive their school environment as equitable and respectful of individual differences;

educational climate, or students' perceptions of how much education is emphasized and valorized within their school; and *security climate*, or students' perceptions security within school.

Perceived school problems. Measures of perceived school problems include perceived frequency of *minor* and *major violence problems* and of *school-related problems.*

Perceived school practices. Measures of perceived school practices include *quality of school disciplinary practices*, or the implementation quality of school rules, students' knowledge of school rules, and consistent application of school rules; *student consultation* (regarding school rules and operations); *teachers' classroom management practices*, or the quality of teachers' pedagogical and behavior management practices; *school extracurricular activities* (quality and availability); *school support mechanisms* (to help students with academic or personal problems); and *quality of school-family collaboration* (information, involvement in decisions, etc.).

ANALYTICAL STRATEGY

Missing Data Replacement

To reduce the amount of missing data, two complementary strategies were used. First, variable scores were computed allowing for 25% to 33% of missing values on scale items. Once this strategy was applied, 0% to 14.82% of the participants still had missing values on the variables studied (*M* = 5.40%; *SD* = 4.19%), although few of them had recurring patterns of missing data. Missing data were replaced with variable means to which a random number was added according to the variables' means and standard deviations[7]. This procedure allows for the correction of the variance restriction problem inherent in simple mean-replacement strategies (Little & Rubin, 2002). For further precision in the missing data replacement process (Allison, 2001), variable means and standard deviations were calculated separately for 32 subgroups on the basis of gender (male, female), age (11-12.49, 12.5-12.99, 13-13.99, 14+), and school[8].

Choosing The Control Variables

Statistical controls were identified using a sequential strategy in which the main objective was to maximally reduce the number of variables included in the analyses in order to maximize statistical power and to limit potential multicollinearity and model specificity problems[9]. First, separate linear regressions were conducted to confirm the predictive role of the controls regarding Time 3 depressive symptoms. Second, these analyses were replicated while controlling for Time 1 depressive symptoms. Some predictors thus became non-significant and were excluded from the remaining analyses. Finally, all of the remaining predictors were entered together as a block in a hierarchical multiple regression analysis in

[7]With the SPSS 10.0 function: IF (MISSING (variable)) variable = RV.NORMAL (MEAN,SD).

[8]The number of subgroups was 32 instead of 40 (gender * age * schools = 2 X 4 X 5 = 40) as nobody from school 5 was over 13 years old and nobody from schools 1-2 was over 14 years old.

[9]As a preliminary attempt to limit the number of variables, exploratory factor analyses were conducted on the controls (as well as predictors). The observed groupings were few and inconsistent, confirming the relative independence of the variables.

which Time 1 depressive symptoms were controlled. This analysis allowed us to retain only the most significant controls.

Answering The Research Question

As the definition of school life used in the present study implied many interrelated predictors, the analytical strategy was again designed to limit the number of variables entered simultaneously in the analyses. The retained sequential strategy allowed us to interpret more clearly the effects of all variables, as well as to limit statistical power, multicollinearity and model specificity problems. Analyses were thus conducted separately to verify the predictive role of the seven dimensions of school life (school-related psychological characteristics, parental school-related educative practices, in-school peer relationships, socialization experiences involving school adults, perceived school climate, perceived school problems, and perceived school practices) evaluated in the present study regarding Time 3 depressive symptoms. First, separate regressions were conducted to evaluate the effects of each predictor on Time 3 depressive symptoms once Time 1 depressive symptoms were taken into account. Second, the remaining significant predictors were entered together as a block in a hierarchical multiple regression analysis in which only Time 1 levels of depressive symptoms were controlled. Once again, non-significant predictors were excluded from subsequent analyses. Third, the remaining significant predictors were entered together as a block in a hierarchical multiple regression analysis in which Time 1 depressive symptoms and background controls were included. Once these analyses were conducted separately for each of the seven sub-dimensions of school life, they were replicated at the dimensional level (school-related psychological characteristics, school-related socialization experiences, and perceived school environment). In these analyses, significant predictors from the preceding analyses were entered together as a block in a hierarchical multiple regression analysis in which Time 1 symptoms and controls were included.

Answering Sub-Questions

In practice, evaluating moderating relationships implies demonstrating that the interaction term composed by the product of both predictors significantly adds to the model over and above the main effects of both variables (Aiken & West, 1991; Jaccard & Turisi, 2003). As interaction terms are obtained through the multiplication of subjects' scores on both variables, which are already included in the model, multicollinearity problems may result from this procedure. To prevent this, all independent variables used in this study were converted to deviation score form by subtracting the variable mean from each individual score (Aiken, & West, 1991; Jaccard & Turisi, 2003). To further limit multicollinearity, interaction effects were tested separately, in independent regressions. In these regressions, the interaction term was entered last, following the main effects of both predictors. In the evaluation of gender-based interactions, students' Time 1 depressive symptoms were controlled[108].

To achieve maximal clarity in decomposing the significant interactions, the effects of each predictor (P) interacting with gender and/or Time 1 depressive symptoms were tested separately at different levels of the moderators (M) (Aiken & West, 1991; Jaccard & Turisi,

[8] The analyses in which the interactions were tested and decomposed were replicated three times, adding additional controls (1- Time 1 depression; 2- Time 1 depression and controls; 3- Time 1 depression, controls, and other variables from the sub-dimension). The results did not change.

2003). Briefly, in multiple regressions in which two-way interaction terms (M * P) are entered after the main effects of both the predictor and the moderator (M and P), the *b* coefficient associated with each predictor (P) represents the slope of the Y (depression) on P regression equation when the moderator (M) equals zero. As each variable was centered at the mean, the *b* coefficient associated with P in regressions, including both M and M * P terms, represents the effect of P on Y at the mean value of M. To obtain an estimate of the effects of P at different values of M, one only has to add or subtract constants to M so that zero represents different values and to compare the relative strength of the resulting *a* (intercept) and *b* coefficients to interpret the interaction. In the decomposition of gender-based interactions, regressions were thus replicated twice to estimate the effect of each predictor in males (males coded 0 and females coded 1) and females (reversed coding: males = 1 and females = 0). In these regressions, only Time 1 levels of depressive symptoms were controlled. For the interactions involving Time 1 depressive symptoms, a similar strategy was employed, but no controls were included. In the decomposition of these interactions, the effects of the predictors were evaluated at three different levels of Time 1 depressive symptoms, following Kessler's (1997) suggestion: (1) asymptomatic (zero reflects the absence of symptoms); (2) symptomatic (one to four symptoms: zero reflects the mid-point, 2.5 symptoms); (3) or clinical (five or more symptoms: zero reflects five symptoms). For the last group, the label "clinical" was preferred to "diagnostic" to account for the fact that full diagnostic criteria were not applied to the delineation of this group.

The Final Model

The most robust predictors of depression development were finally identified in three separate hierarchical multiple regressions, one for each dimension of school life. In these regressions, four blocks of predictors were entered sequentially: (1) Time 1 depressive symptoms; (2) background controls; (3) significant predictors (main effects) from the preceding analyses; and (4) significant interaction terms from the preceding analyses. The significant predictors from these three separate analyses were then entered together in a final regression to estimate the total contribution of school life to depression development.

Results

Normality and Multivariate Outliers

Inspection of the skewness and kurtosis of the different variables revealed that few of them showed normal distributions (i.e., most values were over twice their standard errors). Still, this assumption is seldom respected in large samples in which the standard error of skewness and kurtosis tend to be reduced (Tabachnick & Fidell, 1996). Additionally, in large samples, deviation from normality seldom affects the results of multivariate analyses, due to the central limit theorem (Lewis-Beck, 1980). Nevertheless, variables with skewness and/or kurtosis values over 1 were transformed and the analyses were replicated with and without these transformations. With one exception, these replications did not change the results. However, for the loneliness scale, the inverse transformation yielded significantly different results. This scale was thus transformed by inversion before its inclusion in the following analyses. The sign of the *r*, *b*, ß, and *t* coefficients associated with this variable thus has to be inversed before interpretation. Furthermore, residuals from all analyses produced normal distributions, which clearly indicate that the multivariate normality assumption of multiple regressions was respected even without transforming the other variables. Further inspection of the residual plots also indicated that the homoscedasticity and linearity assumptions of the regressions were respected.

Multivariate outliers were identified by examining bivariate scatterplots of subjects' Cooks' Distances, Leverages, and Mahalnobis' D^2 (Tabachnick & Fidell, 1996). This procedure identified 14 potential multivariate outliers. Additional analyses revealed that these subjects differed from the others by exhibiting a more severe pattern of psychosocial adaptation problems. As more seriously affected students were already lost through the attrition process, we decided to keep the multivariate outliers in the analyses. However, the analyses were first replicated with and without these subjects and the results did not significantly change.

Choosing the Control Variables

Results from the analyses designed to reduce the number of control variables are reported in Table 2. The first set of analyses confirmed that all of the proposed controls represented significant predictors of depression development. It should also be noted that the relationship between Time 1 and Time 3 depressive symptoms was quite strong ($\beta = 0.460$, $t = 17.698$, $p = 0.000$, $R^2 = 0.211$).

Table 2. Relationships between controlled variables and Time 3 depressive symptoms.

	Univariate effects			Univariate effects, depression control			Multivariate effects, depression control		
	Beta	t	p	Beta	t	p	Beta	t	p
Age	0.095	3.257	0.001	0.083	3.189	0.001	0.023	0.796	0.426
Gender	0.112	3.864	0.000	0.041	1.551	0.121	0.002	0.059	0.953
Neuroticism	0.304	10.883	0.000	0.150	5.390	0.000	0.029	0.898	0.369
Self-esteem	-0.271	-9.611	0.000	-0.176	-6.728	0.000	-0.107	-3.570	0.000
Body image	-0.187	-6.510	0.000	-0.109	-4.139	0.000	-0.044	-1.568	0.117
Anxiety	0.294	10.494	0.000	0.136	4.859	0.000	0.064	2.113	0.035
Behavioral disorders	0.152	5.261	0.000	0.087	3.320	0.001	0.012	0.430	0.667
Pubertal development	0.162	5.604	0.000	0.102	3.906	0.000	0.049	1.667	0.096
Stressful life events	0.202	7.030	0.000	0.108	4.100	0.000	0.031	1.091	0.275
Past personal difficulties	0.062	2.110	0.035	0.031	1.181	0.238			
Parental monitoring	-0.083	-2.852	0.004	-0.034	-1.295	0.196			
Rules legitimacy	-0.116	-4.001	0.000	-0.037	-1.389	0.165			
Parental punishment	0.090	3.089	0.002	0.016	0.617	0.537			

	Univariate effects			Univariate effects, depression control			Multivariate effects, depression control		
	Beta	t	p	Beta	t	p	Beta	t	p
Familial attachment	-0.118	-4.069	0.000	-0.050	-1.896	0.058			
Familial instability	0.087	2.991	0.003	0.070	2.705	0.007	0.023	0.879	0.380
Familial daily hassles	0.257	9.073	0.000	0.158	5.982	0.000	0.088	3.192	0.001
Communication with friends	0.201	7.008	0.000	0.108	4.075	0.000	0.086	3.100	0.002
R^2 change									0.065

When the analyses were replicated while controlling for previous levels of depressive symptoms, most of the family-related variables, with the exception of familial instability and daily hassles, became non-significant predictors of depressive symptoms. Most of the other variables, however, remained significant predictors of depressive symptoms, with the exception of exposure to past personal difficulties. It should be noted that although gender became a non-significant predictor of Time 3 depressive symptoms when Time 1 symptoms were controlled, we decided to keep this variable as a control in subsequent analyses due to later testing of gender-based interactions. Finally, when all of the previously identified significant predictors were considered together in a hierarchical multiple regression analysis, only four of the purported control variables still predicted Time 3 depressive symptoms: anxiety, self-esteem, familial daily hassles, and communication with friends. Together, these variables explained 6.5% of Time 3 depressive symptoms' variance. When this analysis was replicated including only significant predictors, the resulting model explained 6% of depressive symptoms' variance.

Correlations among Predictors and Controls

The correlations between the variables used in the present study are reported in Table 3. An analysis of these correlations confirms the adequacy of the selected controls, including Time 1 depressive symptoms, as these variables all shared significant relationships with various aspects of students' school life. These correlations also confirm the interrelated character of the different aspects of students' school life. Indeed, most of the school life variables shared low to moderate correlations with each other. However, these correlations are generally low enough to justify their separate consideration in the analyses. The only exception was found among aspects of students' perceptions of their school environment where 12 of the observed correlations were higher than 0.5 (only three of these correlations were higher than 0.6 and none exceeded 0.7, which would have indicated a potential multicollinearity and redundancy problem). Since such interrelations were already postulated in Janosz, Georges *et al.*'s (1998) theoretical model, since validation analyses of the SEQ confirmed the existence of distinct and interrelated factors, and since different forms of preventive interventions would be needed to act on these different variables, the decision was made to keep them separate in subsequent analyses. The selected strategy ensured that no problems of multicollinearity resulted from this decision.

Table 3. Zero-order correlations among predictors and controls.

	COMF	ANX	SE	FDH	D	AA	AINV	ASE	EXI	ISB	FAMS	FAMP	TP	LS (I)
ANX	0.125*													
SE	-0.018	-0.259*												
FDH	0.118*	0.248*	-0.243*											
D	-0.030	0.067*	-0.217*	0.095*										
AA	0.105*	-0.026	0.205*	-0.084*	-0.267*									
AINV	0.014	-0.060*	0.237*	-0.171*	-0.241*	0.245*								
ASE	0.009	-0.057	0.254*	-0.103*	-0.209*	0.376*	0.294*							
EXI	-0.015	0.037	0.050	-0.030	-0.023	0.030	0.162*	0.026						
ISB	0.041	0.101*	-0.181*	0.185*	0.339*	-0.308*	-0.428*	-0.257*	-0.052					
FAMS	-0.016	-0.064*	0.177*	-0.158*	-0.149*	0.064*	0.413*	0.184*	0.103*	-0.290*				
FAMP	0.040	0.086*	-0.069*	0.165*	-0.014	-0.080*	-0.081*	-0.110*	0.020	0.058*	-0.188*			
TP	-0.016	0.125*	-0.235*	0.060*	-0.030	-0.032	-0.083*	-0.051	-0.080*	-0.035	-0.070*	0.074*		
LS (I)	0.062*	-0.130*	0.215*	-0.103*	-0.029	0.083*	0.074*	0.063*	0.073*	0.000	0.081*	-0.071*	-0.521*	
PDH	0.069*	0.224*	-0.230*	0.218*	0.072*	-0.041	-0.142*	-0.029	-0.019	0.119*	-0.089*	0.108*	0.295*	-0.378*
FSA	0.061*	-0.059*	0.203*	-0.177*	-0.345*	0.280*	0.467*	0.256*	0.111*	-0.412*	0.321*	-0.095*	-0.036	0.077*
MINV	0.097*	0.208*	-0.167*	0.151*	0.063*	-0.068*	-0.098*	-0.106*	-0.018	0.228*	-0.065*	0.101*	0.164*	-0.204*
MAJV	0.031	0.131*	-0.152*	0.150*	0.144*	-0.073*	-0.132*	-0.170*	0.034	0.345*	-0.143*	0.014	0.024	-0.089*
SEXV	0.052	0.091*	-0.101*	0.129*	0.132*	-0.109*	-0.106*	-0.158*	0.018	0.325*	-0.089*	-0.037	-0.039	0.000
SDH	0.093*	0.301*	-0.267*	0.279*	0.118*	-0.157*	-0.282*	-0.184*	-0.055	0.304*	-0.176*	0.133*	0.144*	-0.165*
TS	0.088*	0.074*	0.047	-0.011	-0.072*	0.167*	0.269*	0.123*	0.147*	-0.140*	0.171*	-0.073*	-0.008	-0.035
TC	0.116*	0.100*	-0.177*	0.189*	0.124*	-0.146*	-0.362*	-0.253*	-0.103*	0.421*	-0.295*	0.204*	0.062*	-0.052
DSH	-0.048	0.095*	-0.144*	0.046	0.124*	-0.127*	-0.064*	-0.133*	0.057	0.115*	-0.106*	0.095*	0.075*	-0.065*
DSE	0.029	0.131*	-0.020	0.050	-0.015	-0.051	-0.071*	-0.062*	0.013	0.080*	-0.040	0.053	0.067*	-0.037
DSAC	0.103*	0.074*	-0.033	0.055	-0.051	-0.009	-0.164*	-0.100*	-0.084*	0.108*	-0.114*	0.027	0.063*	-0.009
DSDC	0.076*	0.063*	-0.069*	0.089*	0.070*	-0.126*	-0.256*	-0.152*	-0.073*	0.248*	-0.144*	0.108*	-0.018	0.017
BC	0.012	-0.093*	0.171*	-0.105*	-0.108*	0.169*	0.345*	0.173*	0.130*	-0.304*	0.203*	-0.077*	-0.131*	0.140*
BSRC	0.057	-0.138*	0.257*	-0.118*	-0.231*	0.135*	0.263*	0.173*	0.115*	-0.264*	0.206*	-0.057	-0.250*	0.277*
TSRC	-0.033	-0.129*	0.162*	-0.082*	-0.177*	0.132*	0.321*	0.163*	0.100*	-0.336*	0.286*	-0.075*	-0.088*	0.073*
EC	0.008	-0.049	0.190*	-0.093*	-0.184*	0.149*	0.407*	0.240*	0.118*	-0.392*	0.289*	-0.057	-0.076*	0.038
JC	-0.035	-0.053	0.133*	-0.101*	-0.144*	0.137*	0.358*	0.224*	0.071*	-0.323*	0.246*	-0.149*	-0.034	0.021
SC	0.028	-0.139*	0.191*	-0.093*	-0.203*	0.191*	0.217*	0.261*	0.057	-0.290*	0.217*	-0.055	-0.067*	0.130*
MINP	0.081*	0.171*	-0.146*	0.148*	0.137*	-0.127*	-0.191*	-0.056	0.001	0.342*	0.114*	0.043	-0.013	-0.050
MAJP	0.036	0.129*	-0.192*	0.154*	0.292*	-0.229*	-0.280*	-0.195*	-0.024	0.484*	-0.226*	0.018	-0.054	0.004

Table 3. (Continued).

	COMF	ANX	SE	FDH	D	AA	AINV	ASE	EXI	ISB	FAMS	FAMP	TP	LS (I)
SCOP	0.052	0.137*	-0.164*	0.088*	0.177*	-0.191*	-0.253*	-0.072*	-0.019	0.343*	-0.132*	0.056	0.013	-0.048
SDP	-0.038	-0.083*	0.123*	-0.140*	-0.051	0.026	0.232*	0.142*	0.051	-0.254*	0.254*	-0.098*	-0.090*	0.076*
SSC	-0.027	-0.042	0.025	-0.018	0.093*	-0.031	0.057*	-0.030	0.052	-0.028	0.029	-0.032	-0.081*	0.042
TCMP	-0.038	-0.085*	0.217*	-0.128*	-0.163*	0.152*	0.337*	0.257*	0.065*	-0.337*	0.330*	-0.129*	-0.087*	0.049
EXAC	0.006	-0.057	0.112*	-0.099*	-0.089*	0.052	0.251*	0.131*	0.245*	-0.243*	0.220*	-0.022	-0.084*	0.079*
SHP	0.036	-0.104*	0.140*	-0.074*	-0.062*	0.040	0.192*	0.112*	0.032	-0.179*	0.156*	-0.094*	-0.093*	0.102*
PSC	0.010	-0.107*	0.103*	-0.089*	-0.073*	0.059*	0.208*	0.087*	0.094*	-0.229*	0.234*	-0.068*	-0.081*	0.026
IDD-L1	0.213*	0.388*	-0.225*	0.234*	0.007	0.024	-0.038	-0.001	0.006	0.083*	-0.093*	0.062*	0.155*	-0.166*

	PDH	FSA	MINV	MAJV	SEXV	SDH	TS	TC	DSH	DSE	DSAC	DSDC
FSA	-0.152*											
MINV	0.220*	-0.089*										
MAJV	0.094*	-0.172*	0.415*									
SEXV	0.075*	-0.146*	0.258*	0.583*								
SDH	0.392*	-0.283*	0.230*	0.103*	0.127*							
TS	0.012	0.257*	0.003	0.057	-0.035	-0.135*						
TC	0.155*	-0.341*	0.208*	0.119*	0.089*	0.416*	-0.264*					
DSH	0.084*	-0.121*	0.069*	0.063*	0.072*	0.146*	-0.031	0.096*				
DSE	0.074*	-0.045	0.042	-0.022	0.028	0.202*	-0.059*	0.192*	0.459*			
DSAC	0.066*	-0.081*	0.086*	0.013	0.029	0.228*	-0.123*	0.225*	0.086*	0.164*		
DSDC	0.048	-0.244*	0.105*	0.056	0.087*	0.196*	-0.247*	0.328*	0.076*	0.115*	0.322*	
BC	-0.170*	0.295*	-0.236*	-0.101*	-0.076*	-0.279*	0.282*	-0.342*	-0.118*	-0.159*	-0.161*	-0.188*
BSRC	-0.254*	0.269*	-0.264*	-0.237*	-0.163*	-0.210*	0.097*	-0.184*	-0.108*	-0.108*	-0.057	-0.04
TSRC	-0.165*	0.283*	-0.220*	-0.150*	-0.129*	-0.262*	0.183*	-0.335*	-0.116*	-0.160*	-0.126*	-0.107*
EC	-0.102*	0.349*	-0.219*	-0.179*	-0.176*	-0.291*	0.205*	-0.382*	-0.148*	-0.170*	-0.159*	-0.174*
JC	-0.060*	0.261*	-0.216*	-0.126*	-0.079*	-0.227*	0.220*	-0.403*	-0.081*	-0.149*	-0.193*	-0.372*
SC	-0.136*	0.268*	-0.231*	-0.225*	-0.182*	-0.201*	-0.044	-0.214*	-0.221*	-0.128*	-0.012	-0.013
MINP	0.156*	-0.177*	0.341*	0.119*	0.052	0.257*	-0.016	0.264*	0.101*	0.085*	0.079*	0.118*
MAJP	0.126*	-0.300*	0.243*	0.306*	0.279*	0.234*	-0.034	0.264*	0.144*	0.036	0.006	0.103*
SCOP	0.157*	-0.219*	0.221*	0.047	0.010	0.246*	-0.054	0.252*	0.116*	0.138*	0.053	0.098*
SDP	-0.102*	0.229*	-0.218*	-0.205*	-0.125*	-0.250*	0.086*	-0.281*	-0.075*	-0.104*	-0.140*	-0.179*
SSC	-0.067*	0.028	-0.153*	0.056	0.048	-0.137*	0.107*	-0.131*	0.061*	-0.067*	-0.084*	-0.114*
TCMP	-0.165*	0.304*	-0.221*	-0.175*	-0.128*	-0.297*	0.227*	-0.452*	-0.173*	-0.234*	-0.184*	-0.201*
EXAC	-0.093*	0.211*	-0.118*	-0.094*	-0.033	-0.173*	0.170*	-0.295*	-0.053	-0.144*	-0.162*	-0.145*
SHP	-0.135*	0.142*	-0.176*	-0.139*	-0.114*	-0.191*	0.066*	-0.225*	-0.147*	-0.164*	-0.101*	-0.137*
PSC	-0.103*	0.205*	-0.144*	-0.075*	-0.041	-0.176*	0.173*	-0.248*	-0.149*	-0.194*	-0.125*	-0.154*
IDD-L1	0.212*	-0.004	0.161*	0.042	0.012	0.265*	0.033	0.142*	0.039	0.077*	0.103*	0.085*

	BC	BSRC	TSRC	EC	JC	SC	MINP	MAJP	SCOP	SDP	SSC	TCMP	EXAC	SHP	PSC
BSRC	0.493*														
TSRC	0.587*	0.570*													
EC	0.629*	0.449*	0.565*												
JC	0.435*	0.245*	0.422*	0.457*											
SC	0.220*	0.275*	0.310*	0.288*	0.221*										
MINP	-0.367*	-0.198*	-0.364*	-0.323*	-0.250*	-0.330*									
MAJP	-0.275*	-0.241*	-0.351*	-0.354*	-0.262*	-0.411*	0.613*								
SCOP	-0.375*	-0.200*	-0.379*	-0.302*	-0.244*	-0.300*	0.694*	0.533*							
SDP	0.329*	0.313*	0.385*	0.417*	0.416*	0.175*	-0.166*	-0.195*	-0.126*						
SSC	0.259*	0.156*	0.197*	0.186*	0.213*	-0.095*	-0.063*	0.030	-0.105*	0.267*					
TCMP	0.554*	0.383*	0.558*	0.583*	0.514*	0.347*	-0.275*	-0.313*	-0.304*	0.401*	0.214*				
EXAC	0.406*	0.288*	0.352*	0.395*	0.320*	0.179*	-0.164*	-0.141*	-0.139*	0.389*	0.230*	0.412*			
SHP	0.393*	0.319*	0.372*	0.408*	0.343*	0.149*	-0.112*	-0.124*	-0.113*	0.397*	0.240*	0.405*	0.338*		
PSC	0.480*	0.298*	0.404*	0.457*	0.365*	0.119*	-0.208*	-0.178*	-0.217*	0.422*	0.340*	0.439*	0.504*	0.399*	
IDD-L1	-0.086*	-0.094*	-0.064*	-0.033	-0.048	-0.029	0.104*	0.028	0.087*	-0.072*	-0.060*	-0.078*	-0.054	-0.064*	-0.062*

Legend. * Correlation is significant at the 0.05 level (2-tailed); *COMF*: Communication with friends; *ANX*: anxiety; *SE*: Self-esteem; *FDH*: Familial daily hassles; *D*: Academic delay; *AA*: Academic achievement; *AINV*: Academic involvement; *ASE*: Academic self-efficacy; *EXI*: Extracurricular involvement; *ISB*: School misbehaviors; *FAMS*: Parental academic support; *FAMP*: Parental academic pressure; *TP*: Transitional difficulties; *LS (I)*: Loneliness at school (inversed); *PDH*: peer-related daily hassles; *FSA*: Friends' school adaptation; *MINV*: Minor victimization; *MAJV*: Major victimization; *SEXV*: sexual or romantic victimization; *SDH*: School-related daily hassles; *TS*: Warm and supportive teacher-student relationships; *TC*: Conflictual teacher-student relationships; *DSH*: dissatisfaction with school help mechanisms; *DSE*: dissatisfaction with school encouragement mechanisms; *DSAC*: dissatisfaction with school academic control; *DSDC*: dissatisfaction with school disciplinary control; *BC*: Bonding climate; *BSRC*: Inter-student relational climate; *TSRC*: teacher-student relational climate; *EC*: Educational climate; *JC*: Justice Climate; *SC*: Security climate; *MINP*: Perceived frequency of minor violence problems; *MAJP*: Perceived frequency of major violence problems; *SCOP*: Perceived frequency of school-related problems; *SDP*: School disciplinary practices; *SSC*: Student consultation practices; *TCMP*: Teachers' classroom management practices; *EXAC*: Extracurricular activities' quality and availability; *SHP*: School help practices; *PSC*: School-family collaboration mechanisms; *IDD-L1*: Time 1 depressive symptoms.

Relationships between School Life and Depression

School-Related Psychological Characteristics

Main effects. Results from the regressions evaluating the effects of school-related psychological characteristics on Time 3 depressive symptoms are reported in Table 4. Results from the first set of regression analyses indicated that most of the variables studied did predict Time 3 depressive symptoms, even when previous levels of depressive symptoms were taken into account. In fact, only participants' levels of extracurricular involvement were found to be unrelated to depression development. These results indicate that students who exhibit higher levels of school misbehaviors or academic delays tend to present higher levels of depressive symptoms at Time 3, whereas students with higher levels of academic achievement, involvement, and self-efficacy tend to present lower levels of depressive symptoms at Time 3. However, when these variables were considered simultaneously in the analyses, only academic self-efficacy and school misbehaviors remained significant predictors of Time 3 depressive symptoms. Furthermore, when controls were partialled out in the analyses, only participants' levels of school misbehaviors still predicted Time 3 depressive symptoms.

Moderating role of gender. Among all the gender-based interactions evaluated, only the school misbehaviors ($ß = 0.083$; $t= 2.519$; $p = 0.012$) and academic involvement ($ß = -0.078$; $t= -2.167$; $p = 0.030$) interactions appeared significant. The decomposition of these interactions indicates that participants' levels of school misbehaviors represent a more potent predictor of depression development for girls ($a = 1.978$; $b = 0.226$; $p = 0.000$) than for boys ($a = 1.658$; $b = 0.111$; $p = 0.000$), while academic involvement predicted Time 3 depressive symptoms among girls only (girls: $a = 1.954$; $b = -0.733$; $p = 0.000$; boys: $a = 1.678$; $b = -0.252$; $p = 0.099$).

Moderating role of Time 1 depressive symptoms. Among the depression-based interactions, only the effects of participants' levels of extracurricular involvement were moderated by Time 1 depressive symptoms ($ß = -0.090$; $t= -3.471$; $p = 0.001$). Decomposing this interaction revealed that participants' levels of extracurricular involvement did not predict depressive symptom development among asymptomatic ($a = 0.527$; $b = 0.141$; $p = 0.161$) and symptomatic ($a = 1.613$; $b = -0.082$; $p = 0.216$) participants but were negatively related to Time 3 depressive symptoms among previously clinical students ($a = 2.698$; $b = -0.305$; $p = 0.000$).

Final model for the dimension. When students' levels of school misbehaviors were entered alone, following controls, in a regression analysis to predict Time 3 depression symptoms, they explained 1.6% of depressive symptoms variance. Adding the significant interaction (i.e., gender * school misbehaviors, gender * academic involvement, and depression * extracurricular involvement) to this regression explained an additional 1% of Time 3 depressive symptoms variance. However, among the interactions, only the Time 1 depressive symptoms by extracurricular involvement interaction remained significant ($ß = -0.074$; $t= -2.978$; $p = 0.003$).

School-Related Socialization Experiences

Results from the regression analyses evaluating the effects of student's school-related socialization experiences on Time 3 depressive symptoms are reported in Table 5.

Main effects of parental school-related educative practices. Results from the first set of regressions indicate that parental academic support and pressure both predicted Time 3 symptoms, even when previous levels of depressive symptoms were taken into account. More precisely, students exposed to a higher level of parental academic pressure and to a lower level of parental academic support tended to present more symptoms at Time 3. However, when both variables were entered together in the analyses, only parental academic pressure remained a significant predictor of depressive symptoms. Finally, following the inclusion of additional controls, the effects of parental academic pressure on depression also became non-significant.

Main effects of in-school peer relationships. In the first set of analyses, most aspects of in-school peer relationships predicted Time 3 depressive symptoms. More precisely, the results indicated that students exposed to higher levels of transitional problems, loneliness at school, peer-related daily hassles, and minor, major, and sexual victimization tended to present more symptoms at Time 3, while students whose friends presented higher levels of adaptation to school exhibited less symptoms. In the next set of regressions, the simultaneous consideration of these variables in the analysis resulted in the disappearance of two of these effects: transitional problems and major victimization became non-significant predictors of Time 3 symptoms. Finally, only two variables still predicted Time 3 depressive symptoms following the inclusion of background controls in the analyses: loneliness at school and minor victimization.

Main effects of socialization experiences involving school adults. Among the varied dimensions of participants' socialization experiences involving school adults, only two were found to significantly predict Time 3 depressive symptoms: school-related daily hassles and conflictual relationships with teachers. Students who perceived their school experiences as more stressful and who had more conflictual relationships with their teachers tended to develop higher levels of depressive symptoms. Furthermore, these relations were unaffected by the simultaneous consideration of both variables and by the inclusion of background controls in the analysis.

Moderating role of gender. The evaluation of gender-based interactions revealed that the effects of four aspects of students' school-related socialization experiences on Time 3 levels of depressive symptoms were moderated by gender: minor victimization ($ß = 0.132$; $t= 4.052$; $p = 0.000$), school-related daily hassles ($ß = 0.133$; $t= 4.011$; $p = 0.000$), conflictual relationships with teachers ($ß = 0.092$; $t= 2.704$; $p = 0.007$), and dissatisfaction with school disciplinary control ($ß = 0.110$; $t= 3.218$; $p = 0.001$). Additionally, the interaction between gender and major victimization was also found to be marginally significant ($ß = 0.055$; $t= 1.775$; $p = 0.076$). The decomposition of these interactions revealed that the first three variables, as well as major victimization, represented more potent predictors of depressive symptoms in girls (minor victimization: $a = 1.990$; $b = 0.257$; $p = 0.000$; major victimization: $a = 1.962$; $b = 0.216$; $p = 0.000$; daily hassles: $a = 1.909$; $b = 1.212$; $p = 0.000$; conflicts with teachers: $a = 1.950$; $b = 0.592$; $p = 0.000$) than in boys (minor victimization: $a = 1.663$; $b = 0.084$; $p = 0.002$; major victimization: $a = 1.673$; $b = 0.087$; $p = 0.025$; daily hassles: $a = 1.683$; $b = 0.395$; $p = 0.003$; conflicts with teachers: $a = 1.675$; $b = 0.228$; $p = 0.011$), while students' dissatisfaction with school disciplinary control predicted Time 3 depressive symptoms only among girls (girls: $a = 1.905$; $b = 0.684$; $p = 0.002$; boys: $a = 1.700$; $b = -0.228$; $p = 0.219$).

Table 4. Relationships between school-related psychological characteristics and Time 3 depressive symptoms.

	Univariate effects, depression control			Multivariate effects, depression control			Multivariate effects, all controls			Final model for the dimension, all controls		
	Beta	t	p	Beta	t	p	Beta	t	p	Beta	t	p
School-related psychological characteristics												
Academic delay	0.073	2.807	0.005	0.010	0.352	0.725						
Academic achievement	-0.057	-2.199	0.028	0.020	0.709	0.479						
Academic involvement	-0.105	-4.053	0.000	-0.028	-0.956	0.339						
Academic self-efficacy	-0.101	-3.916	0.000	-0.061	-2.162	0.031	-0.029	-1.091	0.276			
Extracurricular involvement	-0.050	-1.909	0.056									
School misbehaviors	0.170	6.621	0.000	0.145	4.837	0.000	0.124	4.706	0.000	0.130	5.047	0.000
R^2 change			NA			0.033			0.016			0.016

Table 5. Relationships between school-related socialization experiences and Time 3 depressive symptoms.

	Univariate effects, depression control			Multivariate, depression control			Multivariate effects, all controls			Final model for the dimension, all controls		
	Beta	t	p	Beta	t	p	Beta	t	p	Beta	t	p
Parental school-related educative practices												
Parental academic support	-0.059	-2.253	0.024	-0.049	-1.838	0.066						
Parental academic pressure	0.064	2.452	0.014	0.055	2.077	0.038	0.034	1.321	0.187			
R^2 change			NA			0.006			0.001			
In-school peer relationships												
Transitional difficulties	0.089	3.380	0.001	0.015	0.502	0.615						
Loneliness at school (inv.)	0.107	4.073	0.000	-0.064	-2.063	0.039	-0.073	-2.653	0.008	-0.084	-3.235	0.001

Table 5. (Continued).

	Univariate effects, depression control			Multivariate, depression control			Multivariate effects, all controls			Final model for the dimension, all controls		
	Beta	t	p	Beta	t	p	Beta	t	p	Beta	t	p
Peer-related daily hassles	0.151	5.770	0.000	0.086	3.040	0.002	0.049	1.763	0.078			
Friends' school adaptation	-0.098	-3.779	0.000	-0.063	-2.417	0.016	-0.044	-1.684	0.092			
Minor victimization	0.176	6.800	0.000	0.134	4.672	0.000	0.109	4.010	0.000	0.106	4.010	0.000
Major victimization	0.090	3.470	0.001	-0.026	-0.797	0.425						
Sexual victimization	0.098	3.807	0.000	0.065	2.083	0.037	0.033	1.283	0.200			
R^2 change			NA			0.055			0.029			
Socialization experiences involving school adults												
School-related daily hassles	0.183	6.905	0.000	0.148	5.170	0.000	0.093	3.168	0.002	0.074	2.542	0.011
Teacher support	-0.006	-0.222	0.824									
Conflicts with teachers	0.141	5.449	0.000	0.084	3.011	0.003	0.066	2.384	0.017	0.059	2.116	0.035
Dissatisfaction: help	0.019	0.721	0.471									
Dissatisfaction: encouragement	0.027	1.017	0.309									
Dissatisfaction: academic control	0.008	0.305	0.760									
Dissatisfaction: discipline	0.028	1.060	0.289									
R^2 change			NA			0.037			0.015			0.034

Table 6. Relationships between perceived school environment and depression development.

	Univariate effects with depression control			Multivariate effects (sub-dimensions), depression control			Multivariate effects (sub-dimensions), all controls			Final model for the dimension, all controls		
	Beta	t	p	Beta	t	p	Beta	t	p	Beta	t	p
Perceived school climate												
Bonding	-0.097	-3.726	0.000	-0.021	-0.582	0.561						
Relational (inter-student)	-0.102	-3.930	0.000	-0.050	-1.526	0.127						
Relational (teacher-student)	-0.100	-3.865	0.000	-0.004	-0.104	0.917						
Educational	-0.093	-3.575	0.000	0.004	0.104	0.917						
Justice	-0.115	-4.471	0.000	-0.076	-2.527	0.012	-0.074	-2.870	0.004	-0.039	-1.282	0.200
Security	-0.118	-4.584	0.000	-0.083	-3.025	0.003	-0.068	-2.579	0.010	-0.044	-1.588	0.113
R^2 change			NA			0.026			0.012			
Perceived frequency of school problems												
Minor violence	0.133	5.145	0.000	0.119	3.033	0.002	0.090	3.503	0.000	0.057	2.103	0.036
Major violence	0.092	3.538	0.000	0.015	0.463	0.643						
School-related	0.097	3.748	0.000	0.007	0.198	0.843						
R^2 change			NA			0.018			0.008			
Perceived quality of school practices												
Disciplinary practices	-0.110	-4.232	0.000	-0.064	-2.091	0.037	-0.053	-1.931	0.054	-0.040	-1.401	0.162
Student consultation	-0.056	-2.167	0.030	-0.020	-0.721	0.471						
Classroom management	-0.127	-4.931	0.000	-0.096	-3.098	0.002	-0.065	-2.343	0.019	-0.023	-0.737	0.461
Extracurricular activities	-0.060	-2.314	0.021	0.010	0.326	0.744						
Support mechanisms	-0.096	-3.700	0.000	-0.040	-1.329	0.184						
School-family collaboration	-0.063	-2.425	0.015	0.023	0.700	0.484						
R^2 change			NA			0.022			0.010			0.016

Moderating role of Time 1 depressive symptoms. Time 1 depressive symptoms were found to moderate the impact of several variables on depression development: transitional difficulties (ß = 0.065; t= 2.494; p = 0.013), minor victimization (ß = 0.062; t= 2.393; p = 0.017), major victimization (ß = -0.084; t= -3.236; p = 0.001), conflictual relationships with teachers (ß = 0.069; t= 2.672; p = 0.008), and dissatisfaction with school encouragement practices (ß = 0.059; t= 2.273; p = 0.023). Additionally, the interaction between Time 1 depressive symptoms and sexual victimization was also found to be marginally significant (ß = -0.048; t= -1.839; p = 0.066). The decomposition of these interactions revealed that experiencing transitional difficulties and conflictual relationships with teachers predicted Time 3 depressive symptoms only among previously symptomatic (transitional difficulties: a = 1.595; b = 0.242; p = 0.013; conflict: a = 1.599; b = 0.317; p = 0.000) and clinically depressed (transitional difficulties: a = 2.641; b = 0.466; p = 0.000; conflict: a = 2.626; b = 0.487; p = 0.000) participants rather than among previously asymptomatic students (transitional difficulties: a = 0.548; b = 0.017; p = 0.910; conflict: a = 0.571; b = 0.146; p = 0.172). Similarly, exposure to minor victimization became more strongly associated with Time 3 depressive symptoms as participants' Time 1 symptoms increased (asymptomatic: a = 0.592; b = 0.080; p = 0.020; symptomatic: a = 1.602; b = 0.128; p = 0.000; clinical: a = 2.611; b = 0.176; p = 0.000) and students' levels of dissatisfaction with school encouragement practices only appeared to predict depressive symptoms among previously clinically depressed adolescents (asymptomatic: a = 0.513; b = -0.253; p = 0.311; symptomatic: a = 1.600; b = 0.116; p = 0.484; clinical: a = 2.688; b = 0.488; p = 0.025). Finally, the effects of major (asymptomatic: a = 0.535; b = 0.247; p = 0.000; symptomatic: a = 1.620; b = 0.142; p = 0.000; clinical: a = 2.704; b = 0.037; p = 0.350) and sexual (asymptomatic: a = 0.528; b = 0.356; p = 0.000; symptomatic: a = 1.613; b = 0.236; p = 0.000; clinical: a = 2.698; b = 0.116; p = 0.162) victimization on Time 3 depressive symptoms were limited to previously asymptomatic and symptomatic students, while they were non-significant among previously asymptomatic youths.

Final model for the dimension. Four variables related to students' school-related socialization experiences were found to significantly and positively predict Time 3 depressive symptoms: loneliness at school, minor victimization, school-related daily hassles and conflictual relationships with teachers. When these four variables were entered together in a multiple regression, following controls, all remained significant predictors of depression development and explained 3.4% of Time 3 depressive symptom variance. Adding the significant interaction terms from the school-related socialization experience dimension to this regression explained an additional 3.1% of Time 3 depressive symptom variance. Among these interactions, six remained significant predictors of Time 3 depressive symptoms in this final model. Three of these interactions involved gender: minor victimization (ß = 0.076; t= 2.143; p = 0.032), school-related daily hassles (ß = 0.075; t= 2.064; p = 0.039), and dissatisfaction with school disciplinary control (ß =0.069; t= 2.012; p = 0.044). The other three interactions involved Time 1 levels of depressive symptoms: minor victimization (ß = 0.074; t= 2.628; p = 0.009), major victimization (ß = -0.086; t= -2.890; p = 0.004), and conflictual relationships with teachers (ß = 0.071; t= 2.700; p = 0.007).

Perceived School Environment

Results from the regression analyses evaluating the effects of student's perceptions of their school environments on Time 3 depressive symptoms are reported in Table 6.

Main effects of perceived school climate. In the first set of regressions, the six aspects of students' school climate perceptions were found to share significant negative relationships with Time 3 symptoms. The simultaneous consideration of these variables in the analysis resulted in the disappearance of four of these effects. Indeed, only students' perceptions of school justice and security climates remained significant predictors of depression development. The inclusion of background controls in the analysis did not change these results.

Main effects of perceived school problems. In the first set of regressions, students' perceptions of the frequency of minor violence, major violence and school-related problems at school were found to share a positive relationship with Time 3 symptoms. When these dimensions were considered together in the analyses, only participants' perceptions of the frequency of minor violence problems remained a significant predictor of their later levels of depression. This relationship remained unaffected by the inclusion of additional controls.

Main effects of perceived school practices. When they were considered alone in analyses in which Time 1 depressive symptoms were controlled, the six aspects of students' perceptions of school practices negatively predicted their Time 3 symptoms. The simultaneous inclusion of these variables in the analyses considerably reduced the number of significant effects. Indeed, only students' perceptions of school disciplinary practices and teachers' classroom management practices still predicted Time 3 symptoms. Moreover, the effects of school disciplinary practices became only marginally significant following the inclusion of additional controls.

Moderating role of gender. The evaluation of gender-based interactions revealed that the effects of four aspects of students' perceptions of their school environment were significantly moderated by gender: security climate (β = -0.085; t= -2.482; p = 0.013), minor violence problems (β = 0.127; t= 3.584; p = 0.000), major violence problems (β = 0.097; t= 2.843; p = 0.005), and school-related problems (β = 0.109; t= 3.070; p = 0.002). The decomposition of these interactions indicated that these four variables predicted Time 3 depressive symptoms only, or mostly, among girls (security climate: a = 1.955; b = -0.632; p = 0.000; minor violence: a = 1.922; b = 0.114; p = 0.000; major violence: a = 1.936; b = 0.176; p = 0.000; school-related: a = 1.890; b = 0.091; p = 0.000) rather than boys (security climate: a = 1.678; b = -0.221; p = 0.041; minor violence: a = 1.690; b = 0.024; p = 0.178; major violence: a = 1.691; b = 0.032; p = 0.340; school-related: a = 1.698; b = 0.011; p = 0.535).

Moderating role of Time 1 depressive symptoms. The evaluation of Time 1 depressive-symptom-based interactions revealed that the effects of several aspects of students' perceptions of their school environment on Time 3 depressive symptoms were moderated by their previous levels of depression: bonding climate (β = -0.091; t= -3.535; p = 0.000), inter-student relational climate (β =- 0.063; t= -2.426; p = 0.015), justice climate (β = -0.087; t= -3.362; p = 0.001), minor violence problem frequency (β = 0.059; t= 2.275; p = 0.023), school disciplinary practices (β =-0.069; t= -2.691; p = 0.007), student consultation practices (β = -0.062; t= -2.382; p = 0.017), teachers' classroom management practices (β = -0.070; t= -2.719; p = 0.007), extracurricular activity quality and availability (β = -0.062; t= -2.376; p = 0.018), and school-family collaboration mechanisms (β = -0.079; t= -3.035; p = 0.002). The decomposition of these interactions revealed that the effects of three of these variables were related to Time 3 depressive symptoms only, or mostly, among students who were clinically depressed at Time 1: student consultation practices (asymptomatic: $a = 0.534$; $b = 0.036$; $p = 0.711$; symptomatic: $a = 1.605$; $b = -0.119$; $p = 0.070$; clinical: $a = 2.676$; $b = -0.273$; $p = 0.001$), extracurricular activity quality and availability (asymptomatic: $a = 0.530$; $b = 0.043$; $p = 0.743$; symptomatic: $a = 1.605$; $b = -0.156$; $p = 0.074$; clinical: $a = 2.681$; $b = -0.355$; $p = 0.001$), and school-family collaboration mechanisms (asymptomatic: $a = 0.539$; $b = 0.096$; $p = 0.506$; symptomatic: $a = 1.609$; $b = -0.187$; $p = 0.053$; clinical: $a = 2.668$; $b = -0.471$; $p = 0.000$). Similarly, the predictive effects of six other variables were limited to symptomatic and clinically depressed students at Time 1: bonding climate (asymptomatic: $a = 0.548$; $b = 0.029$; $p = 0.828$; symptomatic: $a = 1.603$; $b = -0.285$; $p = 0.000$; clinical: $a = 2.649$; $b = -0.598$; $p = 0.000$), inter-student relational climate (asymptomatic: $a = 0.552$; $b = -0.123$; $p = 0.430$; symptomatic: $a = 1.603$; $b = -0.367$; $p = 0.000$; clinical: $a = 2.655$; $b = -0.611$; $p = 0.000$), justice climate (asymptomatic: $a = 0.548$; $b = -0.050$; $p = 0.687$; symptomatic: $a = 1.606$; $b = -0.316$; $p = 0.000$; clinical: $a = 2.665$; $b = -0.582$; $p = 0.000$), minor violence problem frequency (asymptomatic: $a = 0.557$; $b = 0.032$; $p = 0.104$; symptomatic: $a = 1.604$; $b = 0.060$; $p = 0.000$; clinical: $a = 2.650$; $b = 0.088$; $p = 0.000$), school disciplinary practices (asymptomatic: $a = 0.540$; $b = -0.149$; $p = 0.468$; symptomatic: $a = 1.603$; $b = -0.509$; $p = 0.000$; clinical: $a = 2.667$; $b = -0.868$; $p = 0.000$), and teachers' classroom management practices (asymptomatic: $a = 0.551$; $b = -0.196$; $p = 0.245$; symptomatic: $a = 1.604$; $b = -0.488$; $p = 0.000$; clinical: $a = 2.657$; $b = -0.781$; $p = 0.000$).

Final model for the dimension. Five variables related to students' perceptions of their school environment significantly predicted Time 3 depressive symptoms: justice and security climates, perceived frequency of minor violence problems, disciplinary practices, and teachers' classroom management practices. When these five variables were entered together in a multiple regression analysis, following controls, they explained a total of 1.6% in Time 3 depressive symptom variance. However, only perceived frequency of minor violence problems remained a significant predictor of depression development. When this regression was replicated including only this variable and background controls, perceived frequency of minor violence problems explained only 0.8% of the variance in Time 3 depressive symptoms. Adding the significant interaction terms from the perceived school environment dimension to this regression explained an additional 2.6% of Time 3 symptoms variance, although no interaction remained significant.

Contribution of School Life to Depression Development

A final regression analysis was conducted to estimate the total contribution of school life to depression development. When all significant predictors from the previous analyses (final models from each of the three dimensions) were entered together following controls, they explained a total of 4.1% of Time 3 depressive symptom variance. In this regression, Time 1 depressive symptoms and background controls explained 21.2% and 6.0% respectively of Time 3 depressive symptom variance. Among the predictors, four remained significant predictors of Time 3 symptoms: school misbehaviors ($ß = 0.091$; $t = 3.199$; $p = 0.001$), loneliness at school (inversed: $ß = -0.093$; $t = -3.579$; $p = 0.000$), minor victimization ($ß = 0.089$; $t = 3.260$; $p = 0.001$), and school-related hassles ($ß = 0.060$; $t = 2.061$; $p = 0.040$). The effect of the other two variables – conflictual relationships with teachers ($ß = 0.027$; $t = 0.919$;

p = 0.358) and perceived frequency of minor violence problems (ß = 0.021; t= 0.756; p = 0.450) – became non-significant. When this regression was replicated including only these four predictors and background controls, they were found to explain 4% of the Time 3 depressive symptom variance. Adding the significant interaction terms from the preceding analyses to this regression explained an additional 3.4% of Time 3 depressive symptom variance. The final model thus explained a grand total of 34.6% of Time 3 depressive symptom variance. Among the interactions, six remained significant predictors of Time 3 depressive symptoms. Two of those involved gender: school-related daily hassles (ß = 0.069; t= 2.070; p = 0.039) and minor victimization (ß =0.066; t= 2.078; p = 0.044). The other four interactions involved Time 1 symptoms: extracurricular involvement (ß = -0.061; t= -2.508; p = 0.012), minor victimization (ß = 0.080; t= 3.013; p = 0.003); major victimization (ß = -0.093; t= -3.569; p = 0.000), and conflictual relationships with teachers (ß = 0.056; t= 2.236; p = 0.026). Only the previous levels of depression * dissatisfaction with school disciplinary control interaction became non-significant (ß = 0.058; t= 1.763; p = 0.078).

Discussion of the Results

Relationships between School Life and Depression

The main objective of this study was to evaluate the relationship between school life and depression development. A summary of the results is presented in Table 7. Perhaps the most important of these results is that the majority of the school life characteristics evaluated did represent significant predictors of depression development among high school students when their effects were considered separately. The fact that many of these factors became non-significant predictors of depression development when they were considered simultaneously does not mean that they should not be targeted in preventive interventions. Indeed, this study suggests that improving various aspects of students' school-related psychological characteristics, in-school socialization experiences and perceptions of their school environment would likely reduce their risk of developing depression following high school transition. However, the simultaneous consideration of multiple aspects of students' school life in the prediction of depression development clearly indicated that some of these variables may be more potent predictors of depression than others. This result may be due to the interrelated character of the multiple facets of school life. For instance, whereas most aspects of students' perceptions of school climate individually predicted their later levels of depression, their simultaneous consideration in the analyses left only justice and security climates as significant predictors of depression development. A parsimonious interpretation of this result could be that the effects of the other aspects of school climate (inter-student and teacher-student relational climates, bonding climate, and educational climate) on students' levels of depression only represented an artifact of their relationships with justice and security climates. Again, this result does not mean that improving, for example, school bonding climates would not help to prevent depression since such an improvement would likely result in the simultaneous enhancement of school justice and security climates. However, more systematic evaluations of the relationships between school life characteristics would be needed to test the plausibility of this hypothesis.

Alternatively, the fact that most aspects of school life appear to be worthy targets for preventive interventions does not mean that they also provide worthy explanations for depression development. Indeed, in the preceding example, most aspects of students' perceptions of school climates were described as potential targets for prevention programs due to their intertwined character. Nevertheless, only justice and security climates represent potential "causes" of depression development as the results suggest that, no matter how problematic other aspects of school climate may be viewed by students, theses perceptions may not increase students' risk of developing depression if they perceive their schools' justice and security climates positively.

Another important result from this study is the fact that the inclusion of students' personal and social background characteristics as controls in the analyses only minimally affected the observed relationships. Indeed, the effects of only five of the predictors became non-significant once these variables were controlled in the analyses: the relationships between depression and students' levels of academic self-efficacy, parental academic pressure, perceived stressfulness of students' relationships with friends and classmates, sexual/romantic victimization, and friends' school adaptation may thus represent an artifact of students' background characteristics. More precisely, students' background characteristics may influence their exposure to these specific in-school factors as well as their risk of developing depression, and thus explain the observed statistical associations. However, a far more important implication of this finding is that school life effects on depression development may be relatively independent from the effects of students' lives outside of school. Youths' lives in and out of school should therefore be seen as complementary targets for preventive interventions. The present results clearly suggest that neither form of intervention is likely to be sufficient to prevent depression.

Among all the school life characteristics evaluated, few may be seen as exerting a determining impact on depression development: (a) school misbehaviors, (b) loneliness at school, (c) minor victimization, (d) conflictual relationships with teachers, (e) perceived stressfulness of school life, (f) justice climate, (g) security climate, (h) school disciplinary practices, (i) classroom management practices; and (j) nor violence problems frequency. Furthermore, in a more integrated predictive model, it appears that the main effects of school life on depression development may only result from the action of four variables: school misbehaviors, loneliness at school, minor victimization, and perceived stressfulness of students' school lives. The disappearance of the other effects should not be surprising since it is highly plausible that these remaining variables act as complete mediators of the relationships between the other variables and depression. For instance, security climates, disciplinary practices, classroom management practices, and minor violence problems frequency all refer to school violence or to school efforts to reduce violence. In this context, it is possible that these variables all converge to augment students' risk of being victimized, and that victimization represents the proximal determinant of depression development involved in their effects. It should be noted that these results lend strong support to the recent societal and scientific claims that school violence prevention programs should be seen as a key priority for modern societies (Gottfredson, 2000). Accordingly, students' negative perceptions of their schools' justice climate and exposure to conflict with teachers may both represent potential contributors to students' perceptions of their schools as stressful places, which may in turn mediate their effects on depression.

Table 7. A summary of the results.

	Main effects					Gender-based variations				Depression-based variations				
	U_CD	M_CD	M_AC	FMD	FM	M	F	FMD	FM	A	S	C	FMD	FM
School-related psychological characteristics														
Academic delay	↑	---	---	---	---									
Academic achievement	↓	---	---	---	---									
Academic involvement	↓	---	---	---	---	---	↓	---	---					
Academic self-efficacy	↓	↓	---	---	---									
Extracurricular involvement	---	---	---	---	---					---	---	↓	↓	↓
School misbehaviors	↑	↑	↑	↑	↑	↑	↑↑	---	---					
School-related socialization experiences : Parental school-related educative practices														
Parental academic support	↓	---	---	---	---									
Parental academic pressure	↑	↑	---	---	---									
School-related socialization experiences : In-school peer relationships														
Transitional difficulties	↑	---	---	---	---					---	↑	↑↑	---	---
Loneliness at school	↑	↑	↑	↑	↑									
Peer-related daily hassles	↑	↑	---	---	---									
Friends' school adaptation	↓	↓	---	---	---									
Minor victimization	↑	↑	↑	↑	↑	↑	↑↑	↑	↑	↑	↑↑	↑↑↑	↑	↑
Major victimization	↑	---	---	---	---	↑	↑↑	---	---	↑↑	↑	---	↑	↑
Sexual victimization	↑	↑	---	---	---					↑↑	↑	---	---	---
School-related socialization experiences : Socialization experiences involving school adults														
School-related hassles	↑	↑	↑	↑	↑	↑	↑↑	↑	↑					
Teacher support	---	---	---	---	---									
Conflicts with teachers	↑	↑	↑	↑	---	↑	↑↑	---	---	---	↑	↑↑	↑	↑
Dissatisfaction: help	---	---	---	---	---									
Dissatisfaction: encour.	---	---	---	---	---					---	---	↑	---	---
Dissatisfaction: acad. control	---	---	---	---	---									
Dissatisfaction: discipline	---	---	---	---	---	---	↑	↑	↑					

Table 7. (Continued).

	Main effects					Gender-based interactions				Depression-based interactions				
	S_CD	M_CD	M_AC	FMD	FM	M	F	FMD	FM	A	S	C	FMD	FM
Perceived school environment: Perceived school climate														
Bonding	↓	---	---	---	---					---	↓	↓↓	---	---
Relational (students)	↓	---	---	---	---					---	↓	↓↓	---	---
Relational (teachers-students)	↓	---	---	---	---									
Educational	↓	---	---	---	---									
Justice	↓	↓	↓	---	---					---	↓	↓↓	---	---
Security	↓	↓	↓	---	---	↓	↓↓	---	---					
Perceived school environment: Perceived frequency of school problems														
Minor violence	↑	↑	↑	↑	---	---	↑	---	---	---	↑	↑↑	---	---
Major violence	↑	---	---	---	---	---	↑	---	---					
School-related	↑	---	---	---	---	---	↑	---	---					
Perceived school environment: Perceived quality of school practices														
Disciplinary practices	↓	↑	↑	---	---					---	↓	↓↓	---	---
Students' involvement	↓	---	---	---	---					---	↓	↓	---	---
Classroom management	↓	↑	↑	---	---					---	↓	↓↓	---	---
Extracurricular activities	↓	---	---	---	---					---	↓	↓	---	---
School support	↓	---	---	---	---									
Parental implication	↓	---	---	---	---					---	↓	↓	---	---

Legend. U_CD: univariate (U) effect of the variable on Time 3 level of depression while controlling (C) for previous levels of depression (D); *M_CD*: effect of the variable on Time 3 level of depression in a multivariate analysis including all predictors from the dimensions and controlling (C) for previous levels of depression (D); *M_AC*: effect of the variable on Time 3 level of depression in a multivariate analysis including all predictors from the dimensions including all (A) controls (C); *FMD*: effect of the variable in the final (F) model (M) for the dimension (D); *FM*: effect of the variable in the final (F) model (M); **M**: effect of the variable among males; *F*: effect of the variable among females; **A**: effect of the variable among asymptomatic subjects at Time 1; **S**: effect of the variable among symptomatic subjects at Time 1; **C**: effect of the variable among clinically depressed subjects at Time 1; **↑**: positive significant relationship (higher levels of the predictor are associated with higher levels of depression); **↓**: negative significant relationship (lower levels of the predictor are associated with higher levels of depression); ↓ or ↑: marginally significant effect; **↑**, **↑↑** and **↑↑↑** (or reversed): comparative importance of the effects; ---: non significant effect.

Some of these results are highly consistent with those from previous studies. For instance, previous studies also generally failed to find significant relationships between depression development and academic achievement (Bandura *et al.*, 1999; Cole *et al.*, 1996; Lewinsohn *et al.*, 1994; Reinherz *et al.*, 1993), parental school-related educative practices (Hilsman, & Garber, 1995; Lewinsohn *et al.*, 1994), and educative climate (Kasen *et al.*, 1990; Roeser & Eccles, 1998; Roeser, Eccles *et al.*, 1998). Previous studies similarly found that students exhibiting school misbehaviors (Austin, & Joseph, 1996; Kaltiala-Heino *et al.*, 1999, 2000; Lewinsohn *et al.*, 1994; Nansel *et al.*, 2001), bullied and/or lonely students (Austin & Joseph, 1996; Hodges & Perry, 1999; Kaltiala-Heino *et al.*, 1999, 2000; Kiesner, 2002; Reinherz *et al.*, 1993; Stein *et al.*, 1996), students feeling more stressed by their school environment (Siddique & D'Arcy, 1984; Turner & Cole, 1994), students with more negative perceptions of their school justice climate (Resnick *et al.*, 1997; Roeser, Eccles *et al.*, 1998), and students negatively evaluating the disciplinary and classroom management practices used in their schools (Eccles *et al.*, 1997; Roeser & Eccles, 1998) presented a higher risk of developing depression.

In some cases, our results appear inconsistent with those found in previous studies. For instance, levels of academic self-efficacy (Bandura *et al.*, 1999; Hilsman & Garber, 1995; Lewinsohn *et al.*, 1994), extracurricular involvement (Gore *et al.*, 2001; Mahoney *et al.*, 2002), stressful peer relationships (Brendgen *et al.*, 2001; Jaffe *et al.*, 2002), affiliation with deviant peers (Cantin *et al.*, 2002) and supportive teacher-student relationships (Roeser and Eccles, 1998; Sim, 2002) were generally found to predict depression development in previous studies. However, it should be noted that this study represents, to our knowledge, the first attempt to systematically evaluate the impact of the different facets of school life in a single study while providing adequate controls for background personal, familial, and friendship characteristics. Since it is well known that personal and familial characteristics exert an impact on individual's exposure to specific environmental characteristics and on the choice of specific school environments and peer groups, it is highly possible that some of the previously found effects of school life dimensions were in reality only an artifact of the lack of control of all relevant variables in the analyses (Mortimore, 1995; Rutter, 1999). Moreover, due to the intertwined character of school life characteristics, it is also possible that some of the effects found in previous studies reflect their general failure to simultaneously consider the full reality of school life. The analytical strategy used in this study allowed us to partially confirm these hypotheses. Indeed, whereas most of the aspects of school life studied were found to predict depression development when they were considered alone in the analyses, many of these effects disappeared altogether when other aspects of school life or background controls were entered in the analyses.

Moderating Role of Gender: Differentiated Impact of School Life on Boys and Girls

The fact that, beginning in early adolescence, girls present higher rates of depression than boys is a well-documented phenomenon in developmental research (Nolen-Hoeksema, 2002). At the theoretical level, a plausible explanation for this result invokes the fact that, due to their earlier pubertal maturation, girls tend to enter adolescence in a state of biopsychosocial dysregulation (Cyranowski *et al.*, 2000). Puberty represents a highly challenging experience for adolescents and may become even more challenging when it simultaneously occurs with other developmental transitions. Due to their earlier pubertal maturation, girls often tend to simultaneously experience pubertal changes and high school transition (Bebbington, 1996). They may therefore be more severely affected than boys by any form of school-related stress and benefit more from school-based support mechanisms. In the present study, we sought to evaluate whether school life did indeed represent a more significant predictor of girls', rather than boys', depression development. Interestingly, many results appear to support this hypothesis. For instance, many school life characteristics were found to predict depression development among girls only: low levels of academic involvement, dissatisfaction with school disciplinary control mechanisms, and the perceived frequency of various forms of school problems (minor violence, major violence, and school-related problems). Other factors, such as school misbehaviors, minor and major victimization, perceived school life stressfulness, conflictual relations with teachers, and security climate perceptions appeared to represent stronger predictors of depression development among girls than among boys. Although it remains to be evaluated, this differential impact may potentially explain the gender differences in depression prevalence rates.

Moderating Role of Previous Depressive Symptoms: Prevention or Intervention Targets?

Following Kessler's (1997) suggestion, the present study also sought to determine whether school life exerted a differential impact on the emergence or aggravation of depressive symptoms. Again, strong evidence was found in favor of such a differentiated impact. Indeed, many aspects of school life were found to represent stronger predictors of depression among previously symptomatic and clinically depressed students rather than among previously asymptomatic students: extracurricular involvement, transitional difficulties, minor victimization, conflictual relationships with teachers, dissatisfaction with school-based encouragement practices, bonding, relational (inter-student) and justice climates, and perceptions of the frequency of minor violence problems and of the quality of school disciplinary practices, student consultation mechanisms, classroom management practices, extracurricular activities, and school-family collaboration mechanisms. These results suggest that these aspects of school life would be worthy targets for school-based treatment programs. Conversely, students' exposure to major and sexual victimization appeared as stronger predictors of depressive symptoms among previously asymptomatic and symptomatic students, rather than clinically depressed ones. Both of these dimensions would appear to be worthy targets for school-based prevention. Interestingly, these results also sustain a dimensional view of depression.

Total Contribution of School Life to Depression Development

In the final model, the most significant predictors of depression development, which were entered together after background controls, were found to explain a grand total of 7.4% of depressive symptom variance (previous levels of depressive symptoms explained 21.2% and background controls explained 6.0%). Three conclusions could be reached from this result.

First, compared with the results from other studies, this percentage is quite low. For instance, Resnick *et al.* (1997) found that 13.1% to 17.6% of the variance in students' levels of depression could be explained by school-level factors. As their study was based on a cross-sectional design, these results are hard to compare with the present ones. However, Roeser and Eccles' (1998) study lends support to Resnick *et al.*'s (1997) results. Indeed, these authors found that school life still explained 14% of depression levels once minimal controls (including previous levels of depression) were included in the analysis. Two reasons may explain this apparent discrepancy with the present results: Roeser and Eccles' (1998) study included only a very limited number of controls in the analyses and was based on a longer term follow-up of students. As we showed in this study, adding controls to the analyses diminished the predictive power of some variables. Moreover, it is also possible that, due to the longer follow-up used in their study, Roeser and Eccles (1998) were able to detect effects which were still unstable in the present study due to the recent school transition. The fact that another one-year follow-up study, in which additional controls were considered, found that school life explained only 3% of the variance in depressive symptoms, lends support to this interpretation (Kuperminc, Leadbeater & Blatt, 2001).

Second, school life was found to contribute as much as students' personal, familial and peer-related background characteristics to depression development. Regardless of the strength of this contribution, this result lends support to the design of school-based prevention programs.

Third, significant interaction terms explained as much variance in depression (3.4%) as the main effects of school life characteristics (4%). This result strongly suggests that school life effects differ according to students' characteristics and thus lends support to the need to rely more often on person-centered analyses in developmental research (Von Eye & Bergman, 2003).

A Note on Controlled Variables

Many of the control variables evaluated represented non-significant predictors of depression development following their simultaneous inclusion in the analyses. Moreover, while the percentage of variance in depressive symptoms explained by previous levels of depression (21.2%) is consistent with what is known about depression stability and continuity (e.g., Kessler, 2002; Lewinsohn & Essau, 2002), background controls were found to explain only 6% of depressive symptom variance. In other studies, individual and familial characteristics were generally found to explain at least twice as much variance (e.g., Chase-Lansdale et al., 1995; Ge, Best, Conger, & Simons, 1996). Many reasons may explain these results. First, many of the variables that became non-significant represented familial characteristics that could already have been present before the onset of the study or were based on retrospective evaluations (past difficulties, stressful life events, and behavioral disorders). Accordingly, if these variables really represented significant predictors of depression, their predictive power could have been offset by the inclusion of Time 1 levels of depressive symptoms in the analyses, which may have themselves been influenced by these variables.

Second, a high level of intercorrelations was observed between Time 1 levels of neuroticism, anxiety, self-esteem and body image satisfaction ($r = -0.132$ to 0.502). This observation, which suggests that these variables may represent overlapping constructs, could explain the disappearance of the effects of neuroticism and body image satisfaction in the multivariate analyses. Previous results strongly support this hypothesis. Indeed, in an article combining a meta-analysis and three studies based on seven samples, Judge, Erez, Bono, and Thoresen (2002) found that self-esteem, neuroticism, locus of control and generalized self-efficacy were best represented as a single higher-order construct.

Third, the disappearance of the effects of age and pubertal development could be explained by a range restriction artifact. Indeed, the present study was based on a sample of seventh graders having just experienced high school transition. Consequently, most students were of similar age and pubertal development status. Fourth, it is also possible that the low predictive power of the control variables regarding depression development reflects the fact that school transition is associated with so many social transitions that it provides a window of opportunity for students to develop in ways that are increasingly independent from their own personal, familial, and friendship backgrounds (Rutter et al., 1997). Only further studies will be able to provide clear answers to this question.

Fifth, the apparent absence of gender differences in rates of depression may seem harder to explain, given the well-documented character of these differences (Nolen-Hoeksema, 2002). However, the fact that the gender effect disappeared following the inclusion of Time 1 levels of depression in the analyses suggests that these differences could have already been present at the beginning of our study. Additional analyses in which age and gender were used to predict Time 1 depressive symptoms support this hypothesis ($ß = 0.163$, $t = 5.591$, $p = 0.000$).

As the main objective of this study was not to evaluate the role of background characteristics in depression development, we did not seek further answers to these questions. The analytical strategy used here was designed to evaluate the contribution of school life to depression development and not to obtain an evaluation of the impact of background characteristics, which were only seen as variables to be controlled in the most parsimonious manner. Alternate strategies may yield different results.

Limitations and Directions for Future Research

Although promising, the results from the present study are plagued by at least four important limitations which should be addressed in future studies. First, we did not conduct mediation analyses, which could have helped to clarify the causal relationships implicated in the present results. For instance, whereas we found a relationship between the perceived quality of classroom management practices and depression development, the reason for this effect remains unclear. Indeed, classroom management practices could diminish the prevalence of conflictual teacher-student relationships or the frequency of students' school misbehaviors, which were both found to significantly predict depression development. However, the present analytical strategy did not allow us to distinguish whether the non-significant variables identified in this study really exerted no impact on depression development or whether their effects were completely meditated by other variables. For example, it remains possible that students exposed to higher levels of parental academic support and to lower levels of parental academic pressure would exhibit lower levels of school misbehaviors which in turn predict depression development.

Second, while the present study tried to identify risk factors for adolescent depression development, no attempt was made to evaluate protective factors or other forms of moderating relationships. Thus, although we know that some factors do not predict depression development, we did not evaluate the possibilities that these factors could protect at-risk students from developing depression or amplify their already elevated risk level. Indeed, previous studies focusing on outcomes other than depression repeatedly found that school-related variables could play a protective role on at-risk students (e.g., Fallu & Janosz, 2003).

Third, the present design did not allow us to evaluate the impact of aggregated and structural characteristics of students' school environments. Ideally, analyzing the impact of aggregated or structural school characteristics on students' development would require the use of multilevel statistical analysis (hierarchical linear modeling) to disentangle the effects of individuals' characteristics on depression development from the effect of generic characteristics of their school environment (Bryk & Raudenbush, 1992). The MADDP did not include a sufficient number of schools to conduct this kind of analysis with sufficient statistical power. However, some previous results indicate that this bias may be smaller than it appears. Indeed, Roeger, Allison, Martin, Dadds, and Keeves (2001) found that almost none of the variance in students' levels of depression (0.87%) could be explained by school-level factors.

Fourth, the research design used in the present study seriously limits the generalizability of the findings. Firstly, this part of the MADDP is based on a short term follow-up of young students following high school transition, a period of known developmental instability. Thus, whether the present results can be generalized to the following grades remains unknown and should be evaluated in further studies. Hopefully, the design of the MADDP would allow us to answer this question as more years of data collection become available. Secondly, the present sample is far from representative of the North American population. Indeed, our desire to maximize the organizational differences between the schools selected for the present study led us to over-sample gifted or academically talented students. Moreover, many of the most problematic students were lost through the attrition process. Fortunately, all subjects had the option to complete, on an in-and-out basis, each of our questionnaires. Consequently, although they were not used in the present analyses, some subjects did complete at least some of the questionnaires, including the last one. Complementary analyses in which pairwise case deletion procedures were used revealed that attrition did not induce systematic biases in the results.

Conclusion

Notwithstanding these limitations, the present study clearly illustrates the need to move beyond single variable designs and ritualistic hypothesis testing (Richters, 1997) in depression development research to better accommodate the full richness and complexity of human development. If the present results were to be replicated in designs built to answer the present limitations, they would strongly suggest that prevention and treatment programs for adolescent depression would do well to simultaneously consider background individual and familial risk factors in conjunction with factors directly related to adolescents' lives at school. Among these factors, school violence and loneliness appear to represent particularly valuable targets for such programs, although more global organizational development programs may also indirectly influence depression development through complex mediating relationships involving, among other factors, school violence and loneliness. Additionally, the fact that school life appears to exert a stronger impact on girls, who also tend to present higher levels of depression than boys, suggests that schools may not be that adapted to girls after all and that similar factors may affect boys' development of conduct disorders and girls' levels of depressive symptoms. Consequently, programs designed to better students' school lives may potentially directly influence depression (girls) and delinquency (boys) and indirectly affect depression development through their impact on school levels of delinquency.

ACKNOWLEDGMENTS

This study was made possible by a grant from the Social Sciences and Humanities Research Council of Canada (SSHRC: second author). The authors wish to thank Isabelle Madore, Jocelyn Morin, Jean Phaneuf, Julien Morizot, and Jean-Sébastien Fallu for invaluable support during chapter preparation, Michel Fournier for his help with the missing data replacement strategy, and every student, school personnel and research assistant involved in the MADDP.

REFERENCES

Ackerson, L. M., Dick, R.W., Manson, S. M., and Baron, A. E. (1990). Properties of the Inventory to Diagnose Depression in American Indian adolescents. *Journal of The American Academy of Child and Adolescent Psychiatry*, 29, 601-607.

Aiken, L., and West, S. (1991). *Multiple regression: Testing and interpreting interactions*. Newbury Park, CA: Sage.

Akiskal, H. S. (2001). Dysthymia and cyclothymia in psychiatric practice a century after Kraeplin. *Journal of Affective Disorders*, 62, 17-31.

Allison, P. D. (2001). *Missing data*. Thousand Oaks, CA: Sage.

American Psychiatric Association (1994). *Diagnostic and Statistical Manual of Mental Disorders, 4th edition* (DSM-IV). Washington, DC: Author.

Anderman, E. M. (2002). School effects on psychological outcomes during adolescence. *Journal of Educational Psychology*, 94, 795-809.

Angold, A., Costello, E. J., and Erkanli, A. (1999). Comorbidity. *Journal of child Psychology and Psychiatry*, 40, 57-87.

Aseltine, R. H. Jr., and Gore, S. (1993). Mental health and social adaptation following the transition from high school. *Journal of Research on Adolescence*, 3, 247-270.

Asher, S.R., Hymel, S., and Renshaw, P.D. (1984). Loneliness in children. *Child Development*, 55, 1456-1464.

Austin, S., and Joseph, S. (1996). Assessment of bully/victim problems in 8 to 11 year-olds. *British Journal of Educational Psychology*, 66, 447-456.

Ayotte, V., Saucier, J. F., Bowen, F., Laurendeau, M. C., Fournier, M., and Blais, J. G. (2003). Teaching multiethnic urban adolescents how to enhance their competencies:

Effects of a middle school primary prevention program on adaptation. *The Journal of Primary Prevention*, 23, 7-24.

Bandura, A., Pastorelli, C., Barbaranelli, C., and Caprara, G.V. (1999). Self-efficacy pathways to childhood depression. *Journal of Personality and Social Psychology*, 76, 258-269.

Baron, P., Joubert, N., and Mercier, P. (1991). Situations stressantes et symptomatologie dépressive chez les adolescents. *Revue Européenne de Psychologie Appliquée*, 41, 173-179.

Bebbington, P. E. (1996). The origins of sex differences in depressive disorder: Bridging the gap. *International Review of Psychiatry*, 8, 295-332.

Beck, A. T., and Steer, R. A. (1993). *Beck Anxiety Inventory manual.* New York, NY: The Psychological Corporation.

Beck, A. T., Steer, R. A., and Brown, G. K. (1996). *Manual for the BDI-II.* San Antonio, TX: Psychological Corporation.

Brendgen, M., Vitaro, F., Bukowski, W. M., Doyle, A. B., and Markiewicz, D. (2001). Developmental profiles of peer social preference over the course of elementary school: Associations with trajectories of externalizing and externalizing behavior. *Developmental Psychology*, 37, 308-320.

Bryk, A. S., and Raudenbush, S. W. (1992). Hierarchical Linear Models: Applications and data analysis methods. Newbury Park, CA: Sage.

Cantin, S., Wanner, B., Brendgen, M., and Boivin, M. (august 2002). *Links between friends' characteristics and children's depressive mood: When misery seeks company.* Paper presented at the 2002 biennial meeting of the ISSBD, Ottawa, Canada.

Chase-Lansdale, P. L., Cherlin, A. J., and Kiernan, K. E. (1995). The long-term effects of parental divorce on the mental health of young adults: A developmental perspective. *Child Development*, 66, 1614-1634.

Cicchetti, D., and Rogosch, F. A. (2002). A developmental psychopathology perspective on adolescence. *Journal of Consulting and Clinical Psychology*, 70, 6-20.

Cicchetti, D., and Toth, S. L. (1998). The development of depression in children and adolescents. *American Psychologist*, 53, 221-241.

Coie, J. D., Watt, N. F., West, S. G., Hawkins, J. D., Asarnow, J. R., Markman, H. J., Ramey, S. L., Shure, M. B., and Long, B. (1993). The science of prevention: A conceptual framework and some directions for a national research program. *American Psychologist*, 48, 1013-1022.

Cole, D. A., Martin, J. M., Powers, B., and Truglio, R. (1996). Modeling causal relations between academic and social competence and depression: A multitrait-multimethod longitudinal study of children. *Journal of Abnormal Psychology*, 105, 258-270.

Cyranowski, J. M., Frank, E., Young, E., and Shear, M. K. (2000). Adolescent onset of the gender difference in lifetime rates of major depression: A theoretical model. *Archives of General Psychiatry*, 57, 21-27.

Dawson, A., and Tylee, A. (2001). *Depression: Social and economic timebomb.* London, U.K.: World Health Organization.

Diekstra, R. F. W. (1995). Depression and suicidal behaviors in adolescence: Sociocultural and time trends. In M. Rutter (Ed.), *Psychosocial disturbances in young people: Challenges for prevention* (pp. 212-243). New York, NY: Cambridge University Press.

Eccles, J. S., Early, D., Frasier, K., Belansky, E., and McCarthy, K. (1997). The relation of connection, regulation, and support for autonomy to adolescents' functioning. *Journal of Adolescent Research, 12*, 263-286.

Eccles, J. S., Midgley, C., Wigfield, A., Buchanan, C. M., Reuman, D., Flanagan, C., and Mac Iver, D. (1993). Development during adolescence: The impact stage-environment fit on young adolescents' experiences in schools and in families. *American Psychologist*, 48, 90-101.

Eccles, J. S., Lord, S., and Midgley, C. (1991). What are we doing to early adolescents? *American Journal of Education*, august, 521-542.

Eysenck, H. J., and Eysenck, S. B. G. (1968). *Manual for the Eysenck Personality Inventory.* San Diego, CA: Educational and Industrial Testing Service.

Fallu, J.-S., and Janosz, M. (2003). La qualité des relations élèves-enseignants à l'adolescence: Un facteur de protection de l'échec scolaire. *Revue de Psychoéducation*, 32, 7-29.

Fergusson, D. M., and Woodward, L J. (2000). Educational, psychosocial, and sexual outcomes of girls with conduct problems in early adolescence. *Journal of Child Psychology and Psychiatry*, 41, 779-792.

Freeston, M. H., Ladouceur, R., Thibodeau, N., Gagnon, F., and Rhéaume, J. (1994). L'inventaire d'anxiété de Beck: Propriétés psychométriques d'une traduction française. *L'Encéphale*, 20, 47-55.

Garnefski, N. (2000). Age differences in depressive symptoms, antisocial behavior and negative perceptions of family, school, and peers among adolescents. *Journal of the American Academy of Child and Adolescent Psychiatry*, 39, 1175-1181.

Gazelle, H., and Ladd, G. W. (2003). Anxious solitude and peer exclusion: A diathesis stress model of internalizing trajectories in childhood. *Child Development*, 74, 257-278.

Ge, X., Best, K. M., Conger, R. D., and Simons, R. L. (1996). Parenting behaviors and the occurrence and co-occurrence of adolescent depressive symptoms and conduct problems. *Developmental Psychology*, 32, 717-731.

Ge, X., Lorenz, F. O., Conger, R. D., Elder, G. H. Jr., and Simons, R. L. (1994). Trajectories of stressful life events and depressive symptoms during adolescence. *Developmental Psychology*, 30, 467-483.

Gore, S., Farell, F., and Gordon, J. (2001). Sports involvement as protection against depressed mood. *Journal of Research on Adolescence, 11*, 119-130.

Gottfredson. D. C. (2000). *Schools and delinquency*. Cambridge: Cambridge University Press.

Haaga, D. A. F., Dyck, M. J., and Ernst, D. (1991). Empirical status of cognitive theory of depression. *Psychological Bulletin*, 110, 215-236.

Hadley-Ives, E., Stiffman, A. R., Elze, D., Johnson, S. D., and Dore, P. (2000). Measuring neighborhood and school environments: Perceptual and aggregated approaches. *Journal of Human Behavior in the Social Environment*, 3, 1-28.

Héroux, G. (1997). *Corrélats des habiletés visuo-spatiales chez les filles et les garçons de 9, 12 et 15 ans: Regard sur les jeux de l'enfance.* Unpublished doctoral thesis, Montreal: University of Montreal.

Hilsman, R., and Garber, J. (1995). A test of the cognitive diathesis-stress model of depression in children: Academic stressors, attributional style, perceived competence, and control. *Journal of Personality and Social Psychology*, 69, 370-380.

Hodges, E. V. E., and Perry, D. G. (1999). Personal and interpersonal antecedents and consequences of victimization by peers. *Journal of Personality and Social Psychology*, 76, 677-685.

Jaccard, J., and Turisi, R. (2003). *Interaction effects in multiple regression*, second edition. Thousand Oaks, CA: Sage.

Jaffe, S. R., Moffitt, T. E., Caspi, A., Fombonne, E., Poulton, R., and Martin, J. (2002). Differences in early childhood risk factors for juvenile-onset and adult-onset depression. *Archives of General Psychiatry*, 59, 215-222.

Janosz, M. (November 2000). The Montreal School Environment Project: The theoretical model and the validity of the School Socioeducational Environment Questionnaire. *Poster presented at the Annual meeting of the American Society of Criminology,* San Francisco.

Janosz, M., Deniger, M.-A., Roy, G., Lacroix, M., Fallu, J. S., Langevin, L., and Le Blanc, M. (2001). *Évaluation de programmes de prévention du décrochage scolaire pour adolescents de milieux défavorisés*. Research report no 98-DS-001 (FCAR). University of Montreal.

Janosz, M., Georges, P., and Parent, S. (1998). L'environnement éducatif à l'école secondaire: Un modèle théorique pour guider l'évaluation du milieu. *Revue Canadienne de Psychoéducation*, 27, 285-306.

Janosz, M., Rondeau, N., and Lacroix, M. (1998, may). *Le passage à l'acte chez le décrocheur: Modèle et instrumentation*. Paper presented at the 66th annual meeting of the ACFAS, Laval, Canada.

Judge, T. A., Erez, A., Bono, J. E., and Thoresen, C. J. (2002). Are measures of self-esteem, neuroticism, locus of control, and generalized self-efficacy indicators of a common core construct? *Journal of Personality and Social Psychology*, 83, 693-710.

Kaltiala-Heino, R., Rimpelä, M., Marttunen, M., Rimpelä, A., and Rantanen, P. (1999). Bullying, depression, and suicidal ideation in Finnish adolescents: School survey. *British Medical Journal*, 319, 348-351.

Kaltiala-Heino, R., Rimpelä, M., Rantanen, P., and Rimpelä, A. (2000). Bullying at school–an indicator of adolescents at risk for mental disorders. *Journal of Adolescence*, 23, 661-674.

Kasen, S., Johnson, J., and Cohen, P. (1990). The impact of school emotional climate on student psychopathology. *Journal of Abnormal Child Psychology*, 18, 165-177.

Kessler, R. C. (2002). Epidemiology of depression. *In* I.H. Gotlib, and C.L. Hammen (Eds.), *Handbook of depression* (pp. 23-42). London, U.K.: Guilford.

Kessler, R. C., Foster, C. L., Saunders, W.B., and Stang, P.E. (1995). Social consequences of psychiatric disorders, I: Educational attainment. *American Journal of Psychiatry*, 152, 1026-1032.

Kiesner, J. (2002). Depressive symptoms in early adolescence: Their relations with classroom problem behavior and peer status. *Journal of Research on Adolescence*, 12, 463-478.

Krause, J., Philipp, M., Maier, W., and Schlegel, S. (1989). A German validation study of the Inventory to Diagnose Depression. *Psychopathology*, 22, 57-64.

Krueger, R. F. (1999). Personality traits in late adolescence predict mental disorders in early adulthood: A prospective-epidemiological study. *Journal of Personality*, 67, 39-65.

Kuperminc, G. P., Leadbeater, B. J., and Blatt, S. J. (1997). School climate and individual differences in vulnerability to psychopathology among middle school students. *Journal of School Psychology*, 39, 141-159.

Kuperminc, G. P., Leadbeater, B. J., Emmons, C., and Blatt, S. J. (1997). Perceived school climate and difficulties in the social adjustment of middle school students. *Applied Developmental Science*, 1, 76-88.

Larose, S., Bernier, A., Soucy, N., and Duchesne, S. (1999). Attachment style dimensions, network orientation, and the process of seeking help from college teachers. *Journal of Social and Personal Relationships*, 16, 227-249.

LeBlanc, M. (1998). MASPAQ: Manuel sur des mesures de l'adaptation sociale et personnelle pour les adolescents québécois, 3ème édition. Montreal: School of psychoeducation and GRAD, University of Montreal.

Lewinsohn, P. M., Allen, N. B., Seeley, J. R., and Gotlib, I. H. (1999). First onset versus recurrence of depression: Differential processes of psychosocial risk. *Journal of abnormal Psychology*, 108, 483-489.

Lewinsohn, P. M., and Essau, C. A. (2002). Depression in adolescents. *In* I.H. Gotlib, and C.L. Hammen (Eds.), *Handbook of depression* (pp. 541-559). London, U.K.: Guilford.

Lewinsohn, P. M., Roberts, R. E., Seeley, J. R., Rohde, P., Gotlib, I. H., and Hops, H. (1994). Adolescent psychopathology: II. Psychosocial risk factors for depression. *Journal of Abnormal Psychology*, 103, 302-315.

Lewinsohn, P. M., Rohde, P., Seeley, J. R., and Fisher, S. A. (1993). Age-cohort changes in the lifetime occurrence of depression and other mental disorders. *Journal of Abnormal Psychology*, 102, 110-120.

Lewis-Beck, M. S. (1980). *Applied regression: An introduction*. Newbury Park, CA: Sage.

Little, R. J. A., and Rubin, D.B. (2002). *Statistical analysis with missing data, 2nd Edition*. New-Jersey: John Wiley and Sons.

Mahoney, J. L., Schweder, A. E., and Stattin, H. (2002). Structured after-school activities as a moderator of depressed mood for adolescents with detached relations to their parents. *Journal of Community Psychology*, 30, 69-86.

Marsh, H. W. (1990). Self-Description Questionnaire-II (SDQ-II): Manual and research monograph. New York, *NY: The Psychological Corporation.*

Morin, A. J. S., and Janosz, M. (August 2002). *School climate and depression in adolescence: A cross-sectional analysis*. Poster presented at the biennial meeting of the ISSBD, Ottawa.

Morin, A. J. S., Janosz, M., and Larivée, S. (submitted). Psychosocial antecedents for child and adolescent depression: A review of the past 12 years. *Psychological Bulletin*.

Mortimore, P. (1995). The positive effects of schooling. *In* M. Rutter (Ed.), *Psychosocial disturbances in young people: Challenges for prevention* (pp. 333-363). New York, NY: Cambridge University Press.

Mrazek, P. J., and Haggerty, R. J. (1994). Reducing risks for mental disorders: Frontiers for preventive intervention research. Washington: National Academy Press.

Murray, C. J. L., and Lopez, A. D. (1996). Evidence-based health policy – lessons from the Global Burden of Disease Study. *Science*, 274, 740-743.

Nansel, T. R., Overpeck, M., Pilla, R. S., Ruan, W. J., Simons-Morton, B., and Scheidt, P. (2001). Bullying behaviors among US youth: Prevalence and association with psychosocial adjustment. *Journal of the American Medical Association*, 285, 2094-2100.

Newcomb, M. D., Huba, G. J., and Bentler, P. M. (1981). A multidimensional assessment of stressful life events among adolescents: Derivation and correlates. *Journal of Health and Social Behavior*, 22, 400-415.

Newman, D. L., Moffitt, T. E., Caspi, A., Magdol, L., Silva, P. A., and Stanton, W. R. (1996). Psychiatric disorder in a birth cohort of young adults: Prevalence, comorbidity, clinical significance, and new cases incidence from ages 11 to 21. *Journal of Consulting and Clinical Psychology*, 64, 552-562.

Nolen-Hoeksema, S. (2002). Gender differences in depression. *In* I.H. Gotlib, and C.L. Hammen (Eds.), *Handbook of depression* (pp. 492-509). London, U.K.: Guilford.

Pariente, P., Smith, M., and Guelfi, J. D. (1989). Un questionnaire pour le diagnostic d'épisode dépressif majeur: L'inventaire pour le diagnostic de la dépression (IDD). Présentation de la version française. *Psychiatrie et Psychobiologie*, 4, 375-385.

Petersen, A. C., Crockett, L., Richards, M., and Boxer, A. (1988). A self-report measure of pubertal status: Reliability, validity, and initial norms. *Journal of Youth and adolescence*, 17, 117-133.

Pianta, R. C., and Steinberg, M. (1992). Teacher-child relationships and the process of adjusting to school. *New Directions for Child Development*, 57, 61-80.

Reinherz, H. Z., Giaconia, R. M., Pakiz, B., Silverman, A. B., Frost, A. K., and Lefkowitz, E. S. (1993). Psychosocial risks for major depression in late adolescence: A longitudinal community study. *Journal of the American Academy of Child and Adolescent Psychiatry*, 32, 1155-1163.

Resnick, M. D., Bearman, P. S., Blum, R. W., Bauman, K. E., Harris, K. M., Jones, J., Tabor, J., Beuhring, T., Sieving, R. E., Shew, M., Ireland, M., Bearinger, L. H., and Udry, J. R. (1997). Protecting adolescents from harm: Findings from the longitudinal study on adolescent health. *Journal of the American Medical Association*, 278, 823-832.

Richters, J. E. (1997). The Hubble hypothesis and the developmentalist's dilemma. *Development and Psychopathology*, 9, 193-229.

Robins, L. N. (1995). Sociocultural trends affecting the prevalence of adolescent problems. *In* M. Rutter (Ed.), *Psychosocial disturbances in young people: Challenges for prevention* (pp. 367-384). New York, NY: Cambridge University Press.

Roeger, L., Allison, S., Martin, G., Dadds, V., and Keeves, J. (2001). Adolescent depressive symptomatology: Improve schools or help students. *Australian Journal of Psychology*, *53*, 134-139.

Roeser, R. W., and Eccles, J. S. (1998). Adolescents' perceptions of middle school: Relation to longitudinal changes in academic and psychological adjustment. *Journal of Research on Adolescence*, 8, 123-158.

Roeser, R. W., Eccles, J. S., and Sameroff, A. J. (1998). Academic and emotional functioning in early adolescence: Longitudinal relations, patterns, and prediction by experience in middle school. *Development and Psychopathology*, 10, 321-352.

Rosenberg, M. (1965). *Society and the adolescent self-image*. Princeton, NJ: Princeton University Press.

Rutter, M. (1999). Psychosocial adversity and child psychopathology. *British Journal of Psychiatry*, 174, 480-493.

Rutter, M., Dunn, J., Plomin, R., Simonoff, E., Pickles, A., Maughan, B., Ormel, J., Meyer, J., and Eaves, L. (1997). Integrating nature and nurture: Implications of person-environment correlations and interactions for developmental psychology. *Development and Psychopathology*, 9, 335-364.

Sakado, K., Sato, T., Uehara, T., Sato, S., and Kameda, K. (1996). Discriminant validity of the inventory to diagnose depression, lifetime version. *Acta Psychiatrica Scandinavica*, 93, 257-260.

Siddique, C. M., and D'Arcy, C. (1984). Adolescence, stress, and psychological well-being. *Journal of Youth and Adolescence*, 13, 459-473.

Siegel, J. M. (2002). Body image change and adolescent depressive symptoms. *Journal of Adolescent Research*, 17, 27-41.

Sim, H.-O. (august 2002). *Gender differences in the cross-lag relations between family, friends, and teachers social support and maladjustment.* Paper presented at the 2002 biennial meeting of the ISSBD, Ottawa, Canada.

Skinner, E. A. (1995). *Perceived control, motivation, and coping.* Thousands Oaks: Sage.

Stein, J. A., Newcomb, M. D., and Bentler, P. M. (1996). Initiation and maintenance of tobacco smoking: Changing personality correlates in adolescence and young adulthood. *Journal of Applied Social Psychology*, 26, 160-187.

Tabachnick, B. G., and Fidell, L. S. (1996). *Using multivariate statistics, third edition.* New York, NY: HarperCollins.

Turner, J. E. Jr., and Cole, D.A. (1994). Developmental differences in cognitive diatheses for child depression. *Journal of Abnormal Child Psychology*, 22, 15-32.

Vallières, E. F. and Vallerand, R. J. (1990). Traduction et validation canadienne-française de l'Échelle d'Estime de Soi de Rosenberg. *International Journal of Psychology*, 25, 305-316.

Vitaro, F., Pelletier, D., Gagnon, C., and Baron, P. (1995). Correlates of depressive symptoms in early adolescence. *Journal of Emotional and Behavioral Disorders*, 3, 241-251.

VonEye, A., and Bergman, L.R. (2003). Research strategies in developmental psychopathology: Dimensional identity and the person-oriented approach. *Development and Psychopathology*, 15, 553-580.

Way, N., and Chen, L. (2000). Close and general friendships among African American, Latino, and Asian American adolescents from low-income families. *Journal of Adolescent Research*, 15, 274-301.

Zaslow, M. J., and Takanishi, R. (1993). Priorities for research on adolescent development. *American Psychologist*, 48, 185-192.

Zimmerman, M., and Coryell, W. (1987 a). The inventory to diagnose depression, lifetime version. *Acta Psychiatrica Scandinavica*, 75, 495-499.

Zimmerman, M., and Coryell, W. (1987 b). The inventory to diagnose depression: A self-report scale to diagnose depression. *Journal of Consulting and Clinical Psychology*, 55, 55-59.

Zimmerman, M., and Coryell, W. (1988). The validity of a self-report questionnaire for diagnosing major depressive disorder. *Archives of General Psychiatry*, 45, 738-740.

Zuckerman, M. (1999). *Vulnerability to psychopathology: A biosocial model.* Washington: American Psychological Association.

In: Perspectives in Psychiatry Research
Editors: Nicole M. Levine and Donna J. Campbell
ISBN: 978-1-61209-236-2

Chapter 6

The Relationship Between Societal Crime and Socio-Economic Status, Income Inequality and Education: A Cross-National Study

Ajit Shah[*]
Ethnicity and Mental Health, University of Central Lancashire, Preston and West London Mental Health NHS Trust, London, United Kingdom.

Abstract

Background

Low socio-economic status, socio-economic inequality and poor educational attainment may be associated with crime.

Methods

The relationship between the percentage of the population victimised by different categories of crime and socio-economic status (measured by per capita gross national domestic product (GDP)), income inequality (measured by the Gini coefficient) and educational attainment (measured by the Education Index) was examined using cross-national data from the World Health Organisation and United Nations Data Banks.

Results

The main findings were: (i) the percentage of the population victimised by most categories of crimes was significantly correlated with the Education Index (negative), male and female life expectancy (negative), male and female child mortality rates (positive), GDP (negative) and Gini coefficient (positive); and, (ii) the percentage of the

[*] Corresponding author: West London Mental Health NHS Trust, Uxbridge Road, Southall, Middlesex, UB1 3EU, United Kingdom, Telephone: 0208 354 8140, Fax: 0208 354 8898, E-mail: ajit.shah@wlmht.nhs.uk

population victimised by the crime of assault was not significantly correlated with any of the measured variables.

Conculsions

The impact of socio-economic factors, socio-economic inequality and educational attainment on crime may occur through interaction with other factors, mediation of the effects of other factors, or by their effects being mediated by other factors, and requires further study. If a causal link can be substantiated then these associations potentially offer strategies for improvement.

Keywords: Crime, soci-economic status, income inequality, education.

Introduction

A negative correlation between different measures of socio-economic status, including per capita gross national domestic product (GDP) and average income, and crime (Kitchen, 2006; Ministry of Justice, 2007), including homicides (Quinney, 1965; Rahav & Jaamdar, 1982; Krahn et al., 1986; Butchart & Engstrom, 2002; Gawryszewski & Costa, 2005), has been reported both in within-country and cross-national aggregate-level studies. However, this relationship has not been consistent (Unnithan & Witt, 1992; Fajnzylber et al., 2000). Moreover, both within-country and cross-national aggregate-level studies have consistently reported a positive correlation between measures of socio-economic inequality, including the Gini coefficient (a measure of income inequality), and homicides (Hseih & Pugh, 1993; Avison & Loring, 1986; Butchart & Engstrom, 2002; Gawryszewski & Costa, 2005). Furthermore, this relationship between socio-economic inequality and homicides was more pronounced in geographical areas with low socio-economic status within individual countries (Gawryszewski & Costa, 2005; Ministry of Justice, 2007) and in countries with low socio-economic status (Butchart & Engstrom, 2002). Also, in an individual-level study of European Americans, psychopathy predicted recidivism for violent crimes in those with lower socio-economic status, but not in those with higher levels of socio-economic status (Walsh & Kosson, 2007).

Crime was positively correlated with lower educational attainment and youths not attending school in a Canadian aggregrate-level study of geographical areas in Ottawa and Saskatoon (Kitchen, 2006). An American review concluded that post-secondary education is the most successful and cost-effective way of reducing recidivism among criminals (Karpowitz & Kenner, 2005). Another study concluded that policies subsidising high school education were more cost effective in reducing crime than imprisonment, particularly if targetted at socio-economically disadvantaged individuals (Gallipoli & Fella, 2006).

Most studies have generally focused on all criminal activity amalgamated together or specifically on homicides. Also, most studies have focused on prevalence rates of all criminal activity or homicides specifically, rather than on the percentage of the population victimised by crime. Therefore, a cross-national study examining the relationship between the percentage of the population victimised by different categories of crime and (i) the Education Index, (ii) male and female life expectancy, (iii) male and female child mortality rates, (iv)

GDP, (v) the Gini coefficient (a measure of income inequality, and (vi) the population size was undertaken.

Methods

1. Data Collection

Data on the percentage of the population victimised by crime were ascertained from the United Nations Development Programme website for the years 1991 to 2001 (median 1999) (www.hdr.undp.org/reports/global/2005/pdf/hdr05_HDI.pdf). The categories of crime included total crime, property crime, robbery, sexual assault (females only), assault and bribery (refers to corruption on part of government officials). This data refers to victimisation as reported in the International Crime Victims Survey conducted in 1992, 1995, 1996-1997 and 2000-2001. Data were available for the whole country for 19 countries and for the main city (usually the captial city) for 35 countries.

Data on the Education Index was ascertained from the United Nations (UN) website (www.hdr.undo.org/hdr2006/statitics/indicators/1.html) for the year 2000. The Education Index is a composite measure of the adult literacy rate, and the combined gross enrollment ratios for primary, secondary and tertiary schools. The Education Index was used as a proxy marker for educational attainment. It is scored on a scale of 0 to 1, with higher scores reflecting greater degree of educational attainment.

The WHO website (www.who.int/countries/en/) provided data on male and female life expectancy, per capita gross national domestic product (GDP), and male and female child mortality rates (i.e mortality before the age of five years). These data were for the year 2002. Per capita GDP was used as a proxy marker of socio-economic status. Life expectancy and child mortality rates were used as proxy measures of the quantity and quality of available healthcare services. The United Nations Development Programme website (www.hdr.undp.org/reports/global/2005/pdf/hdr05_HDI.pdf) provided data on a measure of income inequality called the Gini coefficient. The Gini coefficient is derived from an income distribution curve where the x-axis represents the number of households and the y-axis percentage of the total income. Perfect equality is seen when the income is equally distributed across all the households and perfect inequality is seen when only one household has all the income. The area between the line of perfect equality and the actual income distribution is the Gini coefficient and is expressed as a percentage ranging form 0 (perfect equality) to 100% (perfect inequality). The Gini coefficient was also used as a proxy measure of socio-economic status.

2. Data Analysis

The relationship between the percentage of the population victimised by all the categories of crime across different countries and (i) the Education Index, (ii) male and female life expectancy, (iii) male and female child mortality rates, (iv) per capita GDP, (v) the Gini coefficient, and (vi) the population size was examined using Spearman's rank correlation coefficient (Rho).

RESULTS

Full data set were available for 54 countries, except for the Gini coefficient where data were only available 43 countries. Table 1 illustrates the relationship between the percentage of the population victimised by different categories of crime and the Education Index, life expectancy for males and females, child mortality rates for males and females, GDP, Gini coefficient and population size. The percentage of the population victimised by all (total) crime was significantly correlated with the Education Index (Rho=-0.31, P=0.025), male life expectancy (Rho=-0.39, P=0.004), female life expectancy (Rho=-0.38, P=0.005), male child mortality rates (Rho=+0.43, P=0.001), female child mortality rates (Rho=+0.41, P=0.002) and GDP (Rho=-0.33, P=0.016). The percentage of the population victimised by property crime was significantly correlated with the Education Index (Rho=-0.32, P=0.018), male life expectancy (Rho=-0.34, P=0.011), female life expectancy (Rho=-0.32, P=0.018), male child mortality rates (Rho=+0.38, P=0.005), female child mortality rates (Rho=+0.35, P=0.01), GDP (Rho=-0.31, P=0.021) and Gini coefficient (Rho=+0.31, P=0.042). The percentage of the population victimised by robbery was significantly correlated with the Education Index (Rho=-0.41, P=0.002), male life expectancy (Rho=-0.61, P<0.00001), female life expectancy (Rho=-0.56, P<0.00001), male child mortality rates (Rho=+0.64, P<0.00001), female child mortality rates (Rho=+0.0.6, P<0.00001), GDP (Rho=-0.54, P<0.00001) and Gini coefficient (Rho=+0.45, P=0.003). The percentage of the population victimised by sexual assault was significantly correlated with the Education Index (Rho=-0.29, P=0.03), male life expectancy (Rho=-0.42, P=0.002), female life expectancy (Rho=-0.39, P=0.003), male child mortality rates (Rho=+0.43, P=0.001), female child mortality rates (Rho=+0.4, P=0.003), GDP (Rho=-0.38, P=0.04) and Gini coefficient (Rho=+0.29, P=0.057). The percentage of the population victimised by bribery and corruption crime was significantly correlated with the Education Index (Rho=-0.61, P<0.00001), male life expectancy (Rho=-0.73, P<0.00001), female life expectancy (Rho=-0.74, P<0.00001), male child mortality rates (Rho=+0.75, P<0.00001), female child mortality rates (Rho=+0.75, P<0.00001) and GDP (Rho=-0.82, P<0.00001). The percentage of the population victimised by the crime of assault was not siginificantly correlated with any of the measured variables.

DISCUSSION

The main findings were: (i) the percentage of the population victimised by most categories of crimes was significantly correlated with the Education Index (negative), male and female life expectancy (negative), male and female child mortality rates (positive), GDP (negative) and Gini coefficient (positive); and, (ii) the percentage of population vicitimed by the crime of assault was not significantly correlated with any of the measured variables.

Methodological issues need consideration. The validity of data from the International Crime Victims Survey is unclear. A limitation of utilising national-level aggregate data is the possibility of missing variations in crime rates in different regions within a country (Butchart & Engstrom, 2002), but uniform data on within country variations are not available. Moreover, data on percentage of the population victimised by crime was only available for the whole country for 19 countries and for the remaining 35 countries this data was available for the main city.

Table 1. Correlation between crime and measures of socio-economic status, health status and education.

Crime	Education Index	Male Life Expectancy	Female Life Expectancy	Male Child Mortality Rates	Female Child Mortality Rates	GDP	Gini Coefficient	Population Size
Total Crime	Rho=-0.31 P=0.025	Rho=-0.39 P=0.004	Rho=-0.38 P=0.005	Rho=+0.43 P=0.001	Rho=+0.41 P=0.002	Rho=-0.33 P=0.016	NS	NS
Property Crime	Rho=-0.32 P=0.018	Rho=-0.34 P=0.011	Rho=-0.32 P=0.018	Rho=+0.38 P=0.005	Rho=+0.35 P=0.01	Rho=-0.31 P=0.02	Rho=+0.31 P=0.042	NS
Robbery Crime	Rho=-0.41 P=0.002	Rho=-0.61 P<0.00001	Rho=-0.56 P<0.0001	Rho=+0.64 P<0.00001	Rho=+0.6 P<0.00001	Rho=-0.54 P<0.0001	Rho=+0.45 P=0.03	NS NS
Sexual Assualt Crime	Rho=-0.29 P=0.03	Rho=-0.42 P=0.002	Rho=-0.39 P=0.003	Rho=+0.43 P=0.001	Rho=+0.4 P=0.003	Rho=-0.38 P=0.04	Rho=+0.29 P=0.057	NS
Assault Crime	NS	NS	NS	NS	NS	NS	NS	NS
Bribery and Corruption	Rho=-0.61 P<0.00001	Rho=-0.73 P<0.00001	Rho=-0.74 P<0.00001	Rho=+0.75 P<0.00001	Rho=+0.75 P<0.00001	Rho=-0.82 P<0.00001	NS	NS

NS = Not significant

Data on socio-economic status and income inequality should also be viewed with caution because: the validity of this data is unclear; some countries may have poor infrastructure for providing accurate financial data; and, their influence on social distribution of risk factors may be complex. These latter concerns are more likely to be observed in low-income countries. The Education Index is a composite measure of adult literacy rates and the combined gross enrollment ratios for primary, secondary and tertiary schools. However, data on the latter two variables should also be viewed with caution because: the validity of this data is unclear; and, some countries may have poor registration facilities and infrastructure for collecting educational data. Nevertheless, data sets were gathered from the WHO and the UN data banks and were the best and the latest available data sets.

The main study variable of percentage of the population vicitimised by crime was different from that used in most studies where the actual prevalence of the crime itself has been examined. The negative correlation between the percentage of the population vitimised by most categories of crime and GDP is consistent with observations in previous within-country and cross-national aggregate-level studies of crime (Kitchen, 2006; Ministry of Justice, 2007), including homicides (Quinney, 1965; Rahav & Jaamdar, 1982; Krahn et al., 1986; Butchart & Engstrom, 2002; Gawryszewski & Costa, 2005). The positive correlation between the percentage of the population victimised by most categories of crime and the Gini coefficient (a measure of income inequality) is consistent with observations in previous within-country and cross-national aggregate-level studies of homicides (Hseih & Pugh, 1993; Avison & Loring, 1986; Butchart & Engstrom, 2002; Gawryszewski & Costa, 2005). This consistency together with a positive correlation between child mortality rates and the percentage of population victimised by most categories of crime, a finding consistent with a Brazilian study of homicides (Gawryszewski & Costa, 2005), supports the validity of the findings.

Although many factors may contribute to criminal behaviour, the combination of poor socio-economic status and socio-economic inequality may significantly contribute to criminal behaviour (Butchart & Engstrom, 2002; Gawryszewski & Costa, 2005). Poor socio-economic status and socio-economic inequality may remove social barriers to violent behaviour, and individuals' frustrations, anger, emotions and perceived needs may be expressed through criminal acts, bringing them gain through criminal means (Butchart & Engstrom, 2002). Moreover, homicide, poor socio-economic status and socio-economic inequality may be affected by availability of public goods and services, and social and physical environments, including less public security, illumination and transportation, thus exposing people to more violence (Gawryszewski & Costa, 2005).

These correlations between the percentage of the population victimised by crime and both socio-economic status and socio-economic inequality cannot be assumed to imply a causal relation because of the cross-sectional study design. However, studies have suggested that both economic development and improving socio-economic inequality may reduce homicides (Butchart & Engstrom, 2002; Gawryszewski & Costa, 2005). Moreover, it has been shown that economic changes may have important impact on homicide rates (Butchart & Engstrom, 2002). Furthermore, in countries with high income inequalities, redistribution of overall wealth without increasing the GDP may produce smaller reduction in homicides than in countries where redistribution of wealth and GDP are both simultaneously improved (Butchart & Engstrom, 2002).

The negative correlation between educational attainment and the percentage of population victimised by crime is also consistent with previous observations (Kitchen, 2006). This correlation should not be assumed to imply a causal relation because of the cross-sectional study design. However, an American review concluded that post-secondary education is the most successful and cost-effective way of reducing recidivism among criminals (Karpwitz & Kenner, 2005). Moreover, another study concluded that policies subsidising high school education were more cost effective in reducing crime than imprisonment, particularly if targetted at socio-economically disadvantaged individuals (Gallipoli & Fella, 2006). Therefore, improving educational attainment at a societal level may have implications for reducing first crime and recidivism.

The findings of this study should be considered cautiously because assumptions about a causal relationship cannot be made due to the cross-sectional study design and may be subject to ecological fallacy. The impact of socio-economic factors, socio-economic inequality and educational attainment on crime may occur through interaction with other factors, mediation of the effects of other factors, or by their effects being mediated by other factors, and requires further study.

Conflict of Interest

Nil

References

Avison, W. R and Loring, P. L. (1986) population diversity and cross-national homocide: the effect of inequality and heterogeneity. *Criminology*, 24, 733-747.

Butchart, A and Engstrom, K (2002) Sex- and age-specific relaitons between economic development, economic inequality and homicide rates in people aged 0-24 years: a cross-sectional analysis. Bull *World Health Organisation*, 80, 797-805.

Fajnzylber, P., Lederman, B. and Loayza, N. (2000) Crime and violence: an economic perspective. *Economia*, 1, 219-302.

Gallipoli, G. and Fella, G. (2006) Education and crime over the life cycle. *Job Market Paper*. www.homepage.ucl.ac.uk/~uctpgga/JMPpaper.pdf. Viewed on 25th June 2007.

Gawryszewski, V. P. and Costa, L. S. (2005) Social inequality and homocide rates in Sao Paulo City, Brazil. *Rev Sau Publica*, 39, 191-197.

Hsieh, C. and Pugh, M. (1993) Poverty, income inequality and violent crime: a meta analysis of recent aggregate studies. *Crim Jus Review*, 18, 182-202.

Karpowitz, D. and Kenner, M. (2005) *Educations crime prevention: the case for reinstating Pell grant eligibility for the incarcerated.* Bard College. www.bard.edu/bpi/pdfs/crime_report.pdf. Viewed 25th June 2007.

Kitchen, P. (2006) Exploring the link between crime and socioeconomic status in Ottawa and Saskatoon: a small-area geographical analysis. *Methdological Series*. Report Prepared for the Department of Justice Canada. Government of Canada. www.justice.gc.ca/en.ps/rs/rep/2006/rr06/index.html. Viewed on 24th June 2007

Krahn, H., Hartnagel, T. F. and Gartrell, J. W. (1986) Income inequality and homicide rates: cross-national data and criminological theories. *Criminology*, 24, 269-295.

Ministry of Justice (2007) New Zealand Crime & Safety Survey 2006 (NZCASS). Key Findings Report. www.courts.govt.nz/media/fact-3-3-april-2006.pdf. Viewed 25th June 2007.

Quinney, R. (1965) Suicide, homocide and economic development. *Social Forces*, 43, 401-406.

Rahav, G. and Jaamdar, S. (1982) Development and crime: a cross-national study. *Dev Change*, 13, 447-462.

Unnithan, N. P. and Witt, H. P. (1992) Inequality, economic development and lethal violence: a cross-national analysis of suicide and homicide. *Int J Com Sociology*, 33, 182-196.

Walsh, Z. and Kosson, D. S. (2007) Psychopathy and violent crime: a prospective study of the influence of socioeconomic status and ethnicity. *Law & Hum Behavior*, 31, 209-229.

In: Perspectives in Psychiatry Research
Editors: Nicole M. Levine and Donna J. Campbell

ISBN: 978-1-61209-236-2

Chapter 7

Development of an Epidemiological Transition Model to Explain Cross-National Variations in Elderly Suicide Rates, Time Trends in Elderly Suicide Rates and Age-Associated Trends in Suicide Rates

***Ajit Shah*[1*] *and Ravi Bhat*[2]**

[1]Ethnicity and Mental Health, University of Central Lancashire, Preston and Consultant Psychiatrist, West London Mental Health NHS Trust, London, United Kingdom.
[2]Centre for Older Persons' Health & School of Rural Health, University of Melbourne, Shepparton, Victoria, Australia.

Abstract

Background

There are cross-national variations in elderly suicide rates, trends over time in elderly suicide rates and age-associated trends in suicide rates.

Methods

A theoretical model with an integrated approach to simultaneously explain the cross-national variations in (i) elderly suicide rates from cross-sectional data, (ii) trends over time for elderly suicide rates from longitudinal data, and (iii) age-associated trends in suicide rates from cross-sectional data was developed upon reviewing the existing literature in the field.

* Corresponding author: John Connolly Unit, West London Mental Health NHS Trust, Uxbridge Road, Southall, Middlesex, UB1 3EU, Telephone: 0208 354 8140, Fax: 0208 354 8898, E-mail: ajit.shah@wlmht.nhs.uk

Results

A developmental model of epidemiological transition for elderly suicide rates with four sequential stages was formulated: (i) low elderly suicide rate-low socio-economic society; (ii) high elderly suicide rate-low socio-economic society; (iii) high elderly suicide rate-high socio-economic society; and (iv) low elderly suicide rate-high socio-economic society.

Conclusions

It is likely that different countries will be at different stages of development within this model. It is envisaged that each country would progress through each of these four developmental stages over time. This model is complimentary to, and does not preclude, other proximal and distil aetiological risk factors for elderly suicides.

Keywords: Elderly suicides, epidemiology, socio-economic factors

INTRODUCTION

There are cross-national and regional variations in elderly suicide rates (De Leo et al., 2001; Kiemo, 2004; Shah et al., 2007a), trends over time in elderly suicide rates (Sartorius, 1995; Shah et al., 2007b) and age-associated trends in suicide rates (Shah, 2007a). Evidence in support of each of these facets is examined with a view to developing a unified explanatory model.

CROSS-NATIONAL VARIATIONS IN ELDERLY SUICIDE RATES

There are wide regional and cross-national variations in elderly suicide rates (De Leo et al., 2001; Kiemo, 2004; Shah et al., 2007a). Elderly suicide rates, ascertained from the World Health Organisation (WHO) data bank for 1992, were low in Malta, Greece, Albania, Armenia, Tajikstan, Uzbekistan, Mexico and Columbia and high in Austria, Belarus, Denmark, Estonia, Finland, France, Hungary, Kazakstan, Latvia, Lithuania, Russia, Slovenia, Switzerland and rural China (Shah & De, 1998). Elderly suicide rates, ascertained from WHO data bank for 2000, were the lowest in Caribbean (Antigua, Barbados, Dominica, Jamiaca, San Martin, St Kitts and Nevis, St Vincent and St Lucia), central American (Belsize, Equador and Guatanmala) and Arabic (Baharain, Eygpt, Kuwait, Qatar and Syria) countries, and the highest in central and east European (Austria, Belarus, Bulgaria, Estonia, Hungary, Kazakstan, Latvia, Lithuania, Moldavia, Russia, Slovenia and Ukraine), some oriental (China, South Korea and Japan), and some west European (France, Finland and Switzerland) countries (Shah et al., 2007a). Elderly suicide rates in a study of 49 medium and high income countries were the highest in the former Soviet Union, and west European, Nordic and east Asian countries, and lowest in south European, north American and south American countries (Kiemo, 2004). Elderly suicide rates in males in 10 European countries were the highest in selected cities in Germany, Hungary, Finland and Austria and the lowest in the United

Kingdom (UK) and Sweden (De Leo et al., 2001); rates in women were the highest in Denmark, Hungary and Germany, but lowest in the UK and Sweden.

Cross-National Variations in Trends Over Time in Elderly Suicide Rates

Elderly suicide rates in both sexes declined in many countries between 1989/1990 and 1992/1993 (Shah & Ganesvaran, 1994). There were exceptions: an increase in elderly suicide rates in both sexes in Denmark, men in Israel, and women in France, Bulgaria, Iceland and Malta; and, there was no change in elderly suicide rates in Norway, Poland and Sweden (Shah & Ganesvaran, 1994). Elderly suicide rates in selected western and eastern European countries between 1987 and 1991/1992 increased in males in Denmark, Sweden and Latvia and in females in Norway, Belarus and Hungary (Sartorius, 1995). Similarly, between 1974 and 1987, elderly suicide rates increased in 13 and 10 of the 21 western countries in males and females respectively (Pritchard, 1992). Moreover, in a study of 13 European countries elderly suicide rates increased in Austria and Umea in Sweden and declined in the UK and Stockholm in Sweden between 1989-1993 (De Leo et al., 2001). Elderly suicide rates declined in 16 high income countries between 1988 and 1995 (Kiemo, 2004). In a recent study of 54 developed and developing countries elderly suicide rates in both sexes either declined or remained unchanged over a ten year period (Shah et al., 2007b); a decline was observed in several European countries and elderly suicide rates remained unchanged in several central and south American countries, eastern European countries and countries emerging from the former Soviet Union (Shah et al., 2007b).

Elderly suicide rates also declined over time in Japan (Watanabe et al., 1995), Singapore (Ko & Kua, 1995; Kua et al., 2003), urban China (Yip et al., 2005), Austria (Etzersdorfer et al., 2007), Germany (Baumert et al., 2005), England and Wales (Gunnell et al., 2003), some east European countries (Sartorius, 1995) and men in the United States (US) (Blazer et al., 1986; McIntosh, 1984). Between 1985 and 1996, in England and Wales, elderly suicide rates declined in both sexes (Hoxey & Shah, 2000; Shah et al., 2001); similar observations were evident between 1979 and 2002 for the whole of the UK (Shah, 2007a).

Age-Associated Trends in Suicide Rates

Traditionally, suicide rates increased with ageing in many countries (Shah & De, 1998). However, exceptions to this observation are emerging. Data from the WHO data bank in 1995 revealed that female suicide rates did not increase with age in Mauritius, Colombia, Albania and Finland (Shah & De, 1998). In a recent study of 62 developed and developing countries suicide rates increased with age in males and females in 25 and 27 countries respectively, and in both sexes in 17 countries, but there was no increase in suicide rates with age in males and females in 31 and 29 countries respectively, and in both sexes in 21 countries (Shah, 2007a). Regional clustering was observed for countries without an increase in suicide rates with age in both sexes (central and south American countries, and eastern European countries and countries emerging from the former Soviet Union), females only (south America) and males only (eastern European countries) (Shah, 2007a). Suicide rates increased with age in 47 of the 49 medium and high income countries (Kiemo, 2004).

Suicide rates for both sexes increased with age in Switzerland (Ajdacic-Gross et al., 2006), Brazil (Mello-Santos et al., 2005), Denmark (Qin & Mortensen, 2001), Australia (Yip et al., 2005), China (Pritchard, 1996; Yip et al., 2000; Qin & Mortensen, 2001), Hong Kong (Yip et al., 1998; Yip & Tan, 1998) and Singapore (Yip & Tan, 1998). Suicide rates for Australian, New Zealand and white American males increased with age, but suicide rates for females initially increased with age, peaking at menopause, and declined thereafter (Skegg & Cox, 1991; Woodbury et al., 1988; Snowdon & Snowdon, 1995). Suicide rates among non-white Americans (Seiden, 1981; Woodbury et al., 1988), Indians (Adityanjee, 1986; Bhatia et al., 1987), Jordanians (Daradekh, 1989) and Indian immigrants to the UK (Raleigh et al., 1990; Needeman et al., 1997), and in some east European countries (Sartorius, 1995) declined with increasing age.

Methodological Considerations

These cross-national variations in elderly suicide rates, trends over time in elderly suicide rates and age-related trends in suicide rates should be viewed with caution because: data are not available from all countries (Moscicki, 1995; Wasserman et al., 2005); the validity of this data is unclear (Diekstra, 1989; Wasserman et al., 2005); the legal criteria for the proof of suicide vary between countries and in different regions within a country (Shah & Ganesvaran, 1994; Wasserman et al., 2005); some countries, particularly low-income countries, may have poor death registration facilities (Shah & Ganesvaran, 1994); cultural and religious factors and stigma attached to suicide may lead to under-reporting of suicides (Wasserman et al., 2005; Abraham et al., 2005); changes in the legal criteria or the international or national classification of suicides over time (Shah & De, 1998; Kiemo, 2004; De Leo, 2007); and, the effect of age, period and cohort on suicide rates were not examined (Shah & De, 1998). Another limitation of utilising national aggregate data is the possibility of missing variations in suicide rates in different regions within a country (Rehkopf & Buka, 2006). However, it has been argued that within individual countries there is internal consistency (Sainsbury, 1983) and such variation is less important when changes in patterns, rather than the prevalence, of suicide rates is concerned (Pritchard, 1992). Furthermore, studies using different methodologies, including those from individual countries and cross-national studies, have observed similar findings in several instances suggesting the many of above findings may be robust; for example, cross-national comparative studies of elderly sucide rates, time trends in elderly sucide rates and age-associated suicide rates ascertained similar findings to those observed in studies of individual countries and other cross-national studies using different methodologies (Shah et al., 2007a,b; Shah, 2007a). Hence, as one author recently concluded "despite limitations, the total epidemiological picture seems to be reliable, and international suicide rates can be compared over time" (Andriessen, 2006).

DEVELOPMENT OF AN EPIDEMIOLOGICAL TRANSITION MODEL FOR ELDERLY SUICIDE RATES

Potential explanations for cross-national variations in elderly suicide rates, trends over time in elderly suicide rates and age-associated suicide rates include cross-national differences in genetic factors predisposing to mental illness and directly to suicidal behaviour (Shah, 2007a), prevalence of mental illness in the elderly (Shah, 2007a), life expectancy (Shah et al., 2007c), socio-economic status (Shah et al., 2007c), income inequality (Shah et al., 2007c), cultural factors (Shah, 2007; Yip, 2001; Kua et al., 2007; Yip et al., 2005), the availability of appropriate healthcare services, public health initiatives to improve identification and treatment of mental illness, mental health and suicide prevention (Shah et al., 2007a; Shah, 2007b), gender effects, and the composite effects of age, period and cohort (Skegg & Cox, 1991; Murphy et al., 1986; Surtees & Duffy, 1989; Snowdon & Snowdon, 1995; Gunnell et al., 2004).

A complimentary theoretical model with an integrated approach to simultaneously explain the cross-national variations in (i) elderly suicide rates from cross-sectional data, (ii) trends over time for elderly suicide rates from longitudinal data, and (iii) age-associated trends in suicide rates from cross-sectional data is developed. Although, a similar model has previously been proposed to explain the cross-national variations in the incidence and prevalence of dementia (Suh & Shah, 2001) and other mental disorders in old age (Shah, 2007c), the current model has been further refined, modified and adapted for elderly suicide rates. The idea of epidemiological transition originally proposed by Omran (1971) has been justifiably criticised for being more of a phenomenological description of demograhic changes rahter than a theoretical explanation (Carolina & Gustavo, 2003) and for downplaying the role of medical factors (Caldwell, 2001) in the evolving population health. In developing the current model of economic and heath transition and its effect on elderly suicide rates it is proposed that countries progresses through four developmental stages during their socio-economic development. Within these stages elderly suicide rates and its known risk factors in any country at a given time is dependent on a complex interplay of availability of healthcare for its citizens, its impact on survival and longevity, and eventually the country's response and adaptation to population ageing and the ability of its older citizens to influence health policies. The model assumes that both elderly suicide rates and socio-economic status of countries can be dichotomised into two groups: high and low; and, makes potentially testable predictions at each stage.

1. Low Elderly Suicide Rate-Low Socio-Economic Society Stage

Positive correlations between gross national domestic product (GDP), a measure of socio-economic status, and suicide rates in both sexes in the general population (Zhang, 1998; Simpson & Conklin, 1989) and men in the age-band 75+ years (Shah et al., 2007c) were observed in large cross-national studies of developed and developing countries. Negative correlations between the Gini coefficient, a measure of income inequality (higher the Gini coefficient higher the income inequality), and suicide rates in the elderly (Shah et al., 2007c) and in the general population (Vijaykumar et al., 2005) were observed in large cross-national studies of developing and developed countries. A study from the US also reported a negative correlation between the suicide rates in the general population and the Gini coefficient and lower household income (Kowalski et al., 1987). Also, other markers of economic adversity, including higher housing loan interest rates, were associated with lower elderly suicide rates in Australia (Berk et al., 2006). These findings collectively suggested that lower socio-economic status and greater income inequality may be associated with lower elderly suicides rates.

Societies with low socio-economic status are likely to have poorly developed healthcare services. This is supported by positive correlations between GDP and proxy markers of the quality and quantity of available healthcare services, including the proportion of GDP spent on health, per capita expenditure on health, the density of mental health workers and available mental health services, and negative correlations between the Gini coefficent and these variables (Shah et al., 2007c; Shah & Bhat, 2007; Shah, 2007c). The amount of expenditure on health is likely to reflect in the degree of development of healthcare services. Poorly developed healthcare services may mediate an increase in child mortality rates by being unable to provide primary preventative measures for diseases in childhood (e.g immunisation programmes) and treatment for diseases that are directly related to low socio-economic status (e.g infectious diseases) (Suh & Shah, 2001). This is supported by the negative correlations between child mortality rates and the proportion of GDP spent on health and per capita expenditure on health (Shah et al., 2007c; Shah, 2007c). Also, child mortality rates were negatively correlated with GDP and positively correlated with the Gini coefficient (Zhang, 1998; Shah et al., 2007c; Shah, 2007c).

Increased child mortality rates will, in turn, reduce the life expectancy. This is supported by negative correlations between child mortality rates and life expectancy (Zhang, 1998; Shah et al., 2007c; Shah, 2007c). Given that suicide rates generally increase with age (Shah & De, 1998), reduced life expectancy will result in fewer people reaching the age of increased risk for suicide in societies with low socio-economic status. This, in turn, will result in a reduced number of elderly suicides in countries with low socio-economic status. This is supported by positive correlations between life expectancy and suicide rates in the elderly (Shah et al., 2007c) and the general population (Zhang, 1998) in large cross-national studies, and by the positive relationship between elderly suicide rates and the proportion of old people in the general population (Kiemo, 2004; Shah et al., 2007c) and elderly dependency ratios (Shah et al., 2007d) in large cross-national studies. Also, selective survival of those at reduced risk of suicide in old age due to genetic or constitutional factors may further compound this trend (Suh & Shah, 2001). Moreover, in societies with low socio-economic status, those who do survive into old age may be at reduced risk of suicide because they may be able to better tolerate additional hardship in old age due to life-long exposure to adversity (Lindesay, 1991; Seiden, 1981), contributing to lower elderly suicide rates. This has been offered as an explanation for the low suicide rate among elderly African Americans and native Americans in the US, who often have a life-long history of socio-economic deprivation (McIntosh, 1984). The positive correlation between elderly suicide rates and the proportion of elderly in the population (Keimo, 2004; Shah et al., 2007c) also supports this hypothesis because increased life expectancy increases the proportion of elderly in the population. Furthermore, correlations between life expectancy and GDP (positive) and Gini coefficient (negative) have also been reported (Zhang, 1998; Kiemo, 2004; Shah et al., 2007c; Shah, 2007c).

The above approach, particularly in societies with low socio-economic status, is consistent with a previously developed model with five sequential stages (Shah et al., 2007c): (i) presence of a low socio-economic status; (ii) low socio-economic status leading to poorly developed healthcare services; (iii) poorly developed healthcare services may interact, mediate and modify other factors and contribute to increased child mortality rates; (iv) increased child mortality rates leading to reduced life expectancy; and, (v) reduced life expectancy leading to fewer people reaching the age of increased risk of suicide, and resulting in low elderly suicide rates in societies with low socio-economic status. This situation could be labelled as a low elderly suicide rate-low socio-economic society stage.

2. High Elderly Suicide Rate-Low Socio-Economic Society Stage

As the socio-economic status of countries improves, the degree of development of healthcare services will also improve. This is supported by positive correlations between GDP and proxy markers of the quality and quantity of available healthcare services, including the proportion of GDP spent on health, per capita expenditure on health, the density of mental health workers and available mental health services, and negative correlations between the Gini coefficent and these variables (Shah et al., 2007c; Shah & Bhat, 2007; Shah, 2007c). The amount of expenditure on health is likely to reflect in the degree of development of healthcare services. Improvement in healthcare services may facilitate reduction in child mortality rates because of improved ability to provide primary preventative measures for diseases in childhood (e.g immunisation programmes) and treatment for diseases that are directly related to low socio-economic status (e.g infectious diseases) (Suh & Shah, 2001). This is supported by the negative correlations between child mortality rates and the proportion of GDP spent on health and per capita expenditure on health (Shah et al., 2007c; Shah, 2007c), and GDP (Zhang, 1998; Shah et al., 2007c).

Reduction in child mortality rates will, in turn, increase the life expectancy. This is supported by significant negative correlations between child mortality rates and life expectancy (Zhang, 1998; Shah et al., 2007c). This is also further supported by positive correlations between life expectancy and GDP, proportion of GDP spent on health, per capita expenditure on health, and negative correlations between life expectancy and the Gini coefficient (Zhang, 1998; Kiemo, 2004; Shah et al., 2007c; Shah, 2007c). There is also other evidence of increasing life expectancy in low income countries (Shah & Mackenzie, 2007). This, in turn, will result in greater number of subjects reaching the age of increased risk of suicide and an increase in elderly suicide rates. This is supported by positive correlations between life expectancy and suicide rates in the elderly (Shah et al., 2007c) and general population (Zhang et al., 1998) in large cross-national studies, and by the positive relationship between elderly suicide rates and the proportion of old people in the general population (Kiemo, 2004; Shah et al., 2007c) and elderly dependency ratios (Shah et al., 2007d) in large cross-national studies. This approach is also consistent with the five stage sequential model described above in the section on Low elderly suicide rates – low socio-economic society stage (Shah et al., 2007c). This will lead to a gradual transition from low elderly suicide rate-low socio-economic society stage to a high elderly suicide rate-low socio-economic society stage.

3. High Elderly Suicide Rate-High Socio-Economic Society Stage

As societies develop they are likely to change from being socio-economically less developed to being socio-economically more developed. This will lead to further improvements in the degree of development of healthcare services. This is supported by positive correlations between GDP and proxy markers of the quality and quantity of available healthcare services, including the proportion of GDP spent on health, per capita expenditure on health, the density of mental health workers and available mental health services, and negative correlations between the Gini coefficent and these variables (Shah et al., 2007c; Shah & Bhat, 2007; Shah, 2007c). The amount of expenditure on health is likely to reflect in the degree of development of healthcare services. Further improvement in healthcare services may facilitate further reductions in child mortality rates because of improved ability to provide primary preventative measures for diseases in childhood (e.g immunisation programmes) and treatment for diseases that are directly related to low socio-economic status (e.g infectious diseases) (Suh & Shah, 2001). This is supported by the negative correlations between child mortality rates and the proportion of GDP spent on health and per capita expenditure on health (Zhang, 1998; Shah et al., 2007c; Shah, 2007c).

Further reductions in child mortality rates will, in turn, further increase the life expectancy. This is supported by significant negative correlations between child mortality rates and life expectancy (Zhang, 1998; Shah et al., 2007c; Shah, 2007c). This is also further supported by positive correlations between life expectancy and GDP, proportion of GDP spent on health, per capita expenditure on health, and negative correlations between life expectancy and the Gini coefficient (Zhang, 1998; Kiemo, 2004; Shah et al., 2007c; Shah, 2007). There is also other evidence of increasing life expectancy in medium and high income countries (Shah & Mackenzie, 2006). This, in turn, will result in increasing number of subjects reaching the age of increased risk of suicide; this is supported by positive correlations between life expectancy and suicide rates in the elderly (Shah et al., 2007c) and general population (Zhang, 1998), and by the positive relationship between elderly suicide rates and the proportion of old people in the general population (Kiemo, 2004; Shah et al., 2007c) and elderly dependency ratios (Shah et al., 2007d) in large cross-national studies. Reduced child mortality rates and increased life expectancy will also lead to reduction in selective survival of those at reduced risk of suicide in old age due to constitutional or genetic factors. Furthermore, the protective effects of life-long adversity on elderly suicide rates (McIntosh, 1984) may be absent in countries with higher socio-economic status. The composite effect of these changes would be an increase in the number of individuals at increased risk of suicide in old age in socio-economically more developed societies. This approach is also consistent with the five stage sequential model described above in the section on Low elderly suicide rates – low socio-economic society stage (Shah et al., 2007c). This will lead to a gradual transition from the high elderly suicide rate-low socio-economic society stage to a high elderly suicide rate-high socio-economic society stage.

4. Low Elderly Suicide Rate-High Socio-Economic Society Stage

Theoretically, in socio-economically well developed societies, due to further reduction in child mortality rates and increase in life expectancy, greater number of people would reach the age of increased of suicide, and consequently lead to higher elderly suicide rates. However, in socio-economically well developed countries, including Italy, Netherlands, Norway, United Kingdom and United States, elderly suicide rates were comparatively low (Shah et al., 2007a) and declined over time (Shah et al., 2007b). The five stage sequential model described above in the section on Low elderly suicide rates – low socio-economic status society stage (Shah et al., 2007c) may not apply to socio-economically well developed socieities. In socio-economically well developed societies, elderly suicide rates may progressively decline over many years due to improved efforts to control the risk factors for elderly suicides, enhance protective factors for elderly suicides, and advances in medical care. Ultimately, this will lead to a gradual transition from a high elderly suicide rate-high socio-economic society stage to a low elderly suicide rate-high socio-economic society stage.

England and Wales could be considered as a society at this developmental stage of epidemiological transition of elderly suicide rates. In England and Wales, elderly suicide rates were higher in areas with high socio-economic deprivation (Whitley et al., 1999; Shah et al., 2002) and high social fragmentation (Whitley et al., 1999). A decline in elderly suicide rates over time in England and Wales was associated with an increase in GDP (Gunnell et al., 2003). Therefore, in socio-economically well developed societies, like England and Wales, further improvement in socio-economic status appears to be an important factor in reducing elderly suicide rates. What is the mechanism for the reduction in elderly suicide rates due to improved socio-economic status?

Almost all elderly suicide victims have mental illness, and up to 90% have depression (Shah & De, 1998). A significant number of elderly suicide victims in western countries consult their general practitioner or psychiatrist or contact mental health services between one week and six months prior to the suicide (Barraclough, 1971; Catell, 1988; Conwell et al., 1990,1991; Catell & Jolley, 1995; Vassilas & Morgan, 1993, 1994). This offers opportunity for identification and treatment of the mental illness. Thus, the availability of appropriate healthcare services may be an important factor contributing to elderly suicide rates. High suicide rates in rural China and Hong Kong, in part, have been attributed to lack of mental health services and poorly developed social welfare and benefit systems (Yip & Tan, 1998; Jianlin, 2000; Yip, 2001; Yip et al., 2000). Socio-economically well developed societies are likely to have well developed healthcare services, and this is supported by the observed positive correlations between GDP and proxy markers of the quality and quantity of available healthcare services, including the proportion of GDP spent on health, per capita expenditure on health, the density of mental health workers and available mental health services, and negative correlations between the Gini coefficient and these variables (Shah et al., 2007c; Shah & Bhat, 2007). The amount of expenditure on health is likely to reflect in the degree of development of healthcare services. Decline in elderly suicide rates in England and Wales was associated with measures of improved healthcare for the elderly (Gunnell et al., 2003; Lodhi & Shah, 2005) including an increase in the number of general practitioners, hospital medical staff, out-patient appointments for mental illness, and field social workers and day centre staff (Lodhi & Shah, 2005). Reduction in elderly suicide rates in Singapore and urban

China have been attributed to improved healthcare and welfare services for the elderly (Kua et al., 2003; Yip et al., 2005).

Socio-economically more developed societies are also more likely to have appropriate healthcare facilities to promptly resusitate those who have attempted suicides, thus further reducing elderly suicide rates. Physical illness is an important risk factor for elderly suicides (Catell, 1988; Catell & Jolley, 1995), and socio-economically well developed societies are more likely to have appropriate healthcare care facilities for the treatment of physical illness, thus helping to reduce elderly suicide rates. Some recent public health initiatives in the UK may be responsible for the improvement in the health structure by improving detection and treatment of individuals at risk of suicide. Such initiatives included legislation encouraging general practitioners to offer annual physical and mental examination to those over the age of 75 years, the Defeat Depression Campaign organised by the Royal College of Psychiatrist and the Royal College of General Practitioners, the governmental "Our Healthier Nation" suicide reduction targets, the National Confidential Enquiry into Suicides and Homicides, the National Service Frameworks for Mental Health and for Older People, and the National Suicide Prevention Strategy (Hoxey & Shah, 2000; Shah et al., 2001; Shah, 2007b). Additionally, a decline in elderly suicide rates in England and Wales was associated with an increase in prescription rates of antidepressants (Gunnell et al., 2003; Lodhi & Shah, 2004), particularly in the category selective serotonin reuptake inhibitors (Lodhi & Shah, 2004); this has also been reported in Sweden (Carlsten et al., 1999) and Australia (Hall et al., 2003). This change may have been a direct result of the various initiatives described above, which may have promoted health-seeking behaviour among patients at risk of suicide and improved prescribing patterns for antidepressants amongst doctors. Furthermore, such public health initiatives are more likely to be instigated in countries at a more advanced stage of socio-economic development because they require substantive funding. Thus, improvement in the social and health structure of society appears to be important in reducing elderly suicide rates in socio-economically well developed societies.

Conclusion

A developmental model of epidemiological transition for elderly suicide rates with four sequential stages is proposed: (i) low elderly suicide rate-low socio-economic society; (ii) high elderly suicide rate-low socio-economic society; (iii) high elderly suicide rate-high socio-economic society; and (iv) low elderly suicide rate-high socio-economic society. It is likely that different countries will be at different stages of development within this model. It is envisaged that each country would progress through each of these four developmental stages over time. This model can be formally tested using two potential approaches. Countries that are currently at the stage of low elderly suicide rates-low socio-economic society could be followed-up over time to observe if they progress through the four developmental stages of the proposed epidemiological transition model. However, such studies may not be practical or realistic because the follow-up period will be over many years (perhaps several decades). This model could also be tested by using the available cross-sectional data on elderly suicide rates and socio-economic status from different countries at different developmental stages of this model. Such an approach could allow segregation of different countries into each of the four developmental stages. This model is complimentary to, and does not preclude, other proximal and distil aetiological risk factors for elderly suicides.

Conflict of Interest

None

References

Abrahams, V. J., Abrahams, S. and Jacob, K. S. (2005) Suicide in the elderly in Kanyambadi block, Tamil Nadu, South India. *International Journal of Geriatric Psychiatry,* 20, 953-955.

Adityanjee, D. R. (1986) Suicide attempts and suicide in India: cross-cultural aspects. *International Journal of Social Psychiatry*, 32, 64-73.

Ajdacic-Gross, V., Bopp, M., Gostynski, M., Lauber, C., Gutzwiller, F. and Rossler, W. (2006). Age-period-cohort analysis of Swiss suicide data, 1881-2000. *European Archives of Psychiatry and Clinical Neurosciences*, 256, 207-214.

Andriessen, K. (2006) Do we need to be cautious in evaluating suicide statistics? *European Journal of Public Health*, 16, 445-447.

Bhatia, S. C., Kahn, M. H. and Medirrata, R. P. (1987) High risk suicide factors across cultures. *International Journal of Social Psychiatry*, 33, 226-236.

Barraclough, B. M. (1971) Suicide in the elderly. *British Journal of Psychiatry*, 6, 87-97.

Baumert, J. J., Erazo, N. and Ladwig, K. H. (2005) *Sex- and age-specific trends in mortality from suicide and undertermined death in Germany* 1991-2002.

Berk, M., Dodd, S. and Henry, M. (2006) The effect of macroeconomic variables on suicide. *Psychological Medicine*, 36, 181-189.

Blazer, D. G., Bachar, J. R. and Manton, K. G. (1986) Suicide in late life – review and commentary. *Journal of the American Geriatric Society*, 13, 743-749.

Caldwell, J. C. (2001) Population health in transition. *Bulletin of the World Health Organisation,* 79, 159-160.

Carlsten, A., Waern, M. and Allebeck, P. (1999) Suicides by drug poisoning among the elderly in Sweden 1969-1996. *Social Psychiatry & Psychiatric Epidemiology*, 34, 609-614.

Carolina, M. S. and Gustavo, L. F. (2003) Epidemiological transition: model or illusion? A look at health problems in Mexico. *Social Science and Medicine*, 57, 539-550.

Cattell, H. (1988) Elderly suicides in London: an analysis of coroner's inquests. *International Journal of Geriatric Psychiatry*, 3, 251-261.

Cattell, H. and Jolley, D. (1995) One hundred cases of suicide in the elderly. *British Journal of Psychiatry,* 166, 451-457.

Conwell, Y., Rotenberg, M. and Caine, E. D. (1990) Completed suicides at age 50 and over. *Journal of the American Geriatric Society*, 38, 640-644.

Conwell, Y., Olsen, K., Caine, E. D. and Flannery, C. (1991) Suicide in later life: psychological autopsy findings. *International Psychogeriatrics*, 3, 59-66.

Daradekh, T. K. (1989) Suicide in Jordan 1980-1985. *Acta Psychiatrica Scandinavica,* 79, 241-244.

De Leo, D. (2007) Suicide mortality data need revision. *Medical Journal of Australia,* 186, 157-158.

De Leo, D., Padoani, W., Scocco, P et al (2001) Attempted and completed suicide in older subjects: results from the WHO/EURO multicentre study of suicidal behaviour. *International Journal of Geriatric Psychiatry*, 16, 300-310.

Diekstra, R. F. W. (1989) Suicide and attemptede suicide: an international perspective. *Acta Psychiatrica Scandinavica,* 80 (Suppl 354), 1-24.

Etsersdorfer, E., Voracek, M., Kapusta, M. and Sonneck, G. (2005) Epidemiology of suicide in Austria 1990-2000: general decrease, but increased suicide risk for older men. Wirn. Klin. *Wochenschr.,* 117, 31-35.

Gunnell, D., Middleston, N., Whitley, E., Dorling, D. and Frankel, S. (2003) Why are suicide rates rising in young men but falling in the elderly? – a time-series analysis of trends in England and Wales 1950-1998. *Social Science and Medicine*, 57, 595-611.

Gunnell, D., Middleston, N., Whitley, E., Dorling, D., Frankel, S. (2004) Influence of cohort effects on paterrns of suicide in England and Wales, 1950-1999. *British Journal of Psychiatry*, 182, 164-170.

Hall, W., Mant, A., Mitchell, P., Rendle, V. A., Hickie, I. B. and McManus, P. (2003) Association between antidepressant prescribing and suicide in Australia, 1991-2000: trend analysis. *British Medical Journal,* 326, 1008-1011.

Hoxey, K. and Shah, A. K. (2000) Recent trends in suicide rates and methods in England and Wales. *International Journal of Geriatric Psychiatry*, 15, 274-279.

Jianlin, J. (2000) Suicide rates and mental health services in modern China. *Crisis,* 21, 118-121.

Kiemo, K. (2004) *Towards a socio-economic and demographic theory of elderly suicides: a comparison of 49 countries at various stages of development.* www.soc.ou.se/publications/fulltext/diss2003-3.pdf. Viewed 2 Febraury 2007.

Ko, S. M. and Kua, E. H. (1995) Ethnicity and elderly suicide rates in Singapore. *International Psychogeriatrics*, 7, 309-317.

Kowalski, G. S., Faupel, C. E. and Starr, P. D. (1987) Urbanisation and suicides: a study of American Counties. *Social Forces*, 66, 85-101.

Kua, E. H., Ko, S. M. and Ng, T. P. (2003) Recent trends in elderly suicide rates in a multi-ethnic Asian city. *International Journal of Geriatric Psychiatry*, 18, 533-536.

Lindesay, J. (1991) Suicide in the elderly. *International Journal of Geriatric Psychiatry*, 6, 355-361.

Lodhi, L. and Shah, A. K. (2004) Psychotropic prescriptions and elderly suicide rates. *Medicne, Science and the Law*, 44, 236-244.

Lodhi, L. and Shah, A. K. (2005) Factors associated with the recent decline in suicide rates in England and Wales. 1985-1998. *Medicne, Science and the Law*, 45, 115-120.

Mello-Santos, C., Bertolote, J. M. and Wang, Y. P. (2005) Epidemiology of suicide in Brazil (1980-2000): characterisation of age and gender rates of suicide. *Rev Bras Psiquiatr*, 27, 131-134.

McIntosh, J. L. (1984) Components of the decline in elderly suicides: suicide in young old and old old by race and sex. *Death Education,* 8, 113-124.

Moscicki, E. K. (1995) North American perspectives: epidemiology of suicide. *International Psychogeriatrics*, 7, 137-148.

Murphy, E., Lindesay, J. and Grundy, E. (1986) 60 years of suicide in England and Wales: a cohort study. *Archive of General Psychiatry*, 43, 969-976.

Neeleman, J., Mak, V. and Wessely, S. (1997) Suicide by age, ethnic group, coroner's verdict and country of birth. A three-year survey in inner London. *Bristish Journal of Psychiatry*, 181, 463-467.

Omran, A. R. (1971) The epidemiologic transition. A theory of the epidemiology of population change. *Milbank Mem Fund Q*, 49, 509-538.

Pritchard, C. (1992) Changes in elderly suicides in the USA and the developed world 1974-1987: comparison with current homocide. *International Journal of Geriatric Psychiatry*, 7, 125-134.

Pritchard, C. (1996) Suicide in the People's Republic of China categorised by age and gender: evidence of the influence of culture on suicide. *Acta Psychiatrica Scandinavica*, 93, 362-367.

Qin, P. and Mortensen, P. B. (2001) Specific characteristics of suicide in China. *Acta Psychiatrica Scandinavica*, 103, 117-121.

Raleigh, V. S., Bulusu, L. and Balarajan, R. (1990) Suicides among immigrants from the Indian subcontinent. *British Journal of Psychiatry*, 156, 46-50.

Rehkopf, D. H. and Buka, S. L. (2006) The association between suicide and the socio-economic characteristics of geographical areas: a systematic review. *Psychological Medicine*, 36, 145-157.

Sainsbury, P. (1983) Validity and reliabity of trends in suicide statistics. *World Health Statistices Quaterly*, 36, 339-348.

Sartorius, N. (1995) Recent changes in suicide rates in selected eatern European and other European countries. *International Psychogeriatrics*, 7, 301-308.

Seiden, R. H. (1981) Mellowing with age: factors affecting the non-white suicide rate. *International Journal of Ageing and Human Development*, 13, 265-284.

Shah, A. K. (2007a) The relationship between suicde rates and age: an analysis of multinational data from the World Health Organisation. *International Psychogeriatrics*. In Press.

Shah, A. K. (2007b) Trends in elderly suicide rates in the United Kingdom over 24 years from 1979 to 2002. *Medicine, Science and Law*, 47, 56-60.

Shah, A. K. (2007c) The importance of socio-economic status of countries for mental disorders in old age: a development of an epidemiological transition model. *International Psychogeriatrics*, 19, 785-787.

Shah, A. K. and Bhat, R. (2007) The relationship between elderly suicide rates and mental health funding, service provision and national policy: a cross-national study. *International Psychogeriatrics*. In Press.

Shah, A. K., Bhat, R., MacKenzie, S. and Koen, C. (2007a). Elderly suicide rates: cross-national comparisons and association with sex and elderly age-bands. *Medicine, Science and the Law,* 47, 244-252.

Shah, A. K., Bhat, R., MacKenzie, S. and Koen, C. (2007b) Elderly suicide rates: crossnational comparison of trends over a ten year time period. *International Psychogeriatrics*. In Press.

Shah, A. K., Bhat, R. MacKenzie, S. and Koen, C. (2007c). A cross-national study of the relationship between elderly suicide rates and life expectancy and markers of socio-economic status and healthcare. *International Psychogeriatrics*. In Press.

Shah, A. K. and De, T. (1998) Suicide and the elderly. *International Journal of Psychiatry in Clinical Practice*, 2, 3-17.

Shah, A. K., Ellanchanny, N. and Collinge, T. (2001) Trends in age band-specific suicide rates in the elderly. *Medicne, Science and the Law*, 41, 102-106.

Shah, A. K. and Ganesvaran, T. (1994) Suicide in the elderly. *In: Functional Psychiatric Disorders of the Elderly (Eds. Chiu E, Ames D).* Cambridge, Cambridge University Press. Pgs 221-244.

Shah, A. K. and MacKenzie, S. (2007) Disorders of ageing across cultures. *In: Textbook of Cultural Psychiatry* (Eds. Bhugra D). Cambridge, Cambridge University Press. In Press.

Shah, A. K., Padayatchi, M. and Das, K. (2007d) The relationship between elderly suicide rates and elderly dependency ratios: a cross-national study using data from the WHO data bank. *International Psychogeriatrics*. In Press.

Shah, R., Uren, Z., Baker, A. and Majeed, A. (2002) Trends in suicide from drug overdose in the elderly in England and Wales, 1993-1999. *International Journal of Geriatric Psychiatry*, 17, 416-421.

Simpson, M. E. and Conklin, G. H. (1989) Socioeconomic development, suicide and religion: a test of Durkhiem's theory of religion and suicide. *Social Forces*, 67, 945-964.

Skeeg, K. and Cox, B. (1991) Suicide in New Zealand 1957- 1986: influence of age, period and birth cohort. *Australia and New Zealand Journal of Psychiatry,* 25, 181-190.

Snowdon, J. and Snowdon, D. (1995) *Suicide in Australia.* Paper presented at the 8th Congress of the International Psychogeriatric Association, Sydney, Australia.

Suh, G. H. and Shah, A.K. (2001) A review of the epidemiological transition in dementia-cross-national comparisons of indices related to Alzheimer's disease and vascular dementia. *Acta Psychiatrica Scandinavica*, 104, 4-11.

Surtees, P. and Duffy, J. C. (1989) Suicide in England and Wales 1946-1985: an age period cohort analysis. *Acta Psychiatrica Scandinavica*, 79, 216-223.

Vassilas, C. A. and Morgan, H. G. (1993) General practitioner's contact with victims of suicide. *British Medical Journal*, 307, 300-301.

Vassilas, C. A. and Morgan, H. G. (1994) Elderly suicides' contact with their general practitioner before death. *International Journal of Geriatric Psychiatry,* 9, 1008-1009.

Vijayakumar, L., Nagaraj, K., Pirkis, J. and Whiteford, H. (2005) Suicide in developing countries (1): frequency, distribution, and association with socio-economic indicators. *Crisis*, 26, 104-111.

Wasserman, D., Cheng, Q. and Jiang, G. X. (2005) Global suicide rates among young people aged 15-19. *World Psychiatry*, 114-120.

Watanabe, N., Hasegawa, K. and Yoshinaga, Y. (1995) Suicide in later life in Japan: urban and rural differences. *International Psychogeriatrics*, 7, 253-261.

Whitley, E., Gunnell, D., Dorling, D. and Smith, G. D. (1999) Ecological study of social fragmentation, poverty, and suicide. *British Medical Journal*, 319, 1034-1037.

Woodbury, M. A., Manton, K. G. and Blazer, D. (1987) Trends in US suicide mortality rates 1968-1982: race and sex differences in age, period and cohort components. *International Journal of Epidemiology*, 17, 356-352.

Yip, P. S. F. (2001) An epidemiological profile of suicides in Beijing, Chine. *Suicide and Life-Threatening Behaviour*, 31, 62-70.

Yip, P. S. F., Callanan, C. and Yuen, H. P. (2000). Urban/rural and gender differences in suicide rates: East and West. *Journal of Affective Disorders*, 57, 99-106.

Yip, P. S. F., Chi, I. and Yu, K. K. (1998) An epidemiological profile of elderly suicides in Hong Kong. *International Journal of Geriatric Psychiatry*, 13. 631-637.

Yip, P. S. F., Liu, K. Y., Hu, J. and Song, X. M. (2005) Suicide rates in China during a decade of rapid social change. *Social Psychiatry and Psychiatric Epidemiology*, 40, 792-798.

Yip, P. S. F. and Tan, R. C. E. (1998) Suicides in Hong Kong and Singapore: a tale of two cities. *International Journal of Social Psychiatry*, 44, 267-279.

Zhang, J. (1998) Suicide in the world: toward a population increase theory of suicide. *Death Studies*, 22, 525-539.

In: Perspectives in Psychiatry Research
Editors: Nicole M. Levine and Donna J. Campbell
ISBN: 978-1-61209-236-2

Chapter 8

PSYCHOTROPIC ANALGESIC NITROUS OXIDE [PAN] FOR SUBSTANCE ABUSE WITHDRAWAL: CURRENT STATUS

Mark A Gillman*
South African Brain Research Institute
Johannesburg, South Africa

ABSTRACT

PAN is high concentrations of oxygen (O_2) plus low concentrations of nitrous oxide (N_2O) individually titrated to an endpoint where the subject is relaxed and at which they are fully conscious and co-operative throughout inhalation of the gases. PAN is not merely administering nitrous oxide/oxygen. It also specifically excludes using nitrous oxide at a fixed preconceived dose. Instead, PAN uses titration to provide the nitrous oxide using the individual clinical response of each patient as the guide to the optimal concentration required. Thus, optimal concentrations of nitrous oxide vary widely from individual to individual. Titrating to the correct endpoint usually requires hands-on training or very careful attention to the instructions given in previous papers or in a textbook dealing with dental conscious sedation with nitrous oxide, because the inhaled concentrations of N_2O required to achieve the correct endpoint varies between 10-70%. Although this technique has been used safely and effectively in South Africa (S.A.) for more than 25 years and in Finland for over a decade, there has been strong published criticisms of the technique, from armchair academic critics in S. A., Finland and Sweden. Despite their widely published opposition on theoretical grounds alone, it took almost 10 years before the Finnish group attempted to replicate the use of PAN for treating alcoholic withdrawal states. However, although they used nitrous oxide, they failed to use the PAN technique correctly. This review will cover the published criticisms and work on PAN for alcohol withdrawal, as well as detailing the latest research supporting its efficacy. Evidence will be presented that the PAN therapy is safe and rapidly effective and can be applied by a trained registered nurse, without direct physician supervision,

* Email: mag@iafrica.com

making PAN an ideal cost-effective method for First and Third World countries, saving unnecessary in-patient admissions. Although more controlled trials using the correct method are needed, evidence will be presented that PAN is an effective treatment of the acute withdrawal state from most substances of abuse including alcohol, opioids, cannabis, cocaine, methaqualone/cannabis combinations, nicotine and polydrug abuse. PAN is recognised by the Health Professions Council of South Africa (official tariff code: 0203/0204) and is therefore accepted by medical insurance organisations in S.A.. Because it has been used safely (with no more than trivial adverse effects) and effectively on thousands of outpatients in S.A. and Finland the review will highlight how potentially large cost-savings can be made because many more patients can be treated safely as outpatients than with the currently favoured sedative therapies because the:

6) Patient improves within minutes of administration and is often well enough to have the next meal;
7) Use of addictive sedative medications such as the benzodiazepines (e.g. diazepam) are reduced by 90% plus. This obviates the danger of secondary addiction in this highly susceptible group;
8) Extreme rapidity of recovery enables nurses/physicians to distinguish those patients requiring intensive inpatient therapy from those that do not; since 90% plus patients respond positively to one administration of the gases, usually on admission;
9) Rapidity of response enables the patient to abandon the sick role speedily (often within an hour of gas treatment) and enter the essential next phase of rehabilitation; usually requiring social, psychological and/or psychiatric therapy;
10) Placebo (oxygen) alone ameliorates withdrawal in approximately 30-50% of patients who require no further pharmacological therapy.

PAN is usually given on one occasion only for inpatients. Depending on the drug of abuse, out-patients may require more than one application of the gases, but usually no more than 2 applications during the first week of withdrawal. PAN has been used successfully on more than 50,000 patients in South Africa, Finland and the USA. The rationale for using PAN, as a gaseous partial opioid agonist will be discussed. The review concludes by placing the PAN method in the wider perspective of substance withdrawal states and craving, dealing with its current status and ending with an appeal for more studies to be done on this promising therapy.

Introduction – Distinguishing between Psychotropic Analgesic Nitrous Oxide and Anaesthetic Nitrous Oxide

Since its first use in the late 18th century, nitrous oxide has had a rather chequered history punctuated by periods of acceptance and rejection [Frost, 1985]. The times when it has fallen into disrepute have usually been caused by ignorance of the biological properties of the gas and false perceptions of how it should be administered [Frost, 1985].

As will be seen below, history has a habit of repeating itself. Thus, to get a balanced picture, any discussion on the current status of nitrous oxide needs to be placed in the context of the existing perceptions, which in certain cases have been divorced from the scientific facts. Unfortunately, it is often perceptions not facts that guide peoples' attitudes on a subject. Surprisingly perhaps, this applies equally to scientists [Gillman, 1996].

The modern history of nitrous oxide is a case in point. A number of prominent and influential people, working in the substance abuse field, have based their perceptions on the use of psychotropic analgesic nitrous oxide (PAN) for treating substance abuse withdrawal states, on misconceptions and not on the scientific facts. Unfortunately, these misconceptions have driven negative attitudes to PAN. I shall present evidence that these individuals are currently attempting to block the clinical use of PAN for ameliorating acute withdrawal states. They are also, by virtue of their prominence, de facto, blocking further research into this potentially useful therapy. These workers have played a significant role in retarding the progress of the use of the PAN therapy and are continuing to do so. No discussion on the current status of PAN is complete, without dealing with this aspect. Many researchers would eschew such a discussion because they are under the illusion that science is free of personal animus and prejudice. Those scientists labour under this misconception, at a cost, not only to themselves but also science [Gillman, 1996]. Furthermore, one of the most important goals of this review is to disabuse those who believe that science is the disinterested and passionless pursuit of knowledge.

The other more obvious key aim of this paper is to highlight the existing scientific knowledge on nitrous oxide in the context of PAN and the treatment of acute substance withdrawal states.

We introduced the term PAN in order to clearly distinguish the psychotropic effects of nitrous oxide from the anaesthetic effects of nitrous oxide [Gillman and Lichtigfeld, 1994a]. We were constrained to do so because when nitrous oxide is mentioned most medical professionals, with the possible exception of dentists, immediately assume that the anaesthetic properties of the gas are under consideration [Gillman and Lichtigfeld, 1994a; Gillman and Lichtigfeld, 2006]. Many health professionals do not realise that the low concentration of nitrous oxide diluted with high concentrations of oxygen, consistent with conscious sedation with nitrous oxide/oxygen (synonymous with PAN), produce very different pharmacological effects as compared to the much higher concentrations that produce surgical anaesthesia [Gillman and Lichtigfeld, 1994a]. Apart from its well-known analgesic and anaesthetic actions PAN also produces emotional changes. These emotional effects, which occur at low concentration of nitrous oxide, where the subject is always conscious, include mood elevation, anti-stress and anti-craving effects, most of which are inextricably involved in PAN's usefulness for ameliorating acute substance abuse withdrawal states [Gillman and Lichtigfeld, 1994a].

In contrast, as higher concentrations of nitrous oxide are given these produce preanaesthetic excitation and as the concentration increases further, unconsciousness and surgical anaesthesia supervene [Malamed, 1989; Gillman and Lichtigfeld, 1994a]. Although the anaesthetic actions of nitrous oxide have been extensively studied, its emotional effects have not. A phenomenon that might well be related to the fact that the use of nitrous oxide has been mainly confined to anaesthesia, where the anaesthesiologist is anxious to anaesthetise the patient as rapidly as possible and therefore keeps the period of consciousness to a minimum [Marshall and Wollman, 1985].

To avoid preanaesthetic excitation [and anaesthesia] and to obtain the goal of relaxation, PAN is always titrated to the requirements of each individual patient and a predetermined dose should *never* be used [Langa, 1976; Bennet, 1978; Skelly, 1998; Malamed, 1989a; Clark and Brunick 2008; Gillman and Lichtigfeld 2004a;b;c; Gillman and Lichtigfeld, 2006]. The array of doses that are effective range from 10% to 70% inhaled, with 70% of patients responding at inhaled concentrations of between 30%-40% [Malamed, 1989]. Skelly [1998] have suggested a range 'between 20% and 40%... ...although the effective sedation concentrations varies considerably between individuals and may occasionally be as low as 5-10% or as high as 60-70% N_2O in oxygen.' My colleague and I [Gillman and Lichtigfeld, 1990], have suggested a similar range to that of Skelly [1998]. The concentration can be as low as 5% or as high as 70% in very rare hyper or hypo responders [Gillman and Lichtigfeld, 1990]. Indeed, as can be seen above, the amount of nitrous oxide consistent with PAN is so variable across a cohort, there is no universal agreement, even among experts[Langa, 1976; Bennet, 1978; Malamed, 1989; Skelly, 1998; Gillman and Lichtigfeld, 1990; Clark et al, 2006; Clark and Brunick, 1999; 2003; 2008], as to what the average dose is.

Crucially, all workers who have a good understanding of the technique of dental conscious sedation with nitrous oxide/oxygen (which is synonymous with PAN) emphasise the importance of titration to the patient's own individual dose.

If a predetermined dose is chosen, some patients will be oversedated and approach or enter stage II of anaesthesia (or the excitation stage of anaesthesia) [Beirne and Smith, 1985; Malamed, 1989]. This is not only potentially dangerous, but unethical. Malamed [1989] states: 'Only procedures of short duration should be contemplated in stage II and then only by persons who have been thoroughly trained in general anesthesia... Because reflexes are hyperactive in this stage... ...laryngospasm may be produced.' Malamed [1989] also indicates that *another* well-trained person should be present to ensure maintenance of the patient's airway. It is therefore not surprising that, 'Anesthesiologists try to reduce the duration and intensity of this stage to the minimum.' [Marshall and Wollman, 1985]. Cohen [1975] goes further '..the duration and the intensity of this stage should be reduced to a minimum for patients in substandard health.' Presumably this includes chronic alcoholics, who are often malnourished and debilitated [Edwards, 1991].

Indeed, the correctly trained practitioner will always titrate PAN slowly to the patient's clinical response and to obtain relaxation. As the point of relaxation is approaching smaller doses of nitrous oxide are added until the clinical endpoint of relaxation is obtained. This clinical endpoint is well before stage II anaesthesia (excitation) and indeed the entire point of hands-on training is to enable the practitioner to obtain the definite but subtle clinical endpoint without straying into the excitation stage of anaesthesia (stage II). This is the case, since the training inculcates the importance of titration to the individual's unique concentration. Furthermore, it would seem that even among individuals, the concentration required may vary from day to day i.e. it is a state rather than a trait phenomenon [Gillman and Lichtigfeld, 1987].

A classical example of the dangers of choosing a predetermined concentration of nitrous oxide, and not titrating to the individual clinical response, is shown in some recent work [Alho et al, 2002; 2003]. These workers refused offers of hands-on training and instead were guided by an anaesthetist on their team who did not understand the PAN technique [Gillman and Lichtigfeld, 1997; Gillman and Lichtigfeld, 2004a]. They assumed wrongly, despite verbal warnings from Reijo Ojutkangas [personal communication, Ojutkangas 1999] and myself that an anaesthetist would not be well schooled in all applications of nitrous oxide.

Unfortunately, under the guidance of this anaesthetist, they not only chose a predetermined concentration of nitrous oxide i.e. 30% end tidal volume [or 60% inhaled] but instead of titrating to the clinical response, they titrated to their predetermined target concentration of nitrous oxide, which they only decreased when the patient was about to fall unconscious [Alho et al, 2002; 2003]. Clearly, almost all the study group within their cohort of 105 patients were held in a state either in, or very close to the excitation stage of anaesthesia. That their patients were not relaxed (which is the hall mark of correctly used PAN) and indeed in the excitation stage (stage II anaesthesia) is recorded in their paper, in that the majority of patients receiving nitrous oxide exhibited increased facial muscle tone as measured by electromyography as compared to controls [Alho et al, 2002]. These patients also showed evidence of increased sympathetic tone [Alho et al, 2002]. Increased muscle tone and sympathetic activity are classical signs of the excitation seen in the vicinity of the excitement stage of anaesthesia (i.e. stage II) [Cohen, 1975]. This must have been extremely uncomfortable and stressful for their patients [Alho et al, 2002; 2003], already suffering from a condition (alcohol withdrawal) characterised by a tense trembling hyperadrenergic state [Lichtigfeld and Gillman, 1982; Gillman and Lichtigfeld, 1983; Edwards, 1991] but is clearly not appropriate in terms of PAN. Thus, it would not surprise the reader that Morris Clark the senior author of the current gold-standard textbook on conscious sedation [Clark and Brunick, 2008] with nitrous oxide wrote, regarding the work of Alho et al [2002; 2003] as follows [Clark et al, 2006]:

> 'It has been the authors' experience that nitrous oxide/oxygen has been commonly misused [Alho et al.,2002; 2003] to achieve desired outcomes for a specific procedure or patient.'

Clark et al [2006] are at pains to emphasise the importance of titrating to the patients' clinical state, using different concentrations of nitrous oxide for each patient [Clark et al, 2006]; a fact stressed in the textbook as well [Clark and Brunick, 1999; 2003; 2008]. Clark and Brunick [1999; 2003; 2008] also highlight the importance of correct training in the technique of conscious sedation with nitrous oxide, which as mentioned earlier is a synonym for the PAN method.

From this, it will be clear to the reader why it is important to have brief hands-on training [Gillman and Lichtigfeld, 1990; Gillman and Lichtigfeld, 1997]. I have deliberately spent considerable time making the distinction between PAN and anaesthetic nitrous oxide in order to forewarn other workers who might be interested in repeating our work [Gillman and Lichtigfeld, 1990; Gillman and Lichtigfeld; 2006], because a wrong technique and dose (like any other medication), guarantees failure [Gillman and Lichtigfeld, 2004a;c].

Needless to say Alho et al [2002, 2003] were unable to repeat our work because their technique was incorrect [Langa, 1976; Bennet, 1978; Malamed, 1989; Clark et al, 2006; Clark and Brunick, 1999; 2003; 2008; Gillman and Lichtigfeld, 2004a,b,c; Gillman and Lichtigfeld, 2006; Gillman et al, 2007] and because they used a predetermined, excessively high concentration of nitrous oxide, which was well above the doses that the majority of subjects would need to achieve concentrations of nitrous oxide consistent with PAN [Skelly, 1998; Gillman et al, 2007].

Clearly, PAN is not just the use of any predetermined concentration of nitrous oxide, but rather a specialised technique [Gillman and Lichtigfeld, 2006]. A technique of using various concentrations of nitrous oxide at concentrations determined by the individual requirements of each patient, slowly and carefully titrated to a clinical endpoint characterised by relaxation and nowhere near stage II anaesthesia.

When the technique is correctly applied in the hands of trained medical professionals, it is possible to rapidly treat acute substance withdrawal states from alcohol [Lichtigfeld and Gillman, 1982; Gillman et al, 2007]; cocaine [Carey et al, 1991; Gillman et al, 2006b] cannabis [Carey et al, 1991; Daynes and Gillman, 1994]; nicotine [Gillman and Shevel, 1988; Daynes and Gillman, 1994; Bayrakdarian, 2000], opioids [Kripke and Hechtman, 1972; Gillman and Lichtigfeld, 1985; Carey et al, 1991] and combinations of cannabis plus methaqualone [Gillman et al, 2006a].

The PAN therapy was first used in South Africa (S.A.) in 1979. Despite considerable opposition from academics [Gagiano, 1994; Emsley, 1994] and others [Openshaw, 1986] it was accepted as a standard therapy for substance abuse withdrawal states by the South African Medical Association and the Health Professionals Council of South Africa. It has an official fee and tariff code and for this reason is accepted for medical aid (insurance) claims in S. A. [Gillman, 2006]. The PAN therapy is therefore not regarded as an experimental technique in S.A. Furthermore, registered nurses who have been trained to use the gas, are able to treat substance withdrawal, without direct medical supervision, once it has been prescribed by a physician [Gillman and Lichtigfeld, 2006] or in the case of nicotine dependence, by a dentist[Gillman, 2008].

How PAN Ameliorates Substance Abuse Withdrawal States

Right from the very first paper we hypothesised that PAN acted on the endogenous opioid system to produce its therapeutic effect in withdrawal states [Lichtigfeld and Gillman, 1982]. Since then, additional experimental evidence has appeared showing that PAN has opioid properties [Gillman and Lichtigfeld, 1994a; Gillman and Lichtigfeld, 2006].

Not long after we published our initial paper [Lichtigfeld and Gillman, 1982], we suggested that mutually antagonistic κ-opioid and μ-opioid systems were involved in the pathogenesis of substance abuse [Gillman and Lichtigfeld, 1984; 1994a; Lichtigfeld and Gillman, 1996]. Experimental evidence from rodents and primates showed that μ-opioid agonists applied to the mesolimbic dopamine system stimulate dopamine release in the nucleus accumbens [Lichtigfeld, and Gillman, 1996]. In contrast, administration of κ-opioid agonists to the mesolimbic dopamine system have the opposite effect, in that dopamine release is inhibited in the nucleus accumbens [Lichtigfeld, and Gillman, 1996].

There is also evidence that PAN activates both κ-opioid and μ-opioid receptor systems [Gillman and Lichtigfeld, 1994a; Lichtigfeld and Gillman, 1996]. Thus, it is possible that PAN, by differentially acting on the μ-opioid and κ-opioid receptor systems interacts to rapidly restore the homeostatic balance that has been disturbed as a result of alcohol abstinence, during the alcoholic withdrawal state [Gillman and Lichtigfeld, 1994a; Lichtigfeld and Gillman, 1996]. This hypothesis could also be invoked to explain the 'minute'[Gillman, 1995] abuse potential of PAN and its lack of secondary abuse potential observed in over 25,000 (now over 50,000) cases of substance abuse treated by us and others, since 1979 [Gillman, 1992; Gillman and Lichtigfeld, 1994a; Lichtigfeld and Gillman, 1996, Gillman, 2006].

It is possible that the modulation of the μ-opioid and κ-opioid receptor systems by PAN underlies its efficacy in ameliorating all forms of acute substance abuse withdrawal including that from alcohol [Lichtigfeld and Gillman, 1982; Gillman et al, 2007]; cocaine [Carey et al, 1991; Gillman et al, 2006b] cannabis [Carey et al, 1991; Daynes and Gillman, 1994]; nicotine [Gillman and Shevel, 1988; Daynes and Gillman, 1994; Bayrakdarian, 2000], opioids [Kripke and Hechtman, 1972; Gillman and Lichtigfeld, 1985; Carey et al, 1991] and combinations of cannabis plus methaqualone [Gillman et al, 2006a].

Above, I have dealt in some detail with the differences of using nitrous oxide for obtaining anaesthesia as opposed to PAN. I have also highlighted the crucial pitfalls that occur, if these differences are not fully understood and the operator does not have the basic theoretical knowledge to appreciate these differences, before embarking on a study of PAN [Alho et al, 2002; 2003; Clark et al; 2006].

Nonetheless, I have not outlined in detail the method of administering it. Details of the technique can be found in various papers [Gillman and Lichtigfeld, 1990; 2006; Clark et al, 2006] and for those interested in repeating the work, in any textbook devoted to the subject [Langa, 1976; Bennet, 1978; Malamed, 1989; Clark and Brunick, 2008].

PAN for Treating Alcohol Withdrawal States

Alcohol Withdrawal States

At the outset I would like to emphasise that all our studies on the alcoholic withdrawal states excluded any patients suffering pre-delirium or worse. We did so because severe alcoholic withdrawal states can have severe sequelae including death, and there are tried and trusted sedative therapies such as the benzodiazepines [Saitz et al, 1994] that should immediately be used in such cases, rather than exposing patients' that are seriously ill to a clinical trial.

Our first study started in 1979, tested the effects of nitrous oxide against oxygen single-blind. Here, the nurse administering the gases was aware of which gas she was giving but not the patient.

Oxygen was first administered to each subject for 20 minutes. Immediately thereafter, nitrous oxide was slowly added to oxygen until the concentration of nitrous had been titrated to achieve levels consistent with PAN. The average time for titration, ranges between 2-12 minutes, depending on the dose required for each patient. I would like to emphasise, once again, that the use of a predetermined dose, as used by Alho et al. [2002; 2003] is totally unsuitable when using PAN [Gillman and Lichtigfeld, 2004a;b;c] because the concentration of nitrous oxide required to achieve relaxation (the goal of using PAN), differs so markedly between subjects [Langa, 1976; Malamed, 1989; Bennet, 1978; Gillman and Lichtigfeld, 1994a; Clark and Brunick, 1999; 2003; 2008].

The reader should note that regardless of the time taken to obtain the correct dose for each patient, all cases received nitrous oxide for a total of 20 minutes, which includes the titration time [Gillman and Lichtigfeld, 1990]. The goal of the PAN and the hallmark of its effects are relaxation of the patient, without signs of sedation [Gillman and Lichtigfeld, 1990]. After the 20 minute period of PAN administration a washout with 100% oxygen was given [Lichtigfeld and Gillman, 1982].

There were ninety eight patients in this first study [Lichtigfeld, and Gillman, 1982]. After the first exposure to oxygen for 20 minutes the initial aggregate symptom score of 518 was reduced to 188. Nonetheless, PAN reduced the after oxygen score of 188 to 57 [Lichtigfeld and Gillman, 1982]. We concluded from this open study that both PAN and placebo gas [oxygen] were therapeutic.

Two later trials examined the effects of placebo gas [medical air] against oxygen [Lichtigfeld Gillman, 1989a] and oxygen and carbogen [95% oxygen plus 5% carbon dioxide] [Gillman and Lichtigfeld, 1991a]. In the latter studies, the placebo response ranged from 30-50% [Lichtigfeld and Gillman, 1989a; Gillman and Lichtigfeld, 1991a]. We observed a difference in the percentage of placebo responders in each study. However, the placebo gases when compared against each other within each trial did not show a statistically different therapeutic effect. Both these trials were undertaken randomised and double-blind. All placebo *non*-responders from each trial were then exposed to PAN, with most of these subjects responding positively to PAN [Lichtigfeld and Gillman, 1989a; Gillman and Lichtigfeld, 1991a].

Our next step, because of the large placebo response [Lichtigfeld and Gillman, 1982; 1989a; Gillman and Lichtigfeld, 1991a] was to try and demonstrate that PAN was statistically better than placebo. We examined 100 patients who had been randomly given either medical air or oxygen double-blind. 48 patients from these 2 groups did not respond to either air or oxygen. These non-responders were then immediately given PAN single-blind. Of these 48 patients, 42 responded positively to PAN, with 6 not responding.

In order to make the statistical analysis as fair as possible, we assumed that at least 50% of the placebo non-responders (that is 24 of the 48 patients) would have improved by 50% (or more) if given an additional 20 minutes of placebo [oxygen or air]. We then conducted the chi-square test on these results. We did this despite knowing, from previous clinical experience, that exposure of placebo non-responders to a further 20 minutes of placebo gas did not ameliorate alcoholic withdrawal states above that achieved by the initial 20 minute exposure [Gillman and Lichtigfeld, 2006]. Even using this statistical assumption, the results of the chi-square test showed PAN to be significantly better than placebo at the 0.01% level [Lichtigfeld and Gillman; 1989b]. Work published latter supported the latter findings [Gillman and Lichtigfeld; 1991a]. We believed that these studies demonstrated that PAN could rapidly, safely and effectively improve mild to moderate alcohol withdrawal states [Lichtigfeld and Gillman, 1982; 1989b; Gillman and Lichtigfeld, 1986; 1991a].

One of the things that struck us from the very first study was that the maximum therapeutic effect occurred extremely rapidly. Indeed, in most cases, the maximum therapeutic response was observed within 60 minutes of initial gas administration and often well before an hour had elapsed [Lichtigfeld and Gillman, 1982; 1989a;b; Daynes, 1989; Ojutkangas, 1991]. We have also found that a single 20 minute exposure to PAN for inpatients, usually on admission, is adequate in more than 90% of cases for the total 7 day in-patient stay [Lichtigfeld and Gillman, 1982; Gillman and Lichtigfeld, 1990]. Later work in an out-patient setting showed that a single gas exposure is usually all that is required for outpatients in more than 85% of patients [Ojutkangas and Gillman, 1994]. These observations have been confirmed by other investigators [Daynes, 1989; Ojutkangas, 1991; Carey et al, 1991].

We soon realised, with our work with nitrous oxide and withdrawal states, that it would be very difficult to compare an agent that exerts its maximal effect within 60 minutes to sedative agents such as the benzodiazepines, which when used in a standard manner usually take a day or two to exert an equal effect [Goldstein, 1983; Gillman and Lichtigfeld, 1991a; Saitz, et al, 1994; Gillman and Lichtigfeld, 2006].

There are also difficulties when trying to compare different physical formats i.e. a tablet format [such as a benzodiazepine] with a mixture of gases such as PAN. Initially we did not believe this to be a problem, because the effect of PAN was so rapid and obviously superior to sedative detoxifications, that at first we thought it unnecessary to conduct a double-blind trial. Indeed, the therapeutic effect was so dramatic that when we had finished our initial trial, we arrived at the detoxification centre to pack up the equipment, believing that the nursing staff would be happy to return to their previous use of the benzodiazepines and other sedatives. We were quite mistaken. While we were packing, the senior nurse and matron, came into the ward and remonstrated with us. They said that the PAN treatment was so superior to anything they had ever used, that they wanted to adopt it as the treatment of choice for their facility (Rand Aid Association, Wedge Gardens, Edenvale Johannesburg, S. A.).

This was a great compliment for the PAN method because some of these nurses at the Wedge Gardens had been in the field of alcoholic detoxification for over 20 years. These very experienced nurses had therefore seen many different therapies come and go. The gamut of treatments for alcoholic withdrawal states that they had observed over the preceding 20 years included intravenous ethanol drips (in the very early days), and later barbiturates, chlormethiazole and then the advent of the benzodiazepines. Despite the vast superiority of the benzodiazepines when compared to the barbiturates and ethanol drips, they now believed that PAN was superior to the benzodiazepines. Their reasoning was as follows [Gillman, 2006] the:

1) most patients improved within minutes of gas treatment and were often well enough to enjoy the next ward meal;
2) use of addictive sedative medications such as the benzodiazepines (e.g. diazepam) are reduced by 90% plus. This obviates the danger of secondary addiction in this highly susceptible group;
3) extreme rapidity of recovery enables nurses/physicians to distinguish those patients requiring intensive inpatient therapy from those that do not; since 90% plus patients respond positively to one administration of the gases, usually on admission. It has been our experience that those who do not respond by an improvement of 50% or more on a withdrawal instrument after the initial administration of PAN, almost always require aggressive inpatient therapy. It therefore would seem to be a unique method of screening those who can safely be treated as outpatients from those who require inpatient therapy;
4) rapidity of the therapeutic response enables the patient to abandon the sick role speedily and enter the essential next phase of rehabilitation; usually requiring social, psychological and/or psychiatric therapy;
5) placebo (O_2) alone ameliorates the withdrawal state in approximately 30-50% of patients who require no further pharmacological therapy. It is therefore the only detoxification treatment as far as I am aware, that maximises the placebo response.

As the benefits of the PAN therapy became more widely known through various scientific publications and university dissertations [Lichtigfeld and Gillman, 1982; Lichtigfeld and Gillman, 1983a;b; Kahn, 1983; de Rooster, 1983; Edwards, 1985; Myles, 1984; 1994; Gillman, 1985; Gillman and Lichtigfeld, 1983; 1986] other clinicians came to Wedge Gardens and availed themselves of the opportunity to view patients being treated with PAN. After observing one or two patients themselves they became convinced that the PAN therapy had a place in the treatment of withdrawal states and deserved to be researched further [Carey et al, 1991; Daynes, 1994; Fourie, 1994; Ojukangas, 1991]. All these practitioners, including one from Finland (Ojutkangas) soon came to Wedge Gardens for the brief hands-on training and then went on to continue using it successfully at their treatment centres. In short, after seeing for themselves the rapidity of the therapeutic response following an hour of PAN and viewing the scientific work on which it was based [Lichtigfeld and Gillman, 1982; Lichtigfeld and Gillman, 1983a;b; de Rooster, 1983; Christian, 1991; Myles, 1984; 1992; Gillman, 1985; Gillman and Lichtigfeld, 1983; 1986] they were convinced. They did not need a double-blind trial to show them that the PAN treatment had merit – the face validity was good enough for them.

Unlike these open-minded clinicians, the academic community in S. A. and Finland refused to come and see for themselves, although by then, PAN was being used at widely dispersed geographical site in South African and in Finland. The academic resistance was led by the President of the Society of Psychiatrists of S.A. [Gagiano, 1994] and his Vice-President [Emsley, 1994] and by the Dean of Medical Education of Helsinki University Mikko Salaspuro [Salaspuro and Alho, 1997; Metheun et al, 1997]. Moreover, it became apparent that none of these academics were prepared to believe the published work of other investigators [Myles, 1984; 1992; de Rooster, 1983; Daynes, 1989 Christian, 1991] and ourselves [Lichtigfeld and Gillman, 1982; Lichtigfeld and Gillman, 1983a;b; Gillman, 1985; Gillman and Lichtigfeld, 1980; 1983; 1986; 1990; 1991a; 1994a].

Naively (as will be discussed later), we assumed that these scientific purists still required a double-blind randomised study, before being convinced that the PAN treatment might have some merit, or to actually visit one of the sites in S. A. where the treatment was being used successfully. We were therefore obliged, to embark on a double-blind study [Gillman and Lichtigfeld, 2002; 2004d] after more than twenty years of safe and successful use of PAN, in many thousands of patients, without significant side-effects, or evidence of secondary addiction to PAN [Gillman and Lichtigfeld, 1990; 1997; 2002; 2006] or sequelae [Gillman and Lichtigfeld, 1990; 1997; 2002; 2006].

Double-blind, Randomised Trials with PAN versus a Benzodiazepine

As discussed above, in order to design randomised double-blind studies we had to overcome the following practical problems arising from the:

1) rapidity of the effects of the gases, which occurred within minutes and certainly within a maximum of 60 minutes, in cases where the gas or gases were effective. The benzodiazepines take much longer to act than an hour [Gillman, 2006; Gillman and Lichtigfeld, 2006];
2) fact that we were testing physically different agents, in this case tablets versus gases [Gillman, 2006; Gillman and Lichtigfeld, 2006].

3) positive effects of the placebo gas, which on its own, produced such a good therapeutic response that exposure to PAN was not required, for between 30-50% of patients [Gillman, 2006; Gillman and Lichtigfeld, 2006];

I will now describe how we overcome these difficulties by randomly assigning the cohort into 2 different groups and administering the gases double blind and randomly.

All patients that signed informed consent for the trial were given placebo gas for 20 minutes, in order to exclude placebo responders. Thus, those who responded by a 50% or more on a modified Gross scale were then excluded from further study. In this way we were able to minimise the effects of the placebo response [Gillman and Lichtigfeld, 2002; 2004d]. Despite this, we cannot exclude the possibility that a placebo response may have played some part in the therapeutic response measured because each group did eventually receive a placebo [Gillman and Lichtigfeld, 2006].

To eliminate the problems of double-blinding a gas and a tablet that acted at such different speeds we measured the therapeutic response at 2 hours after the start of treatment and we randomly assigned each group (using a random number table) as follows:

1) the one group received carefully titrated placebo gas [oxygen] and active benzodiazepine tablets (diazepam) and;
2) the other group received active gas (carefully titrated PAN) and placebo tablets (dummy tablets, identical in all other respects to the active tablets).

As mentioned above, only non-placebo responders were entered into the double-blind randomised stage of the trial. These patients were given the gases, through identical gas flowmeters (MDM Qauntiflex Matrx, Medical) marked 'A' and 'B'. The gas supply to each flowmeter was hidden, so that neither the administering nurse nor the patient were able to identify which treatment was given. The diazepam and placebo tablets were identical in appearance. One of these flowmeter heads was modified so that the nitrous oxide port at the rear of the machine was connected to the oxygen supply, so that both ports received oxygen.

All subjects entering the trial met the DSM-IV [1994] criteria for alcohol dependence and were actively withdrawing. Patients were excluded if they were suffering from delirium tremens or any of the following; chronic obstructive pulmonary pathology; or any other severe chronic organic or psychiatric pathology [Gillman and Lichtigfeld, 2002; 2004d].

The South African Medical Research Council (MRC) granted ethical approval for the studies and all subjects provided written informed consent.

In the first study [Gillman and Lichtigfeld, 2002] we observed 23 patients who were admitted fairly early on the day of the trial and were given no medication until the double-blind phase of the trial.

The code was broken only after all the data had been collated and analysed.

Of the total of 23 subjects, 11 had been given gas A (PAN plus placebo tablets) and 12 gas B (placebo gas and active tablet). In the group that received PAN plus placebo tablet, 10 subjects responded positively, while the group that received placebo gas plus active diazepam, 8 responded positively.

Despite the small sample used (n=23) PAN was significantly more effective than the benzodiazepine at p=0.05 level when compared at 120 minutes.

After the initial 120 minutes all patients were followed up for the full remainder of the 7-day inpatient detoxification program. Patients who had responded positively to PAN required small doses of oxazepam (30 mgs) nocte on the first and second day only. The remaining patients (i.e. those who had received placebo gas and active tablet), including the single patient who had not responded to PAN, were given a standard benzodiazepine detoxification i.e. diazepam 5 mgs tds for day 1-3; 5mg bd for day 2-5 and 5 mg once only for day 6. Oxazepam nocte was required for all the latter patients [Gillman and Lichtigfeld, 2002].

In the second study [Gillman and Lichtigfeld, 2004d] we pooled the above results with 28 subjects who had received diazepam the previous night, because they had arrived at the alcohol facility too late to be entered into the trial that day. We did so in order to see whether an extra dose of diazepam would make a significant difference to the result of the first study [Gillman and Lichtigfeld, 2002].

After the code had been broken, 23 subjects of the 51 had received PAN plus placebo tablet and 28 placebo gas plus active diazepam.

21 subjects responded positively to active gas plus placebo tablet, while 19 responded positively to placebo gas and active tablet.

There were 10 positive responses in the group who had been given PAN and who had not received diazepam the prior night and 1 negative response. Those in the PAN group who did receive a benzodiazepine the previous night, showed 11 positive and 1 negative responses. Thus in the PAN plus placebo tablet cohort, a total of 21subjects manifested a positive response while 2 had a negative response.

In the other cohort (i.e placebo gas plus diazepam) those not receiving a benzodiazepine the prior night had 8 positive and 4 negative responses. Those in this group that had received a benzodiazepine the night before showed 11 positive and 5 negative responses. Thus in this cohort there were 19 positive and 9 negative responses.

We found that even with an additional dose of diazepam the previous night, superimposed on the same protocol as in the first study [Gillman and Lichtigfeld, 2002], PAN plus placebo tablet is superior to placebo gas plus active diazepam at p=0.05 level [Gillman and Lichtigfeld, 2004d].

As was the case with the patients in the earlier study [Gillman and Lichtigfeld, 2002] all patients were followed up for 7 days. Those patients, who had responded positively to PAN, needed no further treatment except oxazepam [30 mgs] for night sedation usually for day 1 and 2 only. All the remaining patients i.e. those consigned to the group who had received placebo and diazepam plus the 2 non-responder to PAN were given a standard benzodiazepine regimen as described above [Gillman and Lichtigfeld, 2002]. All those detoxified with benzodiazepines required night sedation with oxazepam for 7 days [Gillman and Lichtigfeld, 2004d].

Our double-blind trials [Gillman and Lichtigfeld, 2002; 2004d] have been criticised as poorly designed and therefore useless, on the basis that 'two hours may not have been a sufficient amount of time for diazepam to exert its full therapeutic effect before symptom assessment.'[Prince and Turpin, 2008]. A criticism that is invalid, since diazepam is 'absorbed rapidly, reaching peak concentrations in about an hour' [Baldessareni, 1996]. Greenblatt and Shader [1985] note that diazepam is one of the most rapidly absorbed oral benzodiazepines 'reaching peak concentrations in the blood within one hour after dosage.'

Thus, there was at least an extra hour to cover pharmacokinetic differences that may have manifested over the cohort, and ensuring that all subjects were exposed to peak active levels of diazepam by the time the ratings were taken [Gillman and Lichtigfeld, 2002; 2004d]. Furthermore, the additional dose of diazepam, given the previous night [Gillman and Lichtigfeld, 2004d], was ignored and therefore was discounted [Prince and Turpin, 2008]. The extra dose is relevant because it is likely to have potentiated the diazepam given two hours before ratings were taken [Gillman and Lichtigfeld, 2004d] since diazepam has a long half-life, which is applicable with a multidosing schedule [Greenblatt and Shader, 1985; Baldessareni, 1996].

Furthermore they [Prince and Turpin, 2008] indicate, wrongly, that no outcome was reported after two hours. As can be seen from the description of these trials above, the benzodiazepine requirements for the PAN group was much reduced as compared to those who had been given placebo gas plus active diazepam [Gillman and Lichtigfeld, 2002; 2004d]. They also wrongly state that 'Oxazepam 30 mg was administered to subjects in both groups at bedtime.' While oxazepam was needed for a night or two for the PAN group, it was required every night for the benzodiazepine group [Gillman and Lichtigfeld, 2002; 2004d]. Prince and Turpin [2008] note that our studies did not address adverse outcomes. A recent Cochrane Review, mentions that the review did not 'indicate any causes for concern that PAN is more harmful than the benzodiazepines' [Gillman et al, 2007], showing that adverse effects of PAN are no worse than those found with benzodiazepines. In agreement with the Cochrane Review [Gillman et al, 2007] our experience with thousands of cases is that adverse effects are trivial. Alho et al [2002] used double the inhaled concentration of nitrous oxide than that would (on average) be required for PAN and yet they also reported only minor side-effects.

Of course, when PAN is used at the correct dose, there is no evidence of excitation, as reported by Alho et al [2002]. Obviously, excitation should be avoided in any tremulous, hyperadrenergic state such as alcohol withdrawal [Gillman and Lichtigfeld, 1983; Edwards, 1985]. The excitation found by Alho et al [2002], which is avoided when PAN is used at the correct dose titrated for each individual patient, was clearly due to the excessively high doses of nitrous oxide used [Alho et al, 2002].

Although Prince and Turpin [2008] note in their review that nitrous oxide is 'commonly used… …in outpatient dentistry'. Nonetheless, rather illogically, they assume that PAN 'is not a practical option in the outpatient treatment of alcohol withdrawal.' The latter assumption flies in the face of the existing evidence where it has been used on outpatients for thousands of cases in S.A. [Carey et al, 1991; Gillman and Lichtigfeld, 2006] and Finland [Gillman and Ojutkangas, 1994].

Prince and Turpin [2008] have also ignored all the other work indicating that PAN is useful for alcohol withdrawal states [Lichtigfeld and Gillman, 1982; Lichtigfeld and Gillman, 1983a;b; de Rooster, 1983; Christian, 1991; Myles, 1984; 1992; Carey et al, 1991; Gillman, 1985; Gillman and Lichtigfeld, 1986; 1990; 2002; 2004d] on the basis that none of these are randomised and double-blind. Face validity does not seem to have a place in their reckoning. Obviously it is better to have double-blind randomised trials, but that does not discount clinical observations. Observations, without such controls are still valid [Gillman and Lichtigfeld, 1997]. For instance '.....it takes only two minutes to establish the mind-blowing effect of cocaine!' [Pfeiffer, 1987]. Furthermore, a Harvard psychiatry professor states 'If something works it certainly is important to study it, but doesn't mean that people should stop using it just because it has not been proven efficacious in a double-blind study., ...' [Liu,

1996] A truth that is even more cogent when examining a treatment that on observation has obvious advantages over the 'gold-standard'. Indeed, it was this very fact, which complicated the search for a suitable double-blind technique [Gillman and Lichtigfeld, 1997; 2002; 2004d]. It is clearly dangerous to be bound slavishly to any phenomenon in medicine including double-blind studies.

Although there is no doubt that further good quality studies on the efficacy of PAN are necessary [Gillman et al, 2007; Prince and Turpin, 2008] it is clearly premature to assert that 'Nitrous oxide should not be used in the treatment of alcohol withdrawal because reputable clinical trials are lacking and its administration requires training and specialized devices.' [Prince and Turpin, 2008]. Furthermore, to assert that any health care intervention 'should not be used' because 'its administration requires training and specialized devices.' would banish much of medicine, including all surgery. This is clearly an overkill as is their concluding statement 'nitrous oxide should be avoided for this indication.' The most that these workers can say is that further work is needed before a decision can be taken on the use of PAN.

The work of Alho et al [2002; 2003] can be discounted because although they used nitrous oxide, their technique does not fulfil the criteria for PAN [Clark et al, 2006; Gillman and Lichtigfeld, 1990; Gillman and Lichtigfeld, 2004a;b;c; Gillman et al, 2007]. Their concomitant use of benzodiazepines in all groups studied [Alho et al., 2002; 2003] also disqualifies this work. By adding daytime diazepam, their study [Alho et al., 2002; 2003] 'became not analgesic nitrous oxide against a placebo, but rather nitrous oxide combined with diazepam versus placebo plus diazepam.'[Gillman and Lichtigfeld, 2004a]. Other workers have also criticised Alho et al [2002; 2003] for this poor design feature, rendering their results meaningless [Prince and Turpin, 2008].

Thus, our double-blind randomised studies [Gillman and Lichtigfeld, 2002; 2004d] supports our earlier work [Lichtigfeld and Gillman, 1982; Gillman and Lichtigfeld, 1986;1990] that PAN 'is a safe, rapid and effective therapy for acute mild to moderately severe withdrawal states' and that there is a reduction in the amount of sedative medication required when PAN is used [Lichtigfeld and Gillman, 2004d].

PAN for Treating Other Substances of Abuse Apart from Alcohol

Opioids

Kripke and Hechtman [1972] were the first workers to report after successfully treating a case of substance abuse withdrawal with concentrations of nitrous oxide consistent with PAN. Although the inhaled concentration of nitrous oxide was consistent with PAN, their technique was different because they did not titrate but rather used a proprietary 50:50 mixture of oxygen and nitrous oxide. Apart from the technique differences, 50% nitrous oxide is at the upper end of concentrations of nitrous oxide that could be considered consistent with PAN. Most subjects will respond at 40% inhaled nitrous oxide or less [Malamed, 1989].

Kripke and Hechtman [1972] described using nitrous oxide/oxygen to wean a patient heavily addicted to pentazocine. The patient had used daily doses of pentazocine ranging from 700-1000mg over 2 years. The rationale for trying nitrous oxide was to treat severe gastro-intestinal problems using the well-known analgesic properties of the gas. PAN was used daily for at least 6 hours per day for 200 days. And for the first 30 days she was given PAN for 24 hours each day, to control the intense dysphoria associated with opioid withdrawal. Apart from good pain control was the incidental finding that the PAN enabled the patient to be withdrawn from her addiction.

Another important, but incidental observation by Kripke and Hechtman [1972], was that despite the chronic exposure of the patient to nitrous oxide for 200 days, there was no sign of agranulocytosis. In fact, she had developed pneumonia during the 200 days of exposure but responded with lymphocytosis in response to the infection. This is suprising because some patients develop signs of dyshaemopiesis following chronic long-term exposures to nitrous oxide [Gillman, 1987], which clearly was not the case with this patient.

The work by Kripke and Hechtman [1972] was the first to demonstrate that relatively low concentrations of nitrous oxide could reduce the signs and symptoms of an abstinence syndrome from an opioid. More recently, these findings have been confirmed by other workers, indicating the usefulness of PAN for treating acute opioid withdrawal states [Gillman and Lichtigfeld, 1985b; Carey et al., 1991; Ojutkangas, 1991].

This work has been repeated at a number of treatment centres under the auspices of the South African. National Council for Alcoholism and Drug Dependence (S.A.N.C.A.). The latter is the largest NGO dealing with the treatment and prevention of substance abuse in S.A. One of their associated centres (Family Outreach) specialises in opioid dependency withdrawal. The Family Outreach treatment facility is located in the centre of South Africa 50 miles north of Graaf Reneit in the Western Cape Province. This facility has been using PAN as the treatment of choice for opioid withdrawal for nearly 3 years and reports high levels of success on patients treated there. Although opioid abuse is an escalating problem in S.A. there are still relatively few cases as compared with other countries [Parry et al, 2002]. As a result, there are relatively few cases on which to report. The preliminary analysis of the results of their work since 2005 follow.

26 patients who came to the Family Outreach treatment facility between August 2005 and May 2008, and were suffering form opioid withdrawal were treated for their acute withdrawal symptoms.

All patients provided written informed consent and the trial was approved by the local human ethical review board.

Each subject was given oxygen for 20 minutes followed by carefully titrated PAN for 20 minutes as described earlier in this paper. This was then followed by a pure oxygen washout.

Three patients were excluded from the analysis because their withdrawal data was incomplete.

The mean age of the sample was 23.9 years, with only 2 patients below 20 years and one above 30 years. There were 23 male and 3 female subjects.

23 patients were Caucasoid and 3 of mixed parentage (so-called coloureds). 24 had never been married , while 1 of each had been divorced or was cohabiting.

All subjects had at least secondary school education, while 14 had completed secondary school with a matriculation certificate (usually qualifying for entrance to a university). 2 subjects had achieved a completed tertiary education.

22 subjects were unemployed, 2 were in part-time employment. The employment status of the other 2 was not recorded.

All subjects were using heroin except 1 who abused dipipanone (tradename; Wellconal). 10 subjects had only used heroin, while the others had a history of using a number of other substances including cannabis, cocaine, methamphetamine, ecstasy and L.S.D. Cannabis was the most common of these other illicit drug used.

Subjects were scored before and after the gases had been administered, using the Subjective Opiate Withdrawal Scale (SOWS) [Handelsman et al, 1987].

The baseline aggregate score for the group was 711 and after oxygen and PAN exposure 300.

Thus there was a 57.8% decrease in the scores following a single application the gases.

This rapid decrease in symptoms after only 40 minutes, usually immediately after admission, results in an almost instant change in the subjects' psychological status, enabling them to rapidly abandon the sick role. They were then able to immediately enter the next stage of the rehabilitation process.

The rapidity of the therapeutic intervention using PAN is a major advantage over other treatments for acute opioid withdrawal states.

The findings at Family Outreach supports previous clinical work showing that nitrous oxide and oxygen mixtures used at doses consistent with PAN can ameliorate opioid withdrawal states [Kripke and Hechtman, 1972; Gillman and Lichtigfeld, 1985; Carey et al, 1991; Ojutkangas, 1991].

Some recent animal work, using a place preference paradigm, has provided further evidence supporting the use of PAN for treating opioid abuse. Although nitrous oxide did not itself induce conditioned place preference it reduced the expression of morphine-induced place preference [Benturquia et al, 2007]. Furthermore, in another study the increase in extracellular levels of dopamine produced by placing rats and mice in a morphine-paired compartment was blocked by nitrous oxide [Benturquia et al, 2008].

Cocaine

Cocaine abuse has only become a problem in South Africa over the last 10 or so years. Until then, it was relatively rare and limited to the rich upper classes. Indeed, by 1988 crack abuse was insignificant in S.A. [Searll, 1989]. However, since then, the proportion of those seeking treatment for cocaine, including crack cocaine, has increased as a proportion of the total demand for treatment for substance abuse in S.A. [Parry et al., 2002]. As a result, those SANCA Societies using PAN have been increasingly using PAN to treat the acute withdrawal state arising from cocaine abstinence. These SANCA Societies have reported good results when using PAN to treat cocaine abstinence syndromes.

A recent single-blind study [Gillman et al, 2006b] examined 33 subjects [25 males; 8 females] with cocaine withdrawal symptoms that were treated at the SANCA Port Elizabeth outpatient clinic with an average age of 28.1 years [range 21-42 years].

Baseline recordings using a withdrawal scale were taken and then 100% oxygen was given to eliminate placebo responders. Carefully titrated PAN was then given for 20 minutes and the withdrawal instrument applied again. A reduction in symptom score of 50% or more was taken to be a positive response, since clinical experience has shown a 50% improvement is synonymous with observed recovery. 31 of the 33 cases responded by a decrease of symptom scores of 50% or more,

5 subjects responded positively to oxygen alone and did not improve further with PAN. 11 subjects did not improve with placebo but did respond positively to PAN. 15 subjects responded positively to Oxygen but then improved by a further 50% or more after breathing PAN. 2 patients failed to respond to either oxygen or PAN. Interestingly, neither of these non-responders was suffering from the most severe withdrawal state amongst those treated. All subjects had abused crack cocaine or cocaine.

Placebo reduced craving, depression, remorse, guilt which was further decreased following PAN. Oxygen plus PAN decreased baseline scores 'by 81%, 89%, 91%, 90% and 87% respectively.' [Gillman et al, 2006b].

Thus 93.9% of the subjects were improved by the use of PAN and /or O_2 alone.

These findings confirm the empirical findings reported by the various centres using PAN to treat acute cocaine withdrawal, which appears to be worth investigating further; in particular with a double-blind randomised trial.

As discussed above, we postulated that during the pathogenesis of substance abuse withdrawal states an inbalance develops between the κ and μ opioid systems [Gillman and Lichtigfeld, 1984; Lichtigfeld and Gillman, 1996]. It is therefore significant that Mash and Staley [1999] have provided evidence that the κ_2 opioid system is upregulated during withdrawal from cocaine. It is therefore possible that PAN restores homeostasis by differentially activating the mu and kappa systems which could account for its beneficial effects during withdrawal states [Lichtigfeld and Gillman, 1996].

There is now further evidence from animal studies indicating that PAN is useful for treating substance abuse. For instance, when rats receive nitrous oxide (in subanaesthetic concentrations) in combination with amphetamine, locomotor sensitization is attenuated [Abraini et al, 2005]. Furthermore, as mentioned above for opioids, a place preference paradigm, has provided further evidence supporting the use of PAN for treating substance abuse, in this case cocaine abuse [Benturquia et al, 2007]. Although nitrous oxide did not itself induce conditioned place preference it reduced the expression of cocaine-induced place preference [Benturquia et al, 2007].

Table 1. PAN for Acute Withdrawal from Cigarettes.

	Before Treatment		After Treatment	
Symptoms	**Group Score**	**Average**	**Group Score**	**Average**
Craving	316	9.02	18	0.51
Headache/ Headpressure	181	16	0	0
Anxiety	155	4.43	0	0
Irritable	202	5.77	0	0
Tension	193	5.51	0	0
Sad/ Tearful	35	1.00	5	0.14
Drowsy	159	4.54	34	0.97
Unable to Concentrate	154	4.4	0	0
Restlessness	157	4.48	0	0
Dizziness	36	1.03	8	0.23
Sweating	46	1.31	0	0
Butterflies in Stomach	57	1.63	0	0

Papers/PAN NOVA Paper submitted Vers 2 2008

Nicotine

There have been reports that PAN can be used to ameliorate the acute nicotine withdrawal state [Shevel and Gillman 1988; Daynes and Gillman, 1994; Bayrakdarian, 2000]. In the first study, which was conducted single-blind, 35 heavy smokers (20 cigarettes/day for a minimum of 10 years), both male and female ceased smoking 24 hours before the trial started. Baseline scores were taken using a nicotine withdrawal instrument [Glassman et al, 1984] prior to titration of PAN. PAN was then titrated and the patients re-rated. All symptoms were greatly reduced (see Table 1).

Daynes and Gillman [1994] have also examined the effects of PAN on craving for tobacco (see below under section dealing with craving).

Bayrakdarian [2000] undertook an open trial to establish whether PAN could reduce cigarette smoking in a small sample (n=7). Urine cotinine samples were taken daily as an objective test of abstinence. Following PAN, cigarette use decreased from 17.1(sd=7.6) before N20 to 2.6(sd=3.42) (t=9.04, df=6, P<0.0001). All subjects reported decreased use, which was well correlated with cotinine levels (spearman r=0.94, p=0.005). 71% of subjects quit smoking completely, while the quit rate was 57% at the end of one month.

Some animal work has indicated that the endogenous opioid [Berrendero et al., 2002] and dopamine systems [Mansvelder and McGehee, 2000] are directly involved in nicotine addiction. This also provide further evidence that there is a final common pathway for addiction [Gillman and Shevel, 1988; Gillman and Lichtigfeld, 1991b] but that PAN could exert its positive effects in ameliorating the nicotine withdrawal state and craving by acting on the endogenous opioid system to restore the homeostatic balance that has been disturbed during the pathogenesis of nicotine use.

Cannabis

Cannabis is the most common illegal substance of abuse in S.A. [Parry et al, 2002]. As a result, there has been a great call on treatment facilities in S.A. to treat patient's requiring acute withdrawal from this agent. Thus, since the early 1990's, all the SANCA facilities that treat acute withdrawal states with PAN have been using it to treat acute cannabis withdrawal states. All of these centres have reported good results.

Daynes and Gillman [1994] examined the effects of PAN on cannabis craving (see below for details in the section on craving).

In a later study, also single-blind, the combination of cannabis and methaqualone was also studied. The latter combination seems to be a problem mainly confined to S.A. [Gillman et al, 2006a]. In S.A. it is colloquially known as 'white pipes'.

A cohort consisting of 101 patients (98 male and 3 female; most of whom under the age of 30) treated consecutively were given 100% oxygen followed by carefully titrated PAN single-blind. A positive response was assumed if the patient improved by 50% or more on a rating instrument [Gillman et al, 2006a].

One case of the 101 was excluded from the analysis because their data was incomplete.

Of the 100 cases analysed, 43 patients improved by a minimum of 50% after oxygen alone. Despite the improvement in 37 of the 43, they were given 20 minutes of PAN with further amelioration. 6 of the 43 did not require PAN because their aggregate rating score was zero after oxygen alone. The improvement obtained by oxygen alone in 4 cases of the 37 was reversed by PAN, possibly because the dose was poorly titrated and was excessive [Gillman et al, 2006a]. In the other 2 cases of the 6, there was an improvement when PAN was added following O_2 by a minimum of 3 points. There was no further improvement following PAN in the 31 remaining cases of the 37. A total of 57 patients did not respond positively to oxygen alone but 44 of these did respond by a 50% or more improvement to PAN on their scores at baseline. 13 patients were recalcitrant either to oxygen or PAN. In total 87 patients benefited either by breathing oxygen alone or oxygen followed by PAN.

Thus, oxygen alone, or followed by PAN was therapeutic in 87% of patients.

It would seem that this work indicates that PAN is useful for treating cannabis and cannabis/methaqualone abuse withdrawal states.

Interestingly, naloxone and naloxonazine both opioid receptor anatagonists block the stimulating effects of heroin and cannabinoids on dopamine release in the nucleus accumbens [Tanda et al, 1997]. An observation that provides some basic experimental evidence that PAN, as an opioid, could act during withdrawal states to stimulate the μ-opioid receptor system which we have proposed is underactive during withdrawal states [Gillman and Lichtigfeld, 1983;1984; Lichtigfeld and Gillman, 1996]. It also gives support further support for the concept that there is a final common pathway in the pathogenesis of substance abuse [Gillman and Shevel, 1988; Gillman and Lichtigfeld, 1991b].

Polydrug Abuse

In 1991 my colleague and I suggested that PAN would be useful for treating polydrug abuse [Lichtigfeld and Gillman, 1991]. Soon after, PAN was used to successfully treat polysubstance abuse withdrawal states caused by a wide range of agents including alcohol, nicotine, cannabis, benzodiazepines, methaqualone, heroin and cocaine [Carey et al., 1991]. The latter physicians' private practice continued to use PAN for treating addictive withdrawal states from all forms of substance abuse and reported excellent results over many additional cases [Carey, unpublished observations].

Further support for the use of PAN for polydrug abuse comes from anecdotal reports from the centres in S.A. treating acute substance abuse withdrawal with PAN. Most of these centres do not have the resources to undertake routine testing for the substances that have been used by those admitted to their facilities. Nonetheless, their staff have established by careful history taking that their clients have admitted to have abused an array of agents, apart from the one that had forced their admission.

All these clinics have found that the PAN produces amelioration of these polydrug abusers' acute withdrawal states. The classical combination of dugs used are cannabis plus alcohol; alcohol plus sedative (usually a benzodiazepine); alcohol plus nicotine and other drug combinations. In such cases, careful observation of the patient is essential, particularly if they have been abusing benzodiazepines or other sedatives. The latter patients may require careful tapering of the benzodiazepine or other sedative, after the initial withdrawal state has been completed.

Anti-Craving Properties of PAN

Alcohol

In a study of 216 patients who were craving alcohol, PAN administered for 20 minutes abolished craving in 85.19%, it was reduced in 11.57% with 3.24% recalcitrant [Daynes and Gillman, 1994].

In a study conducted in Finland, PAN was found to useful in reducing craving between relapses in 20 alcoholic outpatients [Ojutkangas and Gillman, 1994].

In more recent work on rodents, the anticraving effects of PAN has as also been demonstrated [Kosobud et al, 2006] supporting the positive clinical findings.

All the above work indicates the potential for using PAN as an outpatient treatment for alcohol withdrawal, and its possible use for relapse prevention for outpatients, which merits further investigation.

Cannabis

In a study of 53 patients craving for cannabis, a 20 minute exposure to PAN reduced craving in 13.21% of patients, abolished it completely in 84.9% and had no effect in 1.89% [Daynes and Gillman, 1994].

Nicotine

Daynes and Gillman [1994] have studied the effects of a 20 minute exposure to PAN on tobacco craving. Of the 211 patients investigated, 82.46% had their craving abolished, 16.59% had their craving reduced and 0.95% were recalcitrant [Daynes and Gillman, 1994].

In an earlier study, of 35 heavy smokers, Gillman and Shevel [1988] found that the group aggregate score of craving was 316 (average per patient 9.02) before PAN. After 20 minutes of PAN this was reduced to 18 (average per patient 0.51).

It would seem that the anticraving effects of PAN for alcohol extend to nicotine and cannabis as well.

Thus, the anticraving effects of PAN may be a major factor in assisting the acute withdrawal state from alcohol, cannabis and nicotine and possibly other substances of abuse including cocaine, methaqualone and opioids [Kripke and Hechtman, 1972; Gillman and Lichtigfeld, 1985; Gillman et al 2006a;b].

Current Status of PAN for Substance Abuse Withdrawal

During our first trial [Lichtigfeld and Gillman,1982] we were very impressed with the speed and the lasting benefit of a single 20 minutes exposure of nitrous oxide given to chronic alcoholic patients during the acute withdrawal state. We also soon realized that the method of giving oxygen before the PAN, enabled approximately 50% to be detoxified with little or no other pharmaceutical intervention, thus maximizing the placebo response [Gillman and Lichtigfeld, 1986; 1990; 2002; 2004; 2006]. Indeed, PAN is the only pharmaceutical intervention for treating substance withdrawal that maximizes the placebo response.

PAN is also extremely safe. After all, clinical experience had shown that PAN is an agent with 'an impeccable safety record that has withstood the test of time' [Clark and Brunick, 2003;2008]. Thus the safety of the agent was not in question even in terms of withdrawal states because much lower doses of nitrous oxide are used for PAN than for anaesthesia. And thousands of alcoholic patients have received nitrous oxide during anaesthesia without any sequelae [Saidman and Hamilton, 1985; Zinn et al, 1985; Gillman, 1987; Everman and Koblin, 1991].

An added safety feature when using PAN for withdrawal, is that those patients who do not respond positively to oxygen or PAN can be placed on a sedative regimen within no more than 40 minutes from the beginning of gas administration [Gillman and Lichtigfeld,1990; 2002; 2004; 2006].

As mentioned earlier, we thought that the PAN therapy would catch on like wildfire because it was economic, safe and rapidly effective [Gillman and Lichtigfeld, 1990]. We were sadly disillusioned.

Almost 30 years after its first use, the PAN treatment although used by clinicians in S.A., Finland and the U.S.A. and possibly elsewhere, has failed to be widely used, despite its advantages and there being a great many publications confirming our findings [Kripke and Hechtman, 1972; Daynes, 1989; Carey et al, 1991; Ojutkangas, 1991;Christian, 1991; Myles, 1984; 1992; Bayrakdarian, 2000; Hall, 2005] and ourselves [Lichtigfeld and Gillman, 1982; Gillman and Lichtigfeld, 1985; 1986; 1990, 1991a; 2002; 2004d; 2006; 2007; Gillman et al, 2006a;b; 2007 Gillman and Shevel, 1988].

Thirty years later, health professionals excuse their disinterest, by saying that if PAN is so good, why is it not more widely used and why have there been so few studies published from institutions in the northern hemisphere.

My late colleague Fred Lichtigfeld and I, puzzled long and hard over this apparent paradox and eventually came up with possible reasons for this peculiar response to a valid and useful treatment that has many advantages over the addictive benzodiazepines for mild to moderate alcohol and other substance abuse withdrawal states [Gillman and Lichtigfeld, 1986; 1990; 2002; 2004d; 2006; Gillman et al, 2007].

We concluded that main obstacles were due to:

1) A credibility gap existing because the PAN treatment seemed on the surface to be too good to be true and this might have been aggravated by the fact that it was discovered by clinicians while researching outside an academic institution. Linked to this credibility gap was the difficulty of explaining to our colleagues, and particularly physicians, that PAN is not merely the use of any arbitrarily chosen subanaesthetic concentration of nitrous oxide in oxygen [Alho et al, 2002; 2003; Gillman and Lichtigfeld, 1990; 1997; 2002; 2004a;b;c;d; 2006; 2007] but rather a specific technique of administering and using nitrous oxide with specific custom-made, but readily available equipment. As discussed in some details in the introduction to this review, PAN is not merely the use of nitrous oxide. It is a specific technique in which the nitrous oxide is titrated in a specific manner to the individual clinical needs of each individual subject.

    In other words, PAN is unlike other pharmacological agents such as a tablet that are used at a specific dose and at a specific time within a multidosing schedule. Instead, PAN is a gaseous pharmaceutical agent usually utilized on one occasion but with a specific technique on custom-made equipment. Thus when PAN is used it is a pharmacological agent inextricably linked to the technique of administration; unlike most other pharmaceutical preparations and agents. Unlike PAN, tablets can usually be prescribed at an average dose and dosing schedule for an entire cohort.

In summary, the technique of using PAN is an integral and essential part of applying this gaseous agent which does not normally apply to non-gaseous medications such as tablets [Gillman and Lichtigfeld, 1990; 1997; 2002; 2004a;b;c;d, 2006], without which it is not PAN [Alho et al, 2002; 2003; Clark and Brunick, 1999; 2003; 2008; Clark et al, 2006; Gillman et al, 2007].

2) The lack of commercial support for research and travel to extend knowledge, research and the actual use of PAN.

I shall now deal with these apparent problems in some detail.

Credibility Gap

The credibility gap has been caused by a combination of factors.

First and foremost, there is a credibility gap because no other agent in medicine produces a lasting effect on withdrawal states within minutes. As mentioned above, PAN correctly given for 20 minutes, rapidly reverses the withdrawal state with lasting effect in 90% of inpatients in a period of less than an hour [Lichtigfeld and Gillman, 1982; Gillman and Lichtigfeld, 1990a].

The gold-standard medication, namely the benzodiazepines take some hours to days before the withdrawal state is reversed [Saitz et al., 1994; Gillman and Lichtigfeld, 2002; 2004d]. Furthermore the pharmacokinetics properties of nitrous oxide are well known. It has very evanescent effects, which for anaethesia, wear off within minutes. Any fair-minded but skeptical scientific observer would naturally be incredulous that an evanescent agent such as nitrous oxide, could have such a profound, rapid and lasting effect on a condition that usually takes hours to days to be reversed by the benzodiazepines.

There is also the linked problem (mentioned in the introduction), namely the inability of physicians, unlike dentists, to understand that PAN cannot be given at any arbitrarily chosen concentration of nitrous oxide.

Most physicians, when discussing nitrous oxide immediately think of anaesthesia and the domain of the anesthesiologists. Unfortunately very few anaesthesiologists that work with nitrous oxide understand the method of administration and indeed the concept of PAN. This is well illustrated by the work of Alho et al [2002; 2003]. The latter investigators chose a 60% inhaled concentration of nitrous oxide, judged by the anaesthetist in their team [personal communication, Darroch] as the target for the titration. Thus they did not titrate to the patients' clinical response but rather to their arbitrarily chosen target concentration. Alho et al [2002; 2003] used nitrous oxide as an isolated pharmacological agent. This indicates that they were unaware of the theoretical and scientific basis of the differences between PAN as a linked agent-technique as opposed to nitrous oxide used as an anesthetic agent [Gillman and Lichtigfeld, 2004a;b;c].

For these (and perhaps others unknown reasons), many of our colleagues simply did not believe us. This was problem enough, but some of them, particularly in academic circles, actually went out of their way to block the progress of the PAN method and spread misinformation, fear and even confusion about it [Gagiano, 1994; Emsley, 1994; Salaspuro and Alho, 1997; Metheun et al, 1997; Gillman and Lichtigfeld, 1997]. This, although they were clearly ignorant of how PAN was used. Their ignorance is encapsulated by their own writings and work on the subject [Gagiano, 1994; Emsley, 1994; Salaspuro and Alho, 1997; Metheun et al, 1997; Gillman and Lichtigfeld, 1997; Alho et al, 2002; 2003; 2004; Berglund et al, 2003]. That their opposition was biased [Gagiano, 1994; Emsley, 1994; Salaspuro and Alho, 1997; Metheun et al, 1997; Gillman and Lichtigfeld, 1997] is demonstrated by the fact that not a single one of these armchair critics ventured to come and see for themselves either in S.A. or Finland, before denigrating the use of PAN. An untenable attitude aggravated by the fact that centres using the gases were widely dispersed geographically in both countries.

It is of some importance to note that when the unsubstantiated criticisms levelled against PAN appeared in the South African Medical Journal (S.A.M.J.) [Gagiano, 1994; Emsley, 1994] so many practitioners wrote into the journal supporting the continued use of PAN for treating substance abuse withdrawal, that the editor published only a few representative examples [Daynes, 1994; Fourie, 1994, Keizan 1994; Gillman, 1994; Gillman and Lichtigfeld, 1994b]. In ending the correspondence, he did however mention that 'The SAMJ has received numerous testimonial letters of support for analgesic nitrous oxide from those who use this to treat alcohol addiction...' [Anonymous, 1994]. Notwithstanding, the letters from Gagiano, who at that stage was President of the Society of Psychiatrists of S.A. and Emsley the Vice-President, did a great deal of damage to the credibility of the PAN therapy both in S.A. and abroad. Indeed, Berglund et al [2001], in Sweden, denigrated the nitrous oxide treatment in a government supported technical document. The latter was compiled ostensibly to inform health professionals and others concerned with the treatment of substance abuse. Berglund et al [2001] used the brief Gagiano letter [1994] as the sole reference in their negative discussion of PAN. These workers neither mentioned the letters of support published simultaneously [Lichtigfeld, 1994; Gillman 1994; Fourie 1994, Keizan, 1994, Gillman and Lichtigfeld 1994, Daynes, 1994] nor any of the numerous published papers available, which showed positive results with PAN. In a subsequent review article Berglund et al, [2003] used the identical tactics to give a one-sided view of the evidence against the use of PAN. Other workers have followed this cue and also used the Gagiano letter [1994] to paint a skewed and negative picture of the use of PAN for substance abuse withdrawal states [Alho et al, 2004; Franck, 2004] indicating how damaging the letter has been and could still be. This propagation and misuse of skewed information from the scientific literature simultaneously illustrates the:

1) power and influence of prominent individuals in medical politics;
2) and the damage that such individuals can cause, if they use their positions of influence to purvey misinformation about treatments and other matters.

Unfortunately, this biased antagonism did not only apply to academics alone. A self-styled expert on substance abuse, who became a media favourite for quotes on the subject of substance abuse, also decided to attempt to use the media to destroy the PAN method. The individual concerned was a general medical practitioner who had no higher qualification in the field, nor scientific publications on the biology of substance abuse. His attack came, despite refusing to visit the facility where the therapy had been pioneered, four years before.

He managed to find a journalist, to write a disparaging article, which was published in the largest circulation evening newspaper in S.A. i.e. 'The Star' [Openshaw, 1986]. Coincidentally, perhaps, the article was published while I was lecturing in the U.S.A. On my return to S.A., I was bombarded by journalists who believed that they were going to be able to release a juicy story on medical malpractice. I soon dampened their enthusiasm by directing them to the scientific publications on the therapy that had already appeared in prestigious medical journals [Gillman, 1986; Lichtigfeld and Gillman, 1982; 1983a;b; Gillman and Lichtigeld, 1980; 1983; 1984; 1985; 1986].

Needless to say, the media physician remained an implacable (and because of his excellent contacts with the media) also a powerful enemy of the PAN treatment. Not only did he try to start an unsuccessful media campaign against the treatment. He also applied a more insidious and destructive strategy by placing obstacles in the way of those wishing to learn more about PAN. When Ojutkangas asked for the writer's telephone number, so that he could get the information directly, he was told that I (Gillman) was too busy to be contacted and that the media expert would be the go-between. Ojutkangas heard nothing further and eventually, after loosing patience with the go-between, Ojutkangas himself phoned from Helsinki. [see below; Ojutkangas, 2005].

It is not difficult to understand that opposition by these high profile academics, regarded by most lay people and the media as being rational and fair-minded has had, and continues to have, very negative effects on the progress of the PAN method, by further widening the credibility gap. The progress of the PAN therapy could also have done without the enmity of a media favourite.

The only really open-minded interest came from clinicians who were faced, with treating this problem in their daily clinical practices [de Rooster, 1983; Myles, 1984; 1992; Carey et al, 1991; Christian, 1991; Ojutkangas, 1991; Fourie, 1994; Bayrakdarian, 2000; Ojutkangas, 2005].

The experience of Ojutkangas as reported at the World Congress of Biological Psychiatry in Vienna [Ojutkangas, 2005] is worth quoting, because it summarises the typical attitude of these armchair academics who have blocked the progress of PAN both in S.A. and Finland. Ojutkangas [2005] states:

> 'As a recovering alcoholic, with years of experience treating alcoholism, I was impressed, but highly sceptical when told that a single 20 min. exposure to PAN rapidly improves mild to moderate alcohol withdrawal states [AWS] with lasting effect'
>
> 'I later, witnessed the PAN treatment and realised this was a true breakthrough.'
>
> 'I tried to contact the pioneers, but was thwarted by the local self-styled SA addiction expert, who although obviously ignorant of PAN's use was nonetheless against it'

Ojutkangas [2005] goes on to say that after receiving the hands-on training he realised that without it, he would have been unlikely to reproduce the published work [Lichtigfeld and Gillman, 1982; Gillman and Lichtigfeld, 1986; 1990]. This is in stark contrast with Alho et al [2002] who despite numerous warnings about the importance of hands-on training [Gillman and Lichtigfeld, 1990; Gillman and Lichtigfeld, 1997; Gillman, 2007] have suggested that my colleague and I have somehow hidden the technique from them by stating 'Gillman et al do not disclose in their publications the exact protocol for administering nitrous oxide that they have used in their studies.' [Alho et al, 2004]. As emphasised repeatedly throughout this chapter, a written description, no matter how good, cannot replace hands-on training, in order to titrate to the correct defined but subtle endpoint, where the patient is relaxed.

To illustrate not only their lack of knowledge about the technique of PAN, but also their unwillingness to make the least effort to understand or learn the technique the experience of some investigators in the U.S.A. is worth mentioning. These workers, who were truly interested in attempting to replicate our work with PAN [Gillman and Lichtigfeld; Gillman and Lichtigfeld, 2006] were able to reproduce our work [Bayrakdarian, 2000; Hall, 2005] by either following the description of the method in our papers [Gillman and Lichtigfeld, 1990] or by consulting one of the numerous textbooks on the technique [Langa, 1976; Bennet; 1978; Malamed, 1989; Clark and Brunick, 1999]. Nonetheless, it is most unusual for workers to be able to use the PAN method without hands-on training by a dentist or other practitioner familiar with the PAN technique, but clearly, it can be done, using the available literature.

Nonetheless, without exception, all the many hundreds of health professionals that I have trained have agreed that they would have had difficulty in reproducing the technique without brief hands-on training.

Ojutkangas [2005] also notes that the PAN therapy attracted heavy armchair criticism by Finnish academics:

> 'in Finland, as in SA, there was strong but unfounded armchair opposition to the use of PAN, culminating in a media conference, at which, an unscientific attack was made by certain academics. Unknown to them, Gillman was present and demolished their attack, resulting in the leader of the team storming out of the conference.' [Ojutkangas, 2005].

Ojutkangas was referring particularly to academics at the Helsinki University Medical School, namely Salaspuro, Alho and colleagues [Salaspuro and Alho, 1997; Metheun et al, 1997].

Similar attacks by Salaspuro, Alho and colleagues began to appear in the lay media in Finland [Tienhaara, 1995] well before their ill-fated attempt to use nitrous oxide [Alho et al, 2002; 2003]. Indeed, these attacks have continued unabated [Järvi, 2005; Gillman, 2007] (see below). This although Alho and colleagues have been informed many times in writing both by Gillman and Lichtigfeld [1997; 2004a;bc;d] and others Clark et al [2006], that the technique they used was incorrect (in terms of PAN) and therefore totally different to the technique used by those who have had positive results with PAN [Kripke and Hechtman, 1972; Daynes, 1989; Carey et al, 1991; Ojutkangas, 1991; Christian, 1991; Myles, 1984; 1992; Bayrakdarian, 2000] and ourselves [Lichtigfeld and Gillman, 1982; Gillman and Lichtigfeld, 1985; 1986; 1990, 1991a; 2002; 2004d; 2006; 2007; Gillman et al, 2006a;b; 2007 Gillman and Shevel, 1988].

Despite this, Alho, Salaspuro and colleagues refuse to admit (except in private; personal communication Darroch, 2006) that their negative findings with nitrous oxide may have been due to their using the wrong technique.

Indeed, unlike most scientists faced with reporting on work where they were unable to reproduce the work of others, they pointedly refuse to mention the possibility that methodological differences could have accounted for their negative findings reported in their published research [Alho et al, 2002; 2003; 2004]. This intransigent attitude remains even though these differences had been spelled out unequivocally before, during and after their work on nitrous oxide was published [Gillman and Lichtigfeld, 2004a;b;c; Gillman, 2007].

These workers continue to state that nitrous oxide for alcohol withdrawal is no better than placebo [Järvi, 2005; Salaspuro, 2006]. Indeed, Alho and colleagues, as done previously [Salaspuro and Alho, 1997] suggest that the use of PAN is not only ineffective but unethical for alcohol withdrawal [Lönnqvist et al, 2007].

These attacks continue unabated, so that in another typical attack by Alho and colleagues in a Finnish lay publication, I was forced to reply to them.

In my reply, I mentioned that Alho and colleagues had refused training although the standard textbook on the use of PAN regarded this as essential [Clark and Brunick, 1999] and that their dosage was approximately double the average dose usually used to treat alcohol withdrawal. Because Alho had submitted a draft of their paper to me before publication, I emailed him as follows [Gillman; 2007]:

> 'Any paper you submit for publication with your present results must explicitly include a statement in your discussion explaining that your technique was done without the necessary training [although it was offered] and that you may have not used the correct technique and that you were not sure what the therapeutic endpoint is. Without such a statement your results are tainted. To take your results and believe that these prove that the N2O does not work in withdrawal is like giving patient cyanide from a bottle marked aspirin and then when the patient dies, publishing a finding that aspirin causes fatalities!'

As mentioned earlier, Alho et al [2002; 2003; 2004] published despite this warning, without any statement indicating their method might have been different to that which produced positive results.

I then took them to task for continuing to purvey misinformation to the Finnish people by claiming that their 'faulty work' disproved the research that demonstrated that PAN was a useful treatment for alcohol withdrawal. In addition, I questioned why they had attacked the PAN therapy for almost 10 years before attempting a clinical trial [Gillman, 2007].

In addition, they falsified the lynchpin methodological reference [Alho et al, 2002] to justify the incorrect method they had used in their original papers [Alho et al, 2002; 2003; Gillman and Lichtigfeld, 2004a;b; Gillman, 2007]. Not satisfied with a single misquote, they went further and falsified another reference [Alho et al, 2004] in response to our rebuttal of their research findings [Gillman and Lichtigfeld, 2004a;b;c].

What I did not mention [Gillman, 2007] was the internal inconsistency in their paper. In their written description they state that 'each subject received the corresponding gas treatment during 30 min'[Alho et al, 2002], but in Fig 2 of the same paper, the graph shows that the time course was more than 40 minutes [Alho et al, 2002].

I also did not mention that Alho et al [2002] had doubled the dose of nitrous oxide approved by the Finnish National Agency for Medicines (NAM). When the trial was registered with NAM in accordance with Finnish Law; they were given permission to use 30% nitrous oxide diluted with 70% oxygen. Darroch wrote to NAM and was informed that the latter had not been informed of this increased dose [personal communication 2008]. By not obtaining permission, Alho et al [2002] clearly broke the law, which calls into question their claim that their work received ethical approval from the University of Helsinki [Alho et al, 2002; 2003]. This is the only conclusion that can be drawn, unless the University of Helsinki provides ethical approval for work that involves infractions of Finnish Law.

It might therefore not surprise the reader to note that the University of Helsinki has instituted a formal inquiry [personal communication, Darroch; 2008; Pilke, 2008] to consider charges of scientific misconduct against those involved in the papers [Alho et al, 2002; 2003]. The formal inquiry followed a lengthy preliminary investigation (lasting almost 18 months) to establish whether there was prima facie evidence of misconduct.

Those cited for formal inquiry are: Alho H., Salaspuro M., Paloheimo M. and Methuen T. The charges were brought by Darroch and some of his colleagues. These charges clearly include the unethical use of human subjects in terms of the Declaration of Helsinki (as modified in 1996), which codifies the ethical use of human subjects. Other charges listed include multiple fabrication of crucial methodological references; the existence of 5 different protocols for their published work (offered to an assortment of parties at different times by some of those cited) and deliberately misinforming the scientific and lay public based on their faulty work [Alho et al, 2002; 2003].

The resistance by Alho and colleagues seems to know no limits even though he and colleagues must by now be fully aware that they have used the nitrous oxide incorrectly in their quest to replicate our findings. To illustrate this point: in February 2008, Alho wrote to the Cochrane Collaboration indicating that if their papers [Alho et al, 2002; 2003] continued to be listed as excluded studies in a Cochrane Review on PAN [Gillman et al, 2007], this would somehow reduce the credibility of the entire Cochrane Collaboration. By now, the reasons for this exclusion from any Cochrane Review on PAN must be patently clear.

To put it beyond doubt, and succinctly, the work of Alho et al [2002; 2003] was excluded [Gillman et al, 2007] because they had chosen an arbitrary (and excessively high) single target concentration of nitrous oxide. They did use nitrous oxide but not PAN, because they did not titrate the concentration of nitrous oxide to each patient's individual clinical needs. The importance of individualising the dose of nitrous oxide is stated in the review as follows:

> 'There is no fixed concentration of nitrous oxide [N2O] or oxygen [O2] because each patient receives a carefully titrated amount of N2O and O2 sufficient only to ameliorate the patient's condition.' [Gillman et al, 2007]

To this day, I cannot explain the obdurate opposition of the various academics (and the S.A. media expert), who have for no apparent scientific reason opposed the use of PAN [Openshaw, 1986; Gagiano, 1994; Emsley, 1994; Salaspuro and Alho, 1997; Methuen et al, 1997; Alho et al, 2002; 2003; 2004; Salaspuro, 2006; Lönnqvist et al, 2007]. Indeed, they seem to be prepared to go out on a limb and stake their very reputations on their false belief that PAN is useless. This, despite the overwhelming published evidence [Kripke and Hechtman, 1972; Lichtigfeld and Gillman, 1982; Gillman and Lichtigfeld, 1985; 1986; 1990, 1991a; Daynes, 1989; Carey et al, 1991; Christian, 1991; Myles, 1984; 1992; Daynes; 1989; Daynes and Gillman, 1994; 1994; Bayrakdarian, 2000; Gillman and Shevel, 1988; Gillman et al, 2006a;b; Gillman et al, 2007; Carey et al, 1991; Ojutkangas, 1991; Ojutkangas and Gillman, 1994] that PAN does ameliorate withdrawal states when correctly used [Gillman et al, 2007].

These critics [Alho et al, 2002; 2003; 2004; Methuen et al, 1997; Alho et al, 2002; 2003; 2004; Salaspuro, 2006; Lönnqvist et al, 2007] seem intent on blocking the use of PAN and also preventing any further research into the technique.

This continued and intransigent resistance to the use of PAN is clearly unfounded scientifically, but is nevertheless a very large stumbling block to the further research and progress of the use of PAN for treating substance abuse withdrawal states.

Lack of Commercial Interest in PAN

As mentioned earlier, there has never been a commercial interest in the use of PAN for treating withdrawal states. After our first publication [Lichtigfeld and Gillman, 1982], we were advised that it was still possible to obtain a patent for nitrous oxide as a new use indication for nitrous oxide. We took no heed of this good advice and did not apply for such a patent.

Our decision not to patent this new use of nitrous oxide seems, in hindsight, to have been a grave blunder. Naively, we believed that the treatment we had discovered belonged to everyone and should not be used for personal enrichment. At that stage, we did not understand that had we patented this new indication, we would have been able to interest the gas manufacturers in supporting further research into PAN, not only by ourselves but by others investigators.

We had no conception at that stage, of the importance of commercial pharmaceutical interests for promoting any novel pharmaceutical agent or new indication of an existing agent. Only later, did we realize the importance of the almost unlimited funding available from a commercial sponsor, which allows and promotes research into the agent or new application of it. It also permits emissaries from universities and other institutions to travel throughout the world informing their peers at scientific meetings of the new product, through their researches on it. It is by these means that new treatments are publicized and gain acceptance for daily use in medical practice.

Such support has been notably lacking in regard to PAN. We have received paltry support from a gas company that manufactures nitrous oxide amounting to less than US$20 000 over 32 years i.e. less than US$750 per annum since we started our researches in 1976.

It is still my considered opinion that the lack of significant research funding which would have been readily available from a commercial interest has been a major handicap.

This lack of funding has conceivably lessened the interest of other workers to attempt to repeat our work on PAN. The only exception were the Finns, who were forced, after nearly 10 years of concerted attacks on PAN in the medical and lay media [Salaspuro and Alho, 1997; Methuen et al, 1997, Tienhaara, 1995] to undertake a study. It is noteworthy that these Finnish workers make no mention of their personal conflict of interest in terms of their heated opposition to the PAN therapy prior to their study that resulted in their publications on nitrous oxide [Alho et al, 2002; 2003; 2004]. This despite the fact that the Journal of Clinical Psychopharmacology specifically required such a statement at the time they submitted their work.

Perhaps unsurprisingly, in view of the above, their studies were defective and add nothing to the debate on the efficacy of PAN for treating withdrawal states [Gillman and Lichtigfeld, 20004;a;b;c;d; Gillman et al, 2007]. Nonetheless, their papers do contribute, in that it underlines the need for hands-on training, or at the very least, a thorough understanding of the theory of the technique, if clinicians wish to replicate our work [Gillman and Lichhtigfeld, 1990; 1997; 2002; 2006].

I have been forced to emphasise the work of Alho, Salaspuro and colleagues [Alho et al, 2002; 2003] and their incorrect use of nitrous oxide to treat alcohol withdrawal states because Alho and Salaspuro are prominent in the field of alcohol research. Thus their negative findings have important political impact in the field of alcohol research and add to the credibility problems. Those who do not know better, may regard their findings as the definitive proof that nitrous oxide is ineffective for treating alcohol withdrawal states or at the very least throw doubt on the work showing positive results. For example in a recent papers referring to the positive results reported [Gillman and Lichtigfeld, 1990; 1994b; 2002], Benturquia et al [2007] state 'However, these findings have not be confirmed by a recent clinical study comparing the effects of N_2O versus placebo' [Alho et al, 2003]. This, particularly as these workers [Alho et al, 2002; 2003], despite being appraised of their incorrect technique [Gillman and Lichtigfeld, 2004a;bc;c;d; Gillman et al, 2007] continue to propagate the idea that their work shows that nitrous oxide is no better than placebo for treating alcohol withdrawal states [Salaspuro, 2006; Lönnqvist et al, 2007].

Conclusion

What of the future? Hopefully those who read this paper and acknowledge the problems with the work of Alho et al [2002; 2003] will discount their work and attempt themselves, after receiving hands-on training, to replicate the use of PAN to treat substance abuse withdrawal states. But that is only one aspect of this fascinating opioid gas [Gillman and Lichtigfeld, 1994a; Gillman and Lichtigfeld, 2006]. The development of the endopepditases, which extend the biological half-life of the endogenous opioids [Roques et al, 1993; Coudoré-Civiale et al, 2001], could be used in combination with PAN to treat substance abuse states. It is also possible, that research will show that the synergism between the endopeptidases [Roques et al, 1993; Coudoré-Civiale et al, 2001], and PAN will produce enough analgesia to enable surgical anaesthesia to be obtained without unconsciousness.

Acknowledgments

I would like to acknowledge a debt of gratitude to the late Frederick J. Lichtigfeld, my scientific partner of many years, who passed away in 2005 and to whose memory this work is dedicated.

References

Abraini, J. H., David, H. N. and Lemaire, M [2005]. Potentially neuroprotective and therapeutic properties of nitrous oxide and xenon. *Annals of the New York Academy of Sciences 1053*: 289-300.

Alho, H., Methuen, T., Paloheimo, M., Strid, N., Seppä, K., Tiainen, J., Salaspuro, M. and Roine, R. [2002]. Long-term effects of and physiological responses to nitrous oxide gas treatment during alcohol withdrawal: a double-blind, placebo-controlled trial. *Alcoholism: Clinical and Experimental Research 26*: 1816-22.

Alho, H., Metheun, T., Paloheimo, M., Seppä, K., Strid, N., Apter-Kaseva, N., Tiainen, J., Salaspuro, M. and Roine, R. [2003]. Nitrous oxide has no effect in the treatment of alcohol withdrawal syndrome: double-blind placebo-controlled randomised trial. *Journal of Clinical Psychopharmacology 23*: 211-14.

Alho, H., Metheun, T., Paloheimo, M., Strid, N., Seppä, K., Tiainen, J., Salaspuro, M., Roine, R. [2004]. Reply: Controlled technique demonstrates no benefit from nitrous oxide gas treatment on alcohol withdrawal. *Journal of Clinical Psychopharmacology 24*: 239-240.

Anonymous [1994]. Editorial note. *South African Medical Journal 84*: 708.

Baldessareni, R. J.[1996]. Psychosis and Anxiety In: J.G. Hardman, Limbird, L.E., Molinoff, P.B, Ruddon, R.W., A. Goodman-Gilman [Eds.], *Goodman & Gilman's The pharmacological Basis of Therapeutics*, [pp. 399-430], 9th Ed, New York: MacMillan.

Bayrakdarian, C. Effectiveness of nitrous Oxide [N_20] in reducing cigarette smoking in subjects with nicotine dependence. *American Psychiatric Association Meeting [Abstract]* May 2000. p.2h.

Bennett, C. R. [1978]. *Conscious-sedation in dental practice*. St Louis: Mosby.

Benturquia N., Le Guen, S., Canestrelli, C., Lagente, V., Apiou, G., Roques, B.P., Noble, F. [2007]. Specific blockade of morphine- and cocaine-induced reinforcing effects in conditioned place preference by nitrous oxide in mice. *Neuroscience 149* :477-86.

Benturquia N, Le Marec T, Scherrmann, J. M. and Noble, F. *Neuroscience*. 2008 May 21. (Epub ahead of print).

Berglund, M., Andréasson, S., Franck, J, Fridell, M., Håkanson, I., Johansson, B.-A., Lindgren, A., Lindgren, B., Nicklasson, L., Rydberg, U., Salaspuro, M., Thelander, S., Andreasson, S. and Ojehagen, A. [2001]. Lustgas in Behandling av alkohol-och narkotikaproblem [Translation: Nitrous oxide in treatment of alcohol and drug abuse] *SBU [Swedish Council of Technology Assessment in Health Care]*.August volume 1: 994-95.

Berglund, M., Thelander, S., Salaspuro, M., Franck, J., Andreasson, S. and Ojehagen, A. [2003] Treatment of alcohol abuse; an evidence-based review. *Alcohol: Clinical and Experimental Research 27*: 1645-1656.

Berrendero, F., Kieffer, B. L. and Maldonado, R. [2002]. Attenuation of nicotine-induced antinociception, rewarding effects, and dependence in mu-opioid receptor knock-out mice. *Journal of Neuroscience 22*: 10935-40.

Carey, C., Clark, A. and Saner, T. [1991]. Analgesic nitrous oxide for addictive withdrawal states in general practice. *South African Medical Journal 79*: 516.

Christian, M. K. [1991]. Analgesic nitrous oxide for management of addictive withdrawal: a successful implementation in a Third World alcohol rehabilitation programme. *36th International Institute on the Prevention and Treatment of Alcoholism [Paper]* Stockholm, June 1991.

Clark, M., Clark A., Campbell., S.A. [2006]. Technique for the administration of nitrous oxide/oxygen sedation to ensure psychotropic analgesic nitrous oxide [PAN] effects. *International Journal of Neuroscience 116*:871-877.

Clark, M., Brunick, A. [1999]. *Handbook of nitrous oxide and oxygen sedation*. 1st Edition, St Louis: Mosby.

Clark, M., Brunick, A. [2003]. *Handbook of nitrous oxide and oxygen sedation*. 2nd Edition, St Louis: Mosby.

Clark, M. and Brunick, A. [2008]. *Handbook of nitrous oxide and oxygen sedation*. 3rd Edition, St Louis: Mosby.

Cohen, P. J.[1975]. Signs and stages of anesthesia. In: L.S. Goodman, A. Gilman, A.G. Gilman, G.E. Koelle [Eds.], *The pharmacological basis of therapeutics*, [pp. 60-65], New York: Macmillan.

Coudoré-Civiale, M. A., Méen, M., Fournié-Zaluski, M.-C., Boucher, M., Bernard P Roques, B. P. and Eschalier. A. [2001]. Enhancement of the effects of a complete inhibitor of enkephalin-catabolizing enzymes, RB 101, by a cholecystokinin-B receptor antagonist in diabetic rats. *British Journal of Pharmacology 133*: 179–185.

Daynes, G. [1989]. The initial management of alcoholism using oxygen and nitrous oxide: a transcultural study. *International Journal of Neuroscience 49*: 83-86.

Daynes, G. [1994]. Nitrous oxide for alcohol withdrawal. South African Medical Journal 84: 708.Daynes, G., Gillman, M.A. [1994]. Psychotropic analgesic nitrous oxide prevents craving after withdrawal for alcohol, cannabis and tobacco. *International Journal of Neuroscience 76*: 13-16.

De Rooster, [1983]. Die effektiwitiet van distikstofksied in die behandeling van die alkohol-onttrekingsindroom [Translation: The effectiveness of nitrous oxide in the treatment of the alcohol withdrawal state]. Thesis accepted in fulfilment of the requirements of M.A. [Clinical Psychology] at Rand Afrikaans University, South Africa.

Edwards, R. [1985]. Editorial. Anaesthesia and alcohol. *British Medical Journal 291*: 423-24.

Emsley, R.[1994]. Untitled. *South African Medical Journal 84*:516.

Everman, B. W. and Koblin, D. D. [1991]. Again, chronic administration of ethanol, and acute exposure to nitrous oxide: effects on vitamin B_{12} and folate status in rats. *Mechanisms of Ageing and Development* 62: 229-243.

Fourie J. Distikstofoksied [Translation: Nitrous oxide]. [1994]. *South African Medical Journal 84*: 516.

Franck J. Expert response to Gillman/Alho. [2004]. *Alcoholism: Clinical and Experimental Research 28*: 1275.

Frost, E. A. M. [1985]. A history of nitrous oxide: In E.I. Eger 11 [Ed.], *Nitrous oxide/N2O* [pp. 1-22]. New York: Elsevier.

Gagiano, C. A. [1994]. Nitrous oxide for alcohol withdrawal and other psychiatric disorders. *South African Medical Journal 84*:359.

Gillman, M. A. [1985]. *Nitrous oxide as an opioid agonist: some experimental and clinical applications*. Thesis accepted in fulfilment of the requirements of DSc at Potchefstroom University for CHO, South Africa.

Gillman, M. A. [1986]. Nitrous oxide, an opioid addictive agent. *American Journal of Medicine 8l*: 97-l02.

Gillman, M. A. [1987]. Editorial. Haematological changes caused by nitrous oxide: cause for concern? *British Journal of Anaesthesia 59*: 143-146.

Gillman,M. A.[1992]. Nitrous oxide abuse in perspective. *Clinical Neuropharmacology 15*: 297-306.

Gillman, M. A [1994]. Analgesic nitrous oxide for addictive withdrawal. *South African Medical Journal 84*: 516.

Gillman, M. A. [1995]. Nitrous oxide has a very low abuse potential. *Addiction 90*: 439.

Gillman, M. A. [1996]. Envy as a retarding force in science. U.K. Aldershot: Avebury.

Gillman, M. A. [2006]. Psychotropic analgesic nitrous oxide for addictive withdrawal. *Chinese Journal of Drug Dependence 14*: 73-4.

Gillman, M. A. [2007]. Ilokaasum oikea käyttö auttaa [Translation: Laughing gas helps when used correctly]. *Suomen Kuvalehti 2*:57.

Gillman M. A. [2008]. Editorial: Tobacco cessation and nitrous oxide/oxygen sedation. *South African Dental Journal 63*: 66.

Gillman, M. A, Harker, N. and Lichtigfeld, F. J. [2006a]. Combined cannabis/methaqualone withdrawal treated with psychotropic analgesic nitrous oxide. *International Journal of Neuroscience 116*: 859 - 869.

Gillman, M. A. Lichtigfeld, F.J. [1980]. Nitrous oxide and treatment of withdrawal symptoms. *Lancet 2*: 803.

Gillman, M. A. and Lichtigfeld, F. J. [1983]. Receptor hypothesis of the alcohol withdrawal state. In Mandel, P., DeFeudis, F.V. [Eds.], *CNS Receptors from Molecular Pharmacology to Behaviour*. Raven Press: New York. pp.405-415.

Gillman, M.A. and Lichtigfeld, F. J. [1984]. The opioid and anti-opioid system in addiction. *South African Medical Journal 66*: 592.

Gillman, M. A. and Lichtigfeld, F. J. [1985]. Analgesic Nitrous Oxide : Adjunct to clonidine for opioid withdrawal. *American Journal of Psychiatry 142*: 784-785.

Gillman, M. A. and Lichtigfeld, F. J. [1986]. Minimal sedation required with nitrous oxide-oxygen treatment of the alcohol withdrawal state. *British Journal of Psychiatry 148*: 604-606.

Gillman, M. A. and Lichtigfeld, F. J. [1987]. Nitrous oxide analgesia is potentiated by low dose of naloxone: More possible evidence of an hyperalgesic opioid system. *South African Journal of Science 83*: 560-563.

Gillman, M. A. and Lichtigfeld, F. J. [1990]. Analgesic nitrous oxide for alcohol withdrawal: a critical appraisal after 10 years' use. *Postgraduate Medical Journal 66*: 543-546.

Gillman, M. A and Lichtigfeld, F. J. [1991a]. Placebo and analgesic nitrous oxide for the alcohol withdrawal state. *British Journal of Psychiatry 159*: 672-675.

Gillman, M. A. and Lichtigfeld, F. J. [1991b]. The opioid effects of analgesic [subanesthetic] nitrous oxide on the alcohol withdrawal state. *Annals of the New York Academy of Sciences 625*: 784-785.

Gillman, M. A. and Lichtigfeld, F. J. [1994a]. Opioid properties of psychotropic analgesic nitrous oxide [laughing gas]. *Perspectives in Biology and Medicine 38*: 125-138.

Gillman, M. A. and Lichtigfeld, F. J. [1994b]. The uses of analgesic nitrous oxide in neuropsychiatry. *South African Medical Journal 84*: 706.

Gillman, M. A. and Lichtigfeld, F. J. [1997]. The current status of analgesic nitrous oxide for treating alcoholic withdrawal states. *Suomen Laakarilehti [Finnish Medical Journal] 52*: 1055-58.

Gillman, M. A. and Lichtigfeld, F. J. [2002]. Randomised double-blind trial of psychotropic analgesic nitrous oxide compared with diazepam for alcohol withdrawal state. *Journal of Substance Abuse Treatmant 22*: 129-134.

Gillman, M. A. and Lichtigfeld, F. J. [2004a]. An incorrect technique guarantees failure. *Alcoholism: Clinical and Experimental Research 28*: 1273-1274.

Gillman, M. A. and Lichtigfeld, F. J. [2004b]. Further comments on the effects of nitrous oxide treatment on alcohol withdrawal. *Journal of Clinical Psychopharmacology 24*: 473-475.

Gillman, M. A. and Lichtigfeld, F. J. [2004c]. Correct use of analgesic nitrous oxide for the alcohol withdrawal state essential. *Journal of Clinical Psychopharmacology 24*: 238-239.

Gillman, M. A. and Lichtigfeld, F. J. [2004d]. Enlarged double-blind randomised trial of benzodiazepines against psychotropic analgesic nitrous oxide for alcohol withdrawal. *Addictive Behaviors 29*: 1183-1187.

Gillman M. A. and Lichtigfeld, F. J. [2006]. Psychotropic analgesic nitrous oxide [PAN] as a probe of the endogenous opioid system in man and for treating substance abuse withdrawal In: L.A. Bennet [Ed.], *New Topics in Substance Abuse Treatment*, [pp. 1-72].New York: Nova Science.

Gillman, M. A. and Lichtigfeld, F. J. , Harker, N. [2006b]. Psychotropic analgesic nitrous oxide for acute cocaine withdrawal in man. *International Journal of Neuroscience 116*: 847-57.

Gillman, M. A. and Lichtigfeld, F. J. , Young, T. [2007]. Psychotropic analgesic nitrous oxide for alcoholic withdrawal states. [Review]. *The Cochrane Library, Issue* 2

Gillman, M. A. and Shevel, J. [1988]. Analgesic nitrous oxide and oxygen for acute withdrawal from cigarette smoking. *Proceedings of Drug and Alcohol Forum*, January 1988. pp. 66-74.

Glassman, A. H., Jackson, W. K., Walsh, B. T. and Roose, S. P. [1984]. Cigarette craving, smoking withdrawal and clonidine. *Science 226*: 864-866.

Greenblatt, D. J. and Shader, R. I. [1985]. Clinical pharmacokinetics of the benzodiazepines. In: D.E. Smith, D.R. Wesson (Eds.). *The benzodiazepines: current standards for medical practice*, (pp.43-58) Lancaster: MTP Press.

Handelsman, L., Cochran, K. J., Aronson, M. J., Ness, R., Rubinstein, K. J. and Kanof, P. D. [1987]. Two new rating scales for opiate withdrawal. *American Journal of Drug and Alcohol Abuse 13*: 293-308.

Hall, M. [2005].Quitting smoking: *A laughing matter with nitrous Oxide.* http://maps.org/news-letters/v12n2/12223hal.html Accessed 2008-05-19.

Järvi, U. [2005]. Harva suuttuu, jos lääkäri kysyy alkoholinkäytöstä. [Translation: Very few become angry, if the doctor asks about alcohol use]. *Suomen Lääkärilehti [Finnish Medical Journal] 60*: 1646.

Kahn, R. S. [1983]. Treatment of alcoholic withdrawal states with oxygen and nitrous oxide. *South African Medical Journal 63*: 65-66.

Keizan, A. [1994]. Analgesic nitrous oxide is a very safe agent. *South African Medical Journal 84*: 516.

Kosobud, A. E. K., Kebabian, C. E. and Rebec, G. V. [2006].Nitrous oxide acutely suppresses ethanol consumption in HAD and P rats. *International Journal of Neuroscience 116*: 835-45 .

Kripke, B. J. and Hechtman, H. B. [1972]. Nitrous oxide for pentazocine addiction and intractable pain. *Anesthesia and Analgesia 51*: 520-526.

Langa, H. [1976]. *Relative Analgesia in Dental Practice: Inhalation Analgesia with Nitrous Oxide*. Philadelphia: W B. Saunders.

Lichtigfeld, F. J. [1994]. Analgesic nitrous oxide for addictive withdrawal. *South African Medical Journal 84*: 513.

Lichtigfeld, F. J., Gillman, M. A. [1982]. The treatment of alcoholic withdrawal states with oxygen and nitrous oxide. *South African Medical Journal 61*: 349-351.

Lichtigfeld, F. J. and Gillman, M. A. [1983a]. Treatment of alcoholic withdrawal states with oxygen and nitrous oxide. *Psychiatry Digest June*: 12-13.

Lichtigfeld, F. J. and Gillman, M. A. [1983b]. The treatment of alcoholic withdrawal states with oxygen and nitrous oxide. *South African Medical Journal 63*: 66.

Lichtigfeld, F. J., Gillman, M. A. [1989a]. The effect of placebo in the alcohol withdrawal state. *Alcohol & Alcoholism 24*: 109-112.

Lichtigfeld, F. J., Gillman, M. A. [1989b]. Analgesic nitrous oxide for alcohol withdrawal is better than placebo. *International Journal of Neuroscience 49*:71-74.

Lichtigfeld, F. J., Gillman, M. A. [1991]. Combination therapy with carbamazepine/ benzodiazepine for polydrug analgesic/depressant withdrawal. *Journal of substance Abuse Treatment 8*: 293-295.

Lichtigfeld, F. J., Gillman, M. A. [1996]. Role of dopamine mesolimbic system in opioid action of psychotropic analgesic nitrous oxide [PAN] in alcohol and drug withdrawal. *Clinical Neuropharmacology 19*: 246-50.

Liu, L. [1996]. Hand waving?, quoting van der Kolk B.A. *The Sciences 36*:13.

Lönnqvist, J., Alho, H., Aro, H., Eriksson, P., Isometsä, E., Kaprio, J., Kiianmaa, K.,Kuoppasalmi, K., Lillsunde, P., Marttunen, M., Partonen, T., Portman, M., Seppälä, T. and Suvisaari, J. [2007]. *Kansanterveyslaitoksen Julkaisuja B* 21/2007:176. National Public Health Institute Department of Mental Health and Alcohol Research Background material for the international evaluation. Accessed 2008-05-20 ww.ktl.fi/attachments/ suomi/julkaisut/julkaisusarja_b/2007/2007b21.pdf

Malamed, S. F. [1989]. *Sedation: A guide to patient management*, 2nd Edition. St Louis: Mosby.

Mansvelder, H. D. and McGehee, D. S. [2000]. Long-term potentiation of excitatory inputs to brain reward areas by nicotine. *Neuron 27*: 349-57.

Marshall, B. and Wollman, H. [1985].History and principles of anesthesiology, In: A. Goodman-Gilman, L.S. Goodman, T.W. Rall, F. Murad, [Eds.], *The pharmacological Basis of Therapeutics*, [pp. 260-275], 7th Ed, New York: MacMillan.

Mash, D. C. and Staley, J. K. [1999]. D3 dopamine and kappa opioid receptor alterations in human brain of cocaine-overdose victims. *Annals of the New York Academy of Sciences 877*: 507-22.

Metheun, T., Poikolainen, K. and Roine, R. P. [1997]. Alkoholin aiheuttamien vieroitusoireiden hoito-mika on ilokaasun asema ? [Translation: Treatment of alcohol withdrawal symptoms – status of nitrous oxide?] *Suomen Laakarilehti [Finnish Medical Journal] 52*: 989-992.

Myles, M. J. [1984].Treatment of the alcohol withdrawal state with nitrous oxide/oxygen. *South African Medical Journal 65*: 948.

Myles, M. J. [1992]. Managing alcohol withdrawal states with oxygen and nitrous oxide. *Nursing RSA 7*: 9-10.

Ojutkangas, R. [1991]. Psychotropic analgesic nitrous oxide: rapid safe therapy for addictive withdrawal. *Postgraduate Medical Journal 67*: 1027-1028.

Ojutkangas, R. and Gillman, M. A.[1994]. Psychotropic analgesic nitrous oxide for treating alcohol withdrawal in an outpatient setting. *International Journal of Neuroscience 76*: 35-39.

Ojutkangas, R. [2005]. Pioneering PAN in Finland for withdrawal states: Success despite biased opposition. *World Journal of Biological Psychiatry 6 [Supplement 1]*:150-151.

Openshaw, J. [11 January 1986]. Call for probe into gas treatment. *The Star*: p.5

Parry, C. D. H., Bhana, A., Pluddermann, A., Myers, B., Siegfried, N., Morojelle, N. K., Flisher, A. J. and Kozell, N. J. [2002]. The South African Community Epidemiology Network on Drug Use [SACENDU]: description, findings [1997-1999] and policy implications. *Addiction 97*: 969-976.

Pfeiffer, C. C. [1987]. *Mental illness and schizophrenia.* Wellingborough, UK: Thorsons,

Pilke, A. [5 July 2008] Krapulahoidoista riitaa Suomen ja Australian välillä. (Translation: Argument between Finland and Australia about hangover treatments). *Helsingin Sanomat* p.A6

Prince, V. and Turpin, K. R. [2008]. Treatment of alcohol withdrawal syndrome with carbemazepine, gabapentin, and nitrous oxide. *American Journal of Health-System Pharmacy 65*: 1039-1047.

Roques, B. P., Noble, F., Daugeâ , V., Fournieâ -Zaluski, M.C., Beaumont, A. [1993]. Neutral endopeptidase 24-11: structure,inhibition and experimental and clinical pharmacology. *Pharmacology Reviews. 45*: 87-146.

Saidman, L. S. and Hamilton, W. K. [1985]. We should continue using nitrous oxide: In E.I. Eger 11 [Ed.], *Nitrous oxide/N2O* [pp. 345-353]. New York: Elsevier.

Saitz, R., Mayo-Smith, M. F., Roberts, M. S., Redmond, H. A., Bernard, D. R. and Calkins, D. R.[1994]. Individualized treatment for alcohol withdrawal. A randomised double-blind controlled trial. *Journal of the American Medical Association 272*: 519-523.

Salaspuro, M. [2006]. Slide 13, 9th international symposium on substance abuse treatment: Finnish Evidence Based guidelines for the Treatment of Alcohol and Drug Abusers. , University of Helsinki. Working group appointed by the Finnish Society of Addiction Medicine. Accessed 2008-05-20 http://www.nad.fi/sat2006/presentations/ Salaspuro.ppt

Salaspuro, M. and Alho, H. [1997]. Lustgasbehandling och medicinska etikens gränser [Translation: Nitrous oxide treatment and the boundaries of medical ethics]. *Suomen Lääkärilehti [Finnish Medical Journal] 52*: 942-43.

Searll, A. [1989]. *It can't happen to me*. [pp.70-80]. Cape Town: Struik Publishers.

Skelly, A. M. [1998]. Dentistry. In: J.G. Whitwam, R.F. McCloy, [Eds.], *Principles and practice of sedation* [pp. 214-19], Oxford: Blackwell.

Smith, R. A. and Beirne, O. R. [1985]. The use of nitrous oxide by dentists. In E.I. Eger 11 [Ed.], *Nitrous oxide/N2O* [pp. 282-304]. New York: Elsevier.

Tanda, G., Pontieri, F. E. and Di Chiara, G. [1997] Cannabinoid and heroin activation of mesolimbic dopamine transmission by a common mu1 opioid receptor mechanism. *Science 276*: 2048- 2050.

Tienhaara, H. [29 January 1995]. Alkoholiprofessori ja menetelmän kehittäjä napit vastakkain. Ilokaasuhoidosta tuli iso riita [Alcohol professor and developer of treatment in argument]. *Iltalehti [Afternoon News]* p.1.

Zinn, S. E., Fairley, H. B. and Glenn, J. D. [1985]. Liver function in patients with mild alcoholic hepatitis, after enflurane, nitrous oxide-narcotic, and spinal anesthesia. *Anesthesia and Analgesia 64*: 487-490.

INDEX

A

Abraham, 200
abstraction, 50, 93, 94, 116, 117, 118, 120, 122, 127, 135
abuse, ix, x, 23, 24, 30, 32, 39, 44, 214, 215, 218, 219, 226, 227, 228, 229, 230, 231, 232, 233, 235, 239, 241, 242, 243, 245, 247
academic motivation, 145
academic problems, 34
academic tasks, 155
access, 2, 3, 5, 10, 11, 51, 68, 121, 135, 155
accessibility, 1, 8, 10, 113
accounting, 62, 80
accuracy, 109, 126
achievement, 69, 106
acne, 151
acoustics, 7
activation, 25, 28, 29, 53, 110, 113, 117, 121, 136, 137
adaptation, 30, 47, 52, 143, 146, 147, 148, 152, 155, 159, 163, 165, 167, 173, 174, 181, 185, 201
ADHD, 20, 22, 23, 26, 35
adjustment, 41, 72, 101, 155, 185, 186
administrators, 10, 11
adolescence, vii, 15, 16, 20, 21, 29, 31
adolescent boys, 32
adolescent development, 187
adolescent psychopathy, 20
adolescents, viii, 20, 24, 32, 33, 141, 142, 143, 144, 146, 147, 148, 150, 155, 169, 177, 180, 181, 182, 183, 184, 185, 186, 187
adult literacy, 191, 194
adulthood, 20, 21, 22, 26, 29, 31, 34, 144, 184, 187
adults, 34, 144, 145, 147, 153, 154, 155, 157, 165, 167, 174, 182, 186
adverse effects, ix, 214, 225
aetiology, 22
affective reactions, 17, 48
Africa, ix, x, 2, 213, 214, 218, 227, 228, 243
African Americans, 202
Afrikaans, 243
age, viii, 16, 19, 24, 26, 28, 31, 32, 34, 35, 38, 98, 104, 119, 123, 126, 133, 144, 148, 150, 156, 179, 191, 195, 197, 198, 199, 200, 201, 202, 203, 204, 205, 206, 207, 208, 209, 210, 227, 228, 230
agencies, 22
agent, 43
aggression, 19, 20, 21, 23, 27, 31, 32, 35, 38
aggressive behavior, 32, 44
aggressiveness, 29
aging, 103, 104
agonist, x, 214, 243
agoraphobia, 38, 41, 42, 44, 65, 71, 72, 75
agranulocytosis, 227
AIDS, 61
Albania, 198, 199
alcohol, 42, 46
alcohol abuse, 242
alcohol consumption, 46
alcohol dependence, 223
alcohol research, 240
alcohol use, 245
alcohol withdrawal, ix, 213, 217, 220, 225, 226, 232, 236, 238, 240, 241, 242, 243, 244, 245, 246, 247
alcoholics, 216
alcoholism, 236, 243
algorithm, 97
alternative, 49, 54, 55, 60, 79, 93, 129
ambivalent, 131
American Psychiatric Association, 11, 40, 44, 70, 181, 242
American Psychological Association, 138, 187
amnesia, 125, 131
amplitude, 65, 102
amygdala, 25, 26, 27, 28, 29, 30

anaesthesiologist, 215
anaesthesiologists, 234
analgesic, 215, 226, 227, 235, 242, 243, 244, 245, 246
anger, 31, 38, 40, 74, 194
animals, 20, 38
antagonism, 235
antidepressant, 208
antidepressants, 206
antisocial acts, 20, 29
antisocial behavior, 33, 35, 183
antisocial children, 34
antisocial offenders, 20
antisocial personality, vii, 18, 19, 20, 21, 22, 23, 24, 29, 31, 32, 33, 34, 35
antisocial personality disorder, vii, 18, 19, 20, 21, 22, 23, 24, 29, 31, 32, 33, 34, 35
anxiety, vii, 10, 20, 21, 37, 38, 39, 40, 41, 42, 43, 44, 45, 46, 47, 48, 49, 50, 51, 52, 53, 54, 55, 56, 57, 58, 59, 60, 61, 62, 63, 64, 65, 66, 67, 68, 69, 70, 71, 72, 73, 74, 75, 143, 148, 149, 150, 160, 163, 178
anxiety disorder, 21, 37, 38, 40, 41, 42, 44, 48, 49, 50, 51, 52, 53, 54, 59, 61, 66, 68, 69, 70, 71, 72, 73, 74, 75
anxiety reaction, 53, 54, 55
APA, vii, 1, 11, 22, 147, 149
apples, 109
appointments, 8, 205
argument, 93, 109, 115, 130
arithmetic, 124
Armenia, 198
arousal, 25, 26, 34, 56
Asian countries, 198
asocial, 16
assault, viii, 71, 74, 190, 191, 192
assertiveness, 67
assessment, 2, 3, 10, 19, 29, 31, 68, 74, 186, 224
assimilation, 123
association, 21, 23, 32, 46, 47, 48, 68
assumptions, 60, 61
asylum, 61
asymptomatic, 158, 164, 169, 171, 175, 177
atmosphere, 155
atoms, 88, 89, 95
attachment, vii, 15, 150, 151, 160
attacks, 41
attention, 20, 27, 28, 30, 32, 51, 52, 53, 54, 55, 56, 63, 109, 116
Attention Deficit Hyperactivity Disorder, 26
attitudes, 60, 71
attribution, 20
Austria, 5, 198, 199, 208
authorities, 4, 31
authority, 22
autogenic training, 63
automatisms, 55
autonomic activity, 34
autonomic nervous system, 26, 27, 30
autonomy, 142, 146, 182
autopsy, 207
avoidance, 19, 25, 42, 46, 48, 52, 53, 54, 55, 56, 58, 66, 68, 69, 75
avoidance behavior, 48, 53, 54, 55, 68
awareness, 123

B

bacterium, 46
bad habits, 54
baggage, 107
ban, 201
banks, 194
Barbados, 198
barbiturates, 221
barriers, 3, 11, 82, 194
base, 75, 94, 125, 164, 242
Bayesian theory, 140
Beck Depression Inventory, 149
beer, 92
behavior, 33, 34, 43, 44, 45, 46, 48, 50, 52, 53, 54, 55, 65, 66, 67, 68, 69, 73, 74, 123
behavior modification, 73
behavior therapy, 54, 55, 65, 66, 67, 68, 69
behavioral disorders, 75, 143, 148, 150, 178
behavioral models, 68
behaviorism, 128
behaviors, 44, 46, 48, 51, 52, 53, 54, 55, 58, 68, 75, 150, 155, 182, 183, 185
Beijing, 211
Belarus, 198, 199
beneficial effect, 229
beneficiaries, 10
benefits, 3, 221
benzodiazepine, 221, 223, 224, 225, 231, 246
bias, 23, 116, 128, 180
biofeedback, 55
biological processes, 56
birth, 27, 31
blame, 20
blasphemy, 43
blindness, 86, 97, 137
blocks, 52
blood, 29, 35, 224
body, 22, 63, 65, 86, 92, 94, 100, 122, 134
body image, 143, 150, 178

bonding, 142, 147, 155, 170, 172, 177
borderline personality disorder, 25, 32
boredom, 18, 19
boys, 26, 32, 33, 35
brain, vii, viii, 15, 16, 17, 25, 26, 27, 28, 29, 32, 33, 34, 53, 77, 78, 79, 80, 81, 82, 85, 89, 90, 91, 92, 93, 94, 95, 96, 97, 98, 99, 100, 102, 108, 112, 114, 115, 117, 119, 120, 125, 126, 127, 130, 131, 132, 134, 135, 136, 137, 138, 140, 246
brain activity, 28
brain damage, 126, 127
brain functioning, 34
brain structure, 16, 25
brainstem, 26, 27
Brazil, 195, 200, 208
breakdown, 142
breathing, 55, 63, 64, 65, 67, 68, 151, 229, 231
buffer, 121
building blocks, 124
Bulgaria, 198, 199
bullying, 144
bun, 125

C

Cairo, 6, 12
Canary Islands, 1, 2, 3, 4, 5, 6, 10, 11, 12
cannabinoids, 231
cannabis, ix, 214, 218, 219, 228, 230, 231, 232, 243, 244
carbamazepine, 246
carbon, 220
carbon dioxide, 220
caregivers, vii, 15, 21
Caribbean, 198
case studies, 5
cast, 84, 104
catalyst, 89
categorization, 112
causal relationship, 179, 195
causality, 125
cell, 121
central nervous system, 79, 138
cerebral function, vii, 15
certificate, 227
challenges, 16, 73, 142
charm, 19
cheese, 102
chemical, 80, 89, 90, 96, 136
Chicago, 72
child maltreatment, 21
child mortality, viii, 189, 190, 191, 192, 194, 202, 203, 204, 205
childhood, 21, 29, 30, 38, 49, 59, 99, 112, 182, 183, 184, 202, 203, 204
children, 20, 21, 22, 23, 24, 26, 29, 31, 32, 34, 42, 118, 119, 124, 138, 143, 144, 148, 181, 182, 183
chimpanzee, 27
China, 198, 199, 200, 205, 208, 209, 211
cigarette smoking, 230, 242, 245
circular flow, 87
circulation, 236
cities, 198, 211
citizens, 2, 201
clarity, 128, 157
classes, 28, 228
classical conditioning, 28, 48
classification, 40, 200
classroom, 124, 147, 148, 154, 156, 163, 170, 171, 173, 176, 177, 179, 184
classroom management, 147, 156, 163, 170, 171, 173, 176, 177, 179
clients, 58, 63, 68, 231
climate, 145, 153, 155, 157, 163, 168, 170, 172, 173, 175, 176, 177, 184, 185
climates, 147, 170, 171, 172, 173, 177
clinical application, 12, 243
clinical psychiatric care, vii, 1
clinical syndrome, 29
clinical trials, 226
closure, 3
clustering, 20, 199
clusters, 99
CNS, 79, 244
cocaine, ix, 214, 218, 219, 225, 228, 229, 231, 232, 242, 245, 246
cocaine abuse, 229
coding, 80, 81, 82, 121, 158
coffee, 46, 78, 80, 82, 84, 85, 99, 100, 101, 102, 107, 110, 111, 112, 113, 115, 117, 120
cognition, viii, 49, 50, 53, 73, 77, 91, 113, 116
cognitive deficit, 34
cognitive development, vii, 15, 16, 31
cognitive domains, 67
cognitive function, 27, 32, 35
cognitive level, 45
cognitive models, 52
cognitive perspective, 70
cognitive process, 34, 50, 53, 54, 57, 61
cognitive psychology, 49, 139
cognitive science, 17, 44
cognitive tasks, 32
cognitive theory, 51, 70, 75, 183
cognitive therapy, 49, 60, 67, 71, 73, 74
cognitive-behavioral therapy, 38
coherence, 117, 128

cohesion, 136
cohort, 31, 33
colds, 38
collaboration, 69, 147, 154, 156, 163, 168, 170, 177
college students, 74
Colombia, 199
color, 7, 54, 80, 88, 115, 130, 133
commercial, 5, 8, 11, 234, 240
communication, vii, 1, 3, 10, 15, 63, 154, 160, 216, 234, 237, 238
communication skills, 63
community, 2, 4, 23, 28, 142, 186, 222
comorbidity, 23, 27, 35, 186
compassion, 18
compatibility, 106, 140
competence, 51
competition, 49, 101, 113, 128, 136, 142
competitiveness, 146
complement, 2
complexity, 123, 180
compliance, 58
complications, 34
components, 18, 25, 26, 66, 67, 68, 69, 88, 100, 113
composites, 122
composition, 118
computation, 86, 123, 125
computed tomography, 28
computer, 8, 117, 120, 121, 122, 124, 125, 126, 127
computer software, 8
computing, 125
conception, 69, 70, 79, 93, 115, 126, 147, 240
conceptualization, 44, 48, 49, 62
concrete, 39, 52, 81, 96, 101, 104, 105, 106, 107, 109, 110, 112, 116, 117, 120, 122
concreteness, viii, 77, 105, 106, 139
conditioning, 16, 26, 27, 28, 47, 48, 49, 52, 56, 64, 68, 74, 75
conduct, 17, 18, 20, 21, 22, 23, 31, 32, 33, 35, 58
conduct disorder, 20, 21, 22, 32, 33, 35, 181
conference, 71, 237
confidence, 56
confidentiality, 9
configuration, 93, 132
conflict, 144, 155, 169, 173, 240
conflict of interest, 240
confusion, 23
congress, 6, 12, 210, 236
conjecture, 95
connectivity, 21, 26, 29
conscious awareness, 123
conscious experiences, 132
conscious perception, 79, 81, 98, 131
conscious sedation, ix, 213, 215, 216, 217
consciousness, viii, 77, 78, 80, 89, 91, 93, 98, 123, 127, 132, 133, 135, 137, 138, 215
consensus, 71
consent, 9, 148, 151, 223, 227
constituents, 18
consulting, 237
consumption, 40, 42, 46, 245
contamination, 43
context, 45, 51, 52, 63
contingency, 45, 46
continuity, 94, 140
contour, 100
control, 19, 23, 24, 26, 27, 28, 40, 41, 49, 51, 53, 54, 55, 61, 63, 65, 67, 72, 111, 114, 128
control group, 23, 27, 128
controlled exposure, 67
controlled studies, 74
controlled trials, ix, 67, 214
convergence, 128
conversations, 42, 117
cooking, 101
cooling, 8
coordination, 8
coping, 47, 54, 55, 57, 58, 61, 63, 66, 67, 68, 73, 74
coping strategies, 54, 55, 58, 61, 63, 66, 67, 68
correlation, 87, 123, 190, 191, 194, 195, 202
correlation coefficient, 191
correlations, 155, 160, 161, 187, 194, 201, 202, 203, 204, 205
corruption, 191, 192
cortex, 23, 26, 27, 28, 29, 79, 98, 125, 134
cost, ix, 17, 34, 125, 190, 195, 214, 215
costs, 74
cotinine, 230
counseling, 72
covering, 149
craving, x, 214, 215, 229, 230, 232, 243, 245
crime, 32, 34
crimes, viii, 189, 190, 192
criminal activity, 190
criminal acts, 194
criminal behavior, 34
criminality, 16, 17, 20, 35
criminals, 24, 190, 195
critical thinking, 27
critical value, 100
criticism, 114, 149, 224, 237
cross-sectional study, 194, 195
cues, 30, 58, 59, 67, 83, 100, 106, 107, 110, 113, 125, 128, 130, 131
culture, 209
curricula, 148
curriculum, 73

cyanide, 238
cycles, 92
Czech Republic, 5

D

damage, 23, 98, 125, 129, 131
damping, 85
danger, ix, 38, 39, 46, 48, 51, 52, 53, 55, 56, 59, 68, 214, 221
dangerousness, 54
data analysis, 182
data collection, 180
data processing, 80
data set, 192, 194
data structure, 120, 121
death, 39, 53
decision task, 28
decision-making process, 30
decisions, 39
decomposition, 158, 164, 165, 169, 170
deductive reasoning, 27
deficiency, 19, 25
deficit, 17, 19, 24, 25, 27, 30, 32
definition, 17, 19, 29, 41, 114
degenerate, 124
delinquency, 17, 19, 21, 32, 181, 183
delirium, 17, 219, 223
delirium tremens, 223
delusions, 43
demand, 28, 131, 132
dementia, 201, 210
demographic characteristics, 145
Denmark, 198, 199, 200
density, 83, 85, 100
dentist, 218, 237
Department of Justice, 195
dependency ratio, 202, 203, 204, 210
depression, viii, 21, 22, 40, 49, 50, 70, 71, 72, 73, 141, 142, 143, 144, 145, 146, 147, 149, 150, 154, 157, 158, 159, 160, 164, 165, 166, 167, 168, 169, 170, 171, 172, 173, 175, 176, 177, 178, 179, 180, 182, 183, 184, 185, 186, 187, 205, 229
depressive symptomatology, 186
depressive symptoms, 144, 148, 156, 157, 158, 159, 160, 163, 164, 165, 166, 169, 170, 171, 177, 178, 179, 181, 183, 187
deprivation, 28, 202, 205
depth, 17, 79, 80, 82, 121
depth perception, 82
deregulation, 29
destruction, 20
detachment, 25
detection, 206
detoxification, 221, 224
developed countries, 202, 205
developing countries, 199, 201, 210
developmental disorder, 20
developmental neurosciences, vii, 15
developmental psychology, 187
developmental psychopathology, 182, 187
deviation, 18, 157, 158
Diagnostic and Statistical Manual of Mental Disorders, 70, 181
diagnostic criteria, 20, 22, 23, 75, 149, 158
diaphragm, 65
diathesis-stress model, 183
differential diagnosis, 42
differentiation, 94, 108
dimensionality, 132
directionality, 25
disability, 16
discomfort, 43
discontinuity, 136
discrimination, 24, 145
diseases, 202, 203, 204
disgust, 38
disorder, vii, 16, 18, 19, 20, 21, 22, 23, 24, 25, 29, 32, 33, 34, 35, 38, 39, 41, 42, 43, 44, 48, 52, 54, 58, 59, 61, 65, 67, 68, 69, 70, 71, 72, 73, 74, 75, 150, 182, 186, 187
disposition, 25
dissatisfaction, 144, 147, 155, 163, 165, 169, 172, 177
dissociation, 25
distortions, 49, 50, 53, 59, 60, 61, 69
distress, 21, 43
distribution, 84, 191, 194, 210
diversity, 21, 145, 195
dizziness, 41, 59, 61
doctors, 206
dogs, 46, 50
domain, 80
dopamine, 218, 228, 230, 231, 246, 247
dorsolateral prefrontal cortex, 28
dosage, 224, 238
dosing, 234
double-blind trial, 221, 222, 224, 244
dough, 101, 112
draft, 238
dream, 127
drug abuse, 242
drug treatment, 66
drug use, 32
drug withdrawal, 246
drugs, 42

DSM, 18, 19, 20, 22, 23, 40, 41, 42, 68, 70, 73, 74
DSM-II, 23, 70, 73
DSM-III, 23, 70, 73
DSM-IV, 18, 20, 40, 41, 42, 68, 70, 74
duration, 39, 67, 91
dynamism, 102
dysphoria, 227

E

eating, 21, 38, 42, 46
eating disorders, 21
economic change, 194
economic development, 194, 195, 196, 201, 206
economic indicator, 210
economic status, vii, viii, 189, 190, 191, 193, 194, 201, 202, 203, 204, 205, 206, 209, 210
ecstasy, 228
education, vii, 11, 49, 66, 138, 148, 150, 156, 190, 193, 195, 227
educational attainment, viii, 189, 190, 191, 195
Egypt, 12
elaboration, 134, 136
elbows, 122
electromagnetic, 89, 137
electromyography, 217
electrons, 89
elementary school, 152, 182
e-mail, 5
emergency, 10, 39
emission, 28, 33, 34
emotion, 18, 24, 25, 28, 29, 30, 32, 33, 34, 38, 39, 46, 48, 49, 52, 53, 55, 62, 68, 70, 71, 73, 135
emotional disorder, 49
emotional distress, 21
emotional experience, 19, 30, 49, 51, 55, 58
emotional expression of psychopathy, vii
emotional information, 26, 28, 29
emotional problems, 18, 66
emotional processes, 25
emotional reactions, 54
emotional responses, 16, 18, 25, 34, 61
emotional state, 40, 68
emotional stimuli, 24, 29
emotional valence, 25
emotional well-being, 147
emotions, vii, 15, 16, 23, 26, 27, 30, 38, 39, 44, 49, 60, 68, 69, 74
empathy, 16, 17, 19, 23, 24, 27, 30, 69
employment, 227
employment status, 227
encoding, 80, 81, 106, 107, 109, 113, 121, 134, 136, 140
encouragement, 147, 153, 155, 163, 167, 169, 177
energy, 11, 79, 85, 86, 89, 95, 96, 102
enforcement, 22
engineering, 138
England, 12, 199, 205, 206, 208, 209, 210
enrollment, 191, 194
environment, viii, 7, 48, 51, 53, 55, 86, 97, 120, 141, 145, 146, 154, 155, 157, 160, 168, 170, 171, 172, 175, 176, 180, 183, 187
environmental aspects, 46
environmental characteristics, 176
environmental conditions, 51
environmental influences, 28
enzymes, 243
epidemiology, 198, 209
epilepsy, 27, 35
episodic memory, 134, 137, 139
equality, 109, 124, 191
equipment, 3, 5, 6, 8, 9, 10, 221, 233
Estonia, 198
ethanol, 221, 243, 245
ethics, 247
ethnicity, 196
etiquette, 10
Europe, 12
European Union, 4
evening news, 236
everyday life, 30
evidence, ix, 24, 29, 31, 33, 66, 116, 126, 140, 144, 177, 203, 204, 209, 214, 215, 217, 218, 222, 225, 228, 229, 230, 231, 235, 239, 242, 244
evolution, 26, 89, 92, 93, 94, 96, 100
exaggeration, 50
excitation, 38, 51, 55, 215, 216, 217, 225
exclusion, 34, 144, 148, 183, 239
executive function, 23, 24, 33
exercise, 42, 51, 58, 59, 62, 64
expertise, 5, 140
explicit memory, 125
exposure, 26, 54, 55, 56, 57, 58, 59, 62, 65, 66, 67, 68, 69, 71, 73, 74, 75, 142, 150, 151, 155, 160, 169, 173, 176, 177, 202, 220, 223, 227, 228, 232, 236, 243
expression, 18, 27, 29, 30, 39, 40, 97
external environment, 5, 53
externalizing behavior, 182
extinction, 28, 54, 56, 57, 58, 65
eye movement, 97
eye-witness phenomena, viii, 77

F

fabric, 117
fabrication, 239
face validity, 222
facial expression, 9, 15, 24, 25, 28, 31, 34
factor analysis, 21
failure, 17, 19, 52, 53, 70, 109, 122
false alarms, 52
false belief, 239
families, 17, 31, 44, 142, 144, 148, 150, 154, 183, 187
family, 21, 29, 30, 32, 34, 57, 73, 117
family environment, 30, 34
family history, 32
family members, 150
family system, 30
fatigue, 46
fear, vii, 16, 24, 25, 26, 27, 28, 30, 31, 34, 37, 38, 39, 40, 41, 42, 45, 46, 47, 48, 49, 51, 52, 53, 55, 56, 57, 58, 60, 62, 65, 67, 68, 71, 72, 235
fears, 38, 39, 40, 44, 46, 51, 53, 62
feedback, 85, 95, 99
feelings, 17, 18, 25, 43, 49, 51, 60, 62, 63, 142, 149, 150, 155
fidelity, 102
field theory, 137, 139
fights, 153
filters, 53, 60, 86, 87
financial, 194
financial data, 194
fine tuning, 108
Finland, ix, x, 198, 199, 213, 214, 222, 225, 232, 233, 235, 236, 237, 246, 247
flashbacks, 39, 42
flexibility, 8, 69
flight, 26, 39, 46, 52, 54
flights, 2
flooding, 57, 58, 71, 73
flow field, 84, 85, 86, 87, 99, 100, 103
focusing, 109
folate, 243
food, 48
force, viii, 77, 93, 95, 102, 106, 132, 243
forecasting, 119
forensic settings, 23
forgetting, 60
formation, 98, 109, 142
formula, 154
foundations, 70, 139
fractal space, 137
France, 5, 15, 198, 199
free recall, 115, 125, 129
friendship, 155, 176, 179
frontal cortex, 23
frontal lobe, 23, 31, 32
functional analysis, 44, 45, 46, 47, 68
functional architecture, 80
functional imaging, 28
funding, 206, 209, 240
furniture, 105, 106, 120

G

gender differences, 146, 177, 179, 211
gender effects, 201
general anesthesia, 216
general practitioner, 2, 3, 4, 5, 205, 206, 210
generalizability, 180
generalization, 63, 119
generalized anxiety disorder, 38, 44, 66, 70, 71, 72, 73, 74, 75
generation, 66, 78, 107
genes, 98
genetic factors, 201, 204
Germany, 198, 199, 207
gestures, 16, 52
gifted, 148, 180
Gini coefficient, viii, 189, 190, 191, 192, 194, 201, 202, 203, 204, 205
glue, 108
goals, 51, 56
goods and services, 194
grades, 144, 151, 152, 155, 180
graph, 238
grass, 85, 99
Greece, 5, 198
gross national domestic product (GDP), viii, 189, 190, 191, 192, 193, 194, 201, 202, 203, 204, 205
grouping, 40
groups, 20, 23, 28, 40, 63, 64, 67
growth, 90, 103, 104, 114
guidance, 2, 216
guidelines, 247
guilt, 16, 17, 18, 19, 20, 30, 42, 149, 229
guilt feelings, 18
guilty, 61, 149, 152
Guyana, 5

H

habituation, 26, 51, 52, 53, 54, 56, 57, 58, 65
hair, 109
half-life, 225, 241
hands, 44, 46, 59, 68, 122

happiness, 40
harm, 19, 43, 55
haze, 88, 90
health, vii, 1, 2, 3, 4, 5, 6, 10, 11, 38, 42, 72, 142, 181, 182, 185, 186, 193, 201, 202, 203, 204, 205, 206, 207, 208, 209, 215, 216, 226, 233, 235, 237
health care, 1, 2, 4, 10, 11, 72, 226
health care professionals, 2
health problems, 2, 207
Health Professions Council of South Africa, ix, 214
health researchers, 142
health services, 1, 3, 4, 5, 6, 11, 38, 202, 203, 204, 205, 208
health status, 193
healthcare delivery, vii, 1
heart rate, 55
height, 104, 151
helplessness, 51, 142
hemisphere, 233
hepatitis, 247
heroin, 228, 231, 247
heterogeneity, 195
high school, viii, 141, 142, 146, 148, 172, 177, 179, 180, 181, 190, 195
high school transition, viii, 141, 142, 146, 148, 172, 177, 179, 180
hippocampus, 27, 33
historical overview, 80
history, 17, 21, 28, 32, 41, 49, 51, 82, 89, 91, 117, 126, 134, 136, 202, 214, 215, 228, 231, 243
hologram, 81, 82, 100, 129
holographic matter-field, viii, 77, 79, 95, 115, 131
homeostasis, 229
homework, 59, 144, 152, 153, 155
homicide, 29, 194, 195, 196
homicide rates, 194, 195, 196
Hong Kong, 200, 205, 211
hormone, 26
hostile acts, 21
house, 25
household income, 202
housing, 202
human, 11, 17, 26, 32, 49, 50, 68, 70, 94, 124, 125, 137, 138, 140, 180, 227, 239, 246
human behavior, 50
human brain, 32, 246
human development, 180
human sciences, 17
human subjects, 26, 239
Hungary, 198, 199
hyperactivity, 22, 32
hypothalamus, 26
hypothesis, 21, 23, 25, 28, 31, 47, 48, 69, 78, 113, 121, 122, 128, 130, 136, 140, 142, 172, 177, 179, 180, 186, 202, 218, 244
hypothesis test, 180

I

iatrogenic, 11
Iceland, 199
ideal, ix, 1, 214
ideas, 41, 43, 60, 68, 134
identification, 20, 24, 33, 44, 45, 55, 134, 201, 205
identity, 120, 142, 143, 187
idiosyncratic, 145, 146
illicit drug use, 228
illumination, 194
illusion, 87, 122, 207, 215
illusions, 78, 87, 97, 140
image, 8, 9, 34, 61, 78, 79, 80, 81, 82, 86, 95, 96, 100, 104, 105, 106, 107, 115, 119, 120, 121, 123, 126, 132, 143, 150, 159, 179, 186, 187
imagery, viii, 23, 25, 29, 30, 77, 101, 104, 105, 106, 107, 108, 119, 121, 122, 135, 136, 137, 138
images, vii, 1, 42, 78, 94, 104, 105, 106, 116, 118, 120, 121, 122, 126
imagination, 27, 56, 57, 79
imitation, 16, 55
immigrants, 200, 209
impairments, 30
imprisonment, 43, 190, 195
improvements, vii, 1, 6, 67, 204
impulses, 11, 17
impulsive, 18, 20, 22
impulsiveness, 19, 23
impulsivity, 18, 19, 21, 23, 33
in transition, 207
in vivo, 57, 58, 59, 71, 75
inattention, 22, 128
incidence, 186, 201
inclusion, 18, 23
income, vii, 187, 189, 190, 191, 194, 195, 198, 199, 200, 201, 203, 204
income distribution, 191
income inequality, vii, 189, 190, 191, 194, 195, 201
independence, 156
independent variable, 157
India, 207
Indians, 200
indication, 66, 97
individual differences, 155, 185
individuals, 2, 5, 16, 17, 19, 23, 25, 28, 31, 34, 50, 51, 52, 53, 74, 143, 147, 180, 190, 194, 195, 204, 206, 215, 216, 235

inequality, vii, viii, 189, 190, 191, 194, 195, 196, 201
inertia, 84, 100, 136
infancy, vii, 15, 16, 20
infants, 20, 24, 123
infection, 227
inferences, 49
infinite, 90, 91, 92, 93, 94, 115
influence, 28, 47, 49, 51, 60, 86, 95, 137
influenza, 38
influenza a, 38
information processing, 44, 47, 122
informed consent, 9, 223, 227
infrastructure, 5, 8, 194
ingredients, 68
inhibition, 30, 113, 247
inhibitor, 243
inmates, 24
inoculation, 62, 71, 73
input, 78, 116
insane, 61
insects, 38
insight, 82, 106
insomnia, 149
inspiration, 65
institutions, 5, 143, 233, 240
integration, 80, 134
integrity, 8
intelligence, 21, 116, 125
intensity, 25, 38, 40, 41, 42, 46, 50, 54, 55, 56, 57
intent, 91
interaction, vii, 15, 16, 21, 29, 52, 74, 138
interaction effect, 157
interactions, vii, 15, 16, 57
interest, 16, 28, 40, 42
interest rates, 202
interference, 17, 81, 82, 95, 109, 110, 113, 125, 127, 128, 129, 130, 132, 133, 136
internal consistency, 150, 154, 200
internalizing, 183
International Classification of Diseases, (ICD), 6, 40, 41, 42, 68, 75
international meetings, 6
interpersonal communication, 63
interpersonal interactions, 66
interpretation, 49, 53, 60
interrelations, 160
interval, 94
intervention, 54, 55, 56, 58, 59, 60, 63, 66, 67, 68, 69, 173, 185, 226, 228, 232
intimacy, 67, 142
invariance laws, viii, 77, 84, 89, 96, 99, 101, 106, 110, 114, 118
invariants, 84, 85, 86, 88, 90, 98, 100, 106, 107, 112, 113, 115, 117, 122, 124, 136
inversion, 119, 158
investment, 5
Ireland, 5, 186
irritability, 39, 42
islands, 2
isolation, 2
Israel, 199
issues, 11, 29, 72, 192
Italy, 205

J

Japan, 198, 199, 210
Jordan, 208
journalists, 236
judgment, 79
justification, 56
juvenile delinquency, 19
juvenile delinquents, 21

K

kindergarten, 144
knowledge, 16, 49, 62, 65, 69, 114, 116, 121, 122, 124
Korea, 198
Kuwait, 198

L

labeling, 45
laboratory tests, 1
lack of control, 176
land, 85
language, 28, 116, 117, 121, 124, 125, 133, 140
laryngospasm, 216
later life, 207, 210
Latvia, 198, 199
law enforcement, 22
laws, viii, 77, 84, 89, 90, 96, 99, 101, 104, 106, 110, 114, 118, 125, 128, 130, 134
Leahy, 57, 60, 61, 63, 64, 65, 68, 69, 73
learning, viii, 27, 35, 44, 47, 48, 52, 55, 56, 58, 61, 65, 68, 69, 70, 73, 75, 77, 101, 102, 104, 105, 113, 117, 119, 124, 128, 131, 132, 133, 136, 137, 139, 140, 146
learning process, 27
legislation, 29, 206
legs, 41, 64
leisure, 39

lens, 93, 126
lesions, 23, 26, 123, 137
lexical decision, 28, 137, 138
life cycle, 195
life expectancy, viii, 189, 190, 191, 192, 201, 202, 203, 204, 205, 210
life quality, 143
lifestyle, 19
lifetime, 37, 91, 92, 149, 182, 185, 187
light, 7, 17, 20, 23, 47, 59, 69, 79, 80, 81, 103
limbic system, 26, 27, 29
linear model, 180
linear modeling, 180
links, 20, 47, 110, 117
liquids, 112, 122
listening, 69
literacy, 191, 194
literacy rates, 194
Lithuania, 198
localization, 98, 125
loci, 125
locomotor, 229
locus, 26, 27, 179, 184
logical implications, 93
logical reasoning, 60
loneliness, 147, 155, 158, 165, 169, 171, 173, 180
longevity, 201
longitudinal study, 33, 146, 148, 182, 186
long-term memory, 110
love, 151
low risk, 22
lying, 19, 63
lymphocytosis, 227

M

Mackintosh, 48, 73
magnetic field, 80
magnetic resonance, 27, 28, 29, 33
magnetic resonance imaging, 27, 28, 29, 33
magnitude, 94, 115
major depression, 182, 186
major depressive disorder, 187
majority, 172, 217
males, 22, 34
maltreatment, 21
man, 48, 50, 53, 61, 100, 245
management, 2, 10, 11, 52, 53, 55, 61, 63, 65, 66, 67, 69, 71, 74, 147, 154, 156, 163, 168, 170, 171, 173, 175, 176, 177, 179, 242, 243, 246
mania, 17, 21
manipulation, 103, 104, 108, 113, 122
mapping, 80
marijuana, 22, 151
marital conflict, 46
Mars, 101, 105, 137, 139
masking, 128
mass, 84, 85, 102, 116
mathematics, 99, 103, 106, 152, 155
matrix, 80, 84, 98, 121, 129
matter, viii, 3, 27, 34, 35, 77, 78, 79, 80, 88, 89, 91, 92, 93, 94, 95, 96, 97, 98, 100, 114, 115, 117, 122, 125, 127, 130, 131, 139, 173, 237, 245
Mauritius, 199
meanings, 38
measurement, 94, 97, 148, 150
measures, 21, 23, 24, 25, 33, 58, 67
media, 196, 235, 236, 237, 239, 240
median, 191
mediation, viii, 179, 190, 195
medical, vii, ix, 1, 2, 5, 9, 11, 12, 38, 41, 61, 72, 201, 205, 214, 215, 218, 220, 235, 240, 245, 247
medical care, vii, 1, 12, 205
medication, 6, 46, 66, 67, 71, 217, 223, 226, 234
medicine, 226, 234
medulla, 26
melody, 125
memory, viii, 27, 28, 29, 42, 77, 78, 79, 81, 89, 90, 91, 92, 96, 97, 98, 99, 101, 102, 103, 104, 105, 106, 107, 108, 109, 110, 112, 113, 114, 115, 116, 117, 118, 121, 122, 123, 125, 126, 127, 128, 129, 130, 131, 132, 133, 134, 135, 136, 137, 138, 139, 140, 241
memory function, 27
memory loss, 131
memory performance, 104, 108, 109, 115, 130, 133
memory retrieval, 78, 97, 128
men, 27, 61
menarche, 151
menopause, 200
mental disorder, 5, 33, 72, 184, 185, 201, 209
mental health, vii, 1, 2, 3, 4, 5, 6, 10, 11, 142, 182, 201, 202, 203, 204, 205, 208, 209
mental illness, 201, 205
mental image, viii, 77, 105, 121, 138
mental imagery, viii, 77, 138
mental representation, 135
meta-analysis, 72, 73, 179, 195
metaphor, 96, 122, 128
Mexico, 198, 207
mice, 80, 121, 228, 242
Minneapolis, 135
minority, 124
misconceptions, 215
misuse, 235
mixing, 115

mobility, 93
models, 19, 30, 31, 44, 47, 49, 52, 55, 68, 69, 86, 113, 116, 126, 129, 131, 171
moderators, 157
modern science, 127
modern society, 38
modifications, 78, 149
modulation pattern, viii, 77, 96, 98, 122, 125, 127, 132
modus operandi, 29
Moldavia, 198
molecules, 80
momentum, 103, 135, 136
Montreal Adolescent Depression Development Project (MADDP), v, viii, 141, 148
Morocco, 2
morphine, 228, 242
mortality, viii, 31, 189, 190, 191, 192, 194, 202, 203, 204, 205, 207, 208, 210
mortality rate, viii, 189, 190, 191, 192, 194, 202, 203, 204, 205, 210
motion, 78, 81, 83, 84, 86, 87, 88, 91, 92, 93, 94, 96, 97, 99, 100, 102, 105, 106, 112, 114, 115, 120, 125, 127, 129, 131, 134, 140
motivation, 51, 143, 144, 145, 147, 187
motor behavior, 46
motor task, 110
mountains, 84
movement, 26, 51, 97, 127
MRI, 28, 35
multidimensional, 186
multi-ethnic, 208
multiple regression, 156, 157, 158, 159, 160, 169, 171, 184
multiple regression analysis, 156, 157, 160, 171
multiplication, 157
multivariate analysis, 175
multivariate statistics, 187
muscles, 63, 64, 85
music, 18, 63, 126

N

narcissism, 19, 30
narcotic, 247
National Institute of Mental Health, 12, 44, 74
national policy, 209
nature of time, 129
nausea, 41
needs, 29, 119, 121, 126
negative attitudes, 215
negative consequences, 30, 48, 56
negative effects, 236
negative reinforcement, 48
negative relation, 143, 145, 170
neocortex, 27
nervous system, 23, 26, 27, 30, 79, 138
nervousness, 17
Netherlands, 70, 73, 205
network, 87, 110, 111
neural network, 30
neurobiological sufficiency, viii, 77, 78
neurobiology, 44
neuroimaging, 28, 32
neuromotor, 34
neurons, 26, 129
neuropsychiatry, 244
neuropsychology, 44, 68
neuroscience, 79, 96
neutral, 7, 25, 28, 45, 47, 48, 68, 153
neutral stimulus, 47, 48
New England, 12
New Zealand, 196, 200, 210
nicotine, ix, 214, 218, 219, 230, 231, 232, 242, 246
nightmares, 39, 42
nitrous oxide, ix, 213, 214, 215, 216, 217, 219, 220, 223, 225, 226, 227, 228, 229, 232, 233, 234, 235, 236, 237, 238, 239, 240, 241, 242, 243, 244, 245, 246, 247
nodes, 53, 110
noise, 56, 115
norepinephrine, 26
normal distribution, 158
North America, 32, 180, 209
Norway, 199, 205
novelty, 19
novelty seeking, 19
nucleus, 26, 218, 231
null, 89, 121, 122, 131
null hypothesis, 121, 122
nurses, ix, 214, 218, 221
nursing, 5, 10, 221

O

obligation, 44
observations, 31, 45, 47
obsessive-compulsive disorder (OCD), 39, 40, 41, 58, 72, 73
obstacles, 39, 51, 233, 236
offenders, 19, 20, 25, 28, 32, 33
officials, 191
old age, 201, 202, 204, 209
operant conditioning, 47, 48, 68
operations, 83, 97, 107, 116, 119, 120, 122, 123, 125, 127, 154, 156

opioids, ix, 214, 218, 219, 229, 232, 241
opportunities, 63
Oppositional Defiant Disorder, 20
organ, 59
organism, 38, 47, 48, 51, 52, 56, 68, 95, 100
organization, 122
organizational development, 181
organize, 52
orientation, 26, 87
oscillation, 85, 96, 119
outline, 119
outpatients, ix, 3, 5, 11, 214, 220, 221, 225, 232
output, 87
overweight, 5
oxygen, ix, x, 213, 214, 215, 216, 217, 219, 220, 223, 226, 227, 228, 229, 230, 231, 232, 233, 238, 239, 242, 243, 244, 245, 246

P

packaging, 123
pain, 45, 48, 74, 227, 245
palate, 64
palpitations, 41
PAN, v, ix, x, 101, 213, 214, 215, 216, 217, 218, 219, 220, 221, 222, 223, 224, 225, 226, 227, 228, 229, 230, 231, 232, 233, 234, 235, 236, 237, 238, 239, 240, 241, 242, 245, 246
PAN therapy, ix, 213, 215, 218, 221, 233, 235, 236, 237, 238, 240
panic attack, 10, 41, 42, 71
panic disorder, 41, 44, 65, 71, 74, 75
parallel, 17, 20, 23, 110
parallelism, 49
paralysis, 39
parameter, 102
parentage, 227
parental pressure, 155
parenting, 21
parents, 142, 144, 147, 148, 150, 151, 152, 185
participants, 7, 9, 107, 109, 148, 149, 150, 154, 155, 156, 164, 165, 169, 170
partition, 89, 90, 92
pathogenesis, 218, 229, 230, 231
pathology, 27, 42, 44, 223
pathways, 32, 182
patient care, 3, 73
Pavlovian conditioning, 74
PCL-R, 18, 19, 25
peer group, 144, 176
peer rejection, 144
peer relationship, 144, 152, 154, 155, 157, 165, 166, 174, 176
per capita expenditure, 202, 203, 204, 205
perceptions, 140
periodicity, 110, 112
permission, 238
permit, 43, 44, 52, 65
perpetrators, 17
perseverance, 27
personal accomplishment, 51
personal communication, 216, 234, 237, 238
personal control, 155
personal development, 38
personal problems, 153, 154, 156
personality, vii, 18, 19, 20, 21, 22, 23, 24, 25, 29, 31, 32, 33, 34, 35, 46, 187
personality disorder, vii, 18, 19, 20, 21, 22, 23, 24, 25, 29, 31, 32, 33, 34, 35
personality traits, 19, 25, 46
person-oriented approach, 187
perspective, 16, 17, 21, 23, 29, 30, 87, 89, 93, 103, 106, 107, 112, 131
pessimism, 20
pharmaceutical, 232, 233, 240
pharmacokinetics, 234, 245
pharmacological treatment, 58, 66, 72, 73
pharmacology, 247
pharmacotherapy, 67
phenomenology, 40, 79
Philadelphia, 245
phobia, 35, 41, 42, 44, 46, 59, 61, 71, 72, 73, 74, 75
physical environment, 194
physicians, ix, 10, 214, 221, 231, 233, 234
physics, 93, 94, 95, 96, 125, 131, 134, 137
physiological arousal, 56
piano, 98
pitch, 84, 112, 135
placebo, 66, 72, 220, 221, 223, 224, 225, 226, 228, 229, 232, 238, 241, 246
planning, 23, 27, 109
plausibility, 172
pneumonia, 227
Poland, 126, 199
police, 22
policy, 185, 209, 247
politics, 235
polydrug abuse, ix, 214, 231
poor, 19, 21, 50, 112
population, viii, 1, 4, 16, 67, 70, 74, 180, 189, 190, 191, 192, 194, 195, 201, 202, 203, 204, 209, 211
population size, 191, 192
positive correlation, 190, 194, 202, 203, 204, 205
positive relationship, 170, 202, 203, 204
positron, 34
positron emission tomography, 34

posttraumatic stress, 71
post-traumatic stress disorder, 39, 42, 44, 67, 75
potato, 113
Potchefstroom, 243
poverty, 210
power, 67, 101, 106
precedent, 64, 130
prediction, 32, 47, 131
predictors, 22, 33
prefrontal cortex, 27, 28, 125
pregnancy, 30, 35
prejudice, 215
preparation, 11, 39, 57, 181
president, 222, 235
pressure, 26, 29
prevention, viii, 20, 31, 55, 56, 61, 63, 67, 68, 69, 141, 142, 147, 173, 177, 178, 180, 181, 182, 185, 186, 195, 201, 227, 232
preventive approach, 31
prima facie, 239
primacy, 89, 91
priming, viii, 77, 101, 110, 112, 113, 128, 133, 136, 137, 139
principle, viii, 77, 78, 87, 89, 93, 94, 98, 99, 100, 108, 109, 115, 126, 129, 130
principles, 101, 114, 134, 246
prisons, 23
private practice, 231
private schools, 148
probability, 51, 53, 55, 100, 103, 104, 122, 132
probe, 103, 245, 247
problem behavior, 184
problem solving, 27, 55, 61, 63, 66
problem-solving skills, 61
production, 49, 54
professionals, vii, 1, 3, 10, 215, 218, 233, 235, 237
program, 58, 63, 70, 72, 74, 98, 124
programming, 80
project, 4, 5, 20, 26, 83, 94, 148
pronunciation, 116
propagation, 235
proportionality, 95
protection, 58, 183
protective factors, 34, 142, 143, 180, 205
protective role, 180
protocol, 75
prototype, 63
PST, 6
psychiatric diagnosis, 44
psychiatric disorders, vii, 31, 49, 68, 184, 243
psychiatric illness, 37
psychiatric patients, 10
psychiatrist, 2, 4, 5, 6, 7, 8, 9, 10, 205
psychiatry, vii, 17, 32, 33, 35, 38, 70, 225
psychological health, 42
psychological problems, 38, 44
psychological processes, 47, 54
psychological well-being, 187
psychology, 29, 30, 44, 49, 68, 72, 98, 134, 136, 137, 139, 187
psychometric properties, 149
psychopathic offenders, 19
psychopathology, 22, 34, 182, 184, 185, 186, 187
psychopaths, 18, 25, 26, 27, 28, 29, 30, 32, 33
psychopathy, vii, 16, 17, 18, 19, 20, 21, 22, 23, 24, 25, 27, 28, 29, 30, 31, 32, 33, 34, 35, 190
Psychopathy Checklist Revised, 18
Psychopathy Screening Device, 20
psychoses, 18, 39
psychosis, 24
psychosocial factors, 27
psychotherapy, 38, 54, 65, 66, 69, 71, 73
PTSD, 42
pubertal development, 150, 179
puberty, 142
public goods, 194
public health, 38, 201, 206
public schools, 148
publishing, 238
punishment, 17, 39, 150, 151, 159
pupil, 17

Q

quality of life, 4
quantum mechanics, 94
quantum state, 80
quarks, 89
questioning, 69
questionnaire, 3, 155, 186, 187

R

race, 116, 128, 136, 208, 210
radius, 99
range, 19, 20, 27, 80, 100, 109
rape, 71
rating scale, 149, 151, 245
ratings, 73, 103, 104
rationality, 59
reaction time, 112
reactions, 17, 21, 25, 27, 38, 40, 41, 45, 47, 48, 52, 53, 54, 56, 64
reactivity, 26, 27, 74
reading, 97, 107, 126

realism, 96, 97, 133
reality, 43, 48, 49, 50, 53, 57, 60, 61, 62, 93, 94, 110, 121, 130, 176
real-time transmission, vii, 1
reasoning, 16, 17, 27, 50, 60, 121, 122, 221
recall, viii, 30, 64, 77, 99, 102, 103, 104, 105, 107, 108, 110, 115, 118, 125, 126, 128, 129, 130, 132, 133, 140
receptive field, 87
recidivism, 190, 195
recognition, 15, 31, 33, 93, 102, 104, 109, 110, 112, 116, 129, 130, 133, 134
recognition phase, 104
recognition test, 104, 110, 133
recommendations, 5
reconstruction, 82, 96, 125, 126, 128, 130, 132
recovery, ix, 42, 70, 136, 214, 221, 228
recurrence, 69, 185
redistribution, 194
reduction, 27, 28, 52, 53, 55, 56, 67, 116, 120
reductionism, 16, 134
redundancy, 160
reflection, 28, 55, 125, 129, 131
reflexes, 26, 216
regression, 156, 157, 158, 160, 164, 169, 170, 171, 181, 184, 185
regression analysis, 156, 157, 160, 164, 171
regression equation, 158
regulation, 26, 29
rehabilitation, x, 214, 221, 228, 242
rehabilitation program, 242
reinforcement, 48
rejection, 21, 34, 144, 214
relapses, 232
relationship, 16, 19, 72, 106
relationships, 26, 30, 42, 49, 69
relatives, 6, 9
relativity, 137
relaxation, 46, 58, 63, 64, 65, 66, 67, 68, 69, 72, 74, 75, 215, 216, 218, 219
relevance, 1, 27, 55, 69
reliability, 5
relief, 46, 52, 66, 120
religion, 43, 210
remembering, 78, 99, 102
remission, 149
remorse, 17, 19, 23, 24, 229
repetitions, 129
reprocessing, 54, 55, 56
requirements, 2, 8, 120, 121, 215, 218, 225, 243
research funding, 240
research institutions, 5
researchers, 13, 109, 142, 215
residuals, 159
resistance, 11, 84, 95, 102, 110, 112, 115, 222, 239
resources, 1, 3, 6, 11, 46, 53, 154, 231
respiratory, 45
respiratory problems, 45
response, ix, x, 16, 17, 23, 24, 25, 26, 28, 30, 31, 32, 42, 44, 46, 47, 55, 56, 57, 67, 68, 101, 102, 105, 110, 111, 112, 113, 128, 132, 133, 201, 213, 214, 216, 217, 220, 221, 222, 223, 224, 227, 228, 230, 232, 233, 234, 238, 243
response time, 110, 111, 112
responsibility, 19
responsiveness, 25
restaurants, 38, 42
restructuring, vii, 1, 54, 60, 61, 66, 67, 68, 75
retention, 78, 126, 134
retina, 79, 82, 83, 84, 85
retrieval, 78, 98, 99, 113, 114, 116, 117, 120, 125, 126, 128, 129, 131, 132, 136, 137, 138, 139
retroactive interference, 133
returns, 99
rewards, 30
rhythm, 64, 65
rights, 38, 42
risk, viii, ix, 21, 22, 26, 30, 32, 35, 39, 57, 58, 63, 141, 142, 143, 144, 145, 146, 147, 150, 172, 173, 176, 180, 184, 185, 194, 198, 201, 202, 203, 204, 205, 206, 207, 208
risk factors, viii, ix, 21, 30, 141, 146, 147, 150, 180, 184, 185, 194, 198, 201, 205, 207
risks, 185, 186
rodents, 218, 232
root, 131
rotation transformation, 115
rotations, 103, 119
rugby, 104
rules, 10, 20, 23, 29, 42, 44, 60, 106, 118, 119, 145, 150, 151, 153, 154, 155, 156
Russia, 198

S

saccades, 97
sadness, 24, 30, 31, 38, 40, 49, 116
safety, 10, 23, 56, 58, 67, 75, 232, 233
sample, 21, 22, 91, 115
sampling, 91, 115
Sartorius, 72, 198, 199, 200, 209
savings, ix, 214
schema, 49, 50, 51, 108, 109
schizophrenia, 17, 247
school, viii, 21, 114, 141, 142, 143, 144, 145, 146, 147, 148, 149, 150, 151, 152, 153, 154, 155, 156,

157, 158, 160, 163, 164, 165, 166, 167, 168, 169, 170, 171, 172, 173, 174, 175, 176, 177, 178, 179, 180, 181, 182, 183, 184, 185, 186, 190, 191, 194, 195, 227
school achievement, 21
school activities, 185
school climate, 145, 153, 155, 157, 168, 170, 172, 173, 175, 185
school failure, 144
school support, 156
schooling, 185
science, 80, 91, 114, 127, 133, 136, 182, 215, 243
scientific knowledge, 44, 215
scientific publications, 221, 235
scientific theory, 131
scope, 87
scores, 19
search, 51, 101, 113, 131, 135, 138
searching, 69
second generation, 65
second language, 117, 133
secondary education, 190, 195
secondary school education, 227
security, 9, 42, 142, 145, 147, 156, 170, 171, 172, 173, 177, 194
sedative, ix, 46, 214, 219, 221, 226, 231, 233
sedative medication, ix, 46, 214, 221, 226
sedatives, 221, 231
segregation, 206
selective serotonin reuptake inhibitor, 206
self, 19, 21, 25, 27, 32, 43, 49, 50, 51, 53, 55, 56, 58, 60, 61, 63, 65, 67, 68, 69, 74, 80, 107, 134
self-confidence, 51, 60, 61
self-control, 65, 67
self-efficacy, 50, 51, 53, 55, 68, 143, 147, 151, 155, 163, 164, 166, 173, 174, 176, 179, 184
self-esteem, 53, 67, 143, 148, 150, 160, 178, 184
self-image, 186
self-monitoring, 27
self-regulation, 51
self-reports, 25, 155
semantic activation, 111
semantic memory, 106, 134, 136
semantic priming, 133, 139
semantics, 125
sensation, 21, 56, 61, 64, 65
sensation seeking, 21
sensations, 63, 64, 65
senses, 19
sensitivity, 20, 52, 133, 149
sensitization, 58, 229
separation, 54, 83
series, 28, 53, 82, 90, 91, 92, 93, 94, 100, 103, 105, 114, 118, 122, 126
serotonin, 206
services, 1, 2, 3, 4, 5, 6, 10, 11, 38, 153, 154, 155, 191, 194, 201, 202, 203, 204, 205, 208
severe stress, 41
severity, 21, 32, 54, 67, 100, 136
sex, 28, 182, 208, 209, 210
sex differences, 182, 210
sexual abuse, 30, 39
shade, 50
shame, 16, 17, 18, 40
shape, 138
shares, 126
sharing, 106, 126
shortage, 1, 2
short-term memory, 110, 133
shoulders, 63, 64
showing, 6, 25, 30, 109, 116, 130, 218, 225, 228, 241
sign, 130
signals, 16, 20, 27, 54, 58, 87, 123, 140
signs, 56, 64, 217, 219, 227
similarity, 114, 116, 136
simulation, 122, 126
Singapore, 199, 200, 205, 208, 211
skewness, 158
skills, 61, 63, 66, 67, 69
skills training, 66, 67
sleep disturbance, 42
smoking, 35, 187, 230, 242, 245
smoothness, 103
social adjustment, 185
social behaviour, 30
social change, 146, 211
social cognitive model, 50
social competence, 182
social competitiveness, 146
social consequences, 42
social exclusion, 34
social interactions, vii, 15, 16, 116
social life, 39
social network, 142, 146
social phobia, 35, 38, 42, 44, 66, 71, 72, 73, 74, 75
social psychology, 44, 68
social regulation, 16
social relations, 39, 146
social relationships, 39, 146
social rules, 23
social situations, 42, 66
social skills, 66
social skills training, 66
social stress, 71
social support, 142, 187

social transition, 179
social welfare, 205
social withdrawal, 46
social workers, 205
socialization, viii, 58, 141, 142, 143, 144, 145, 147, 149, 150, 151, 154, 155, 157, 164, 165, 166, 169, 172, 174
society, ix, 17, 29, 38, 198, 203, 204, 205, 206
socio-economic inequality, viii, 189, 190, 194, 195
socioeconomic status, 195, 196
Socrates, 69
software, 8
solitude, 183
solution, 78, 96, 130
South Africa, ix, x, 213, 214, 218, 222, 223, 227, 228, 235, 242, 243, 244, 245, 246, 247
South Korea, 198
Soviet Union, 198, 199
space-time, 89, 90, 94, 137
Spain, 1, 2, 5
special education, 148
specialists, 3, 10
species, vii, 37, 54
specificity, 29, 62, 101, 104, 105, 106, 108, 109, 113, 134, 139
spectrum, 96
speed, 87, 90
spelling, 107
spinal anesthesia, 247
stability, 19, 33, 140, 178
stages, 15, 116
standard deviation, 156
standard error, 158
standards, 42
state, ix, 6, 40, 42, 45, 46, 51, 53, 56, 62, 63, 65, 68, 89, 91, 93, 94, 95, 96, 97, 99, 100, 119, 125, 127, 129, 131, 132, 145, 147, 176, 214, 216, 217, 218, 221, 225, 228, 229, 230, 231, 232, 234, 238, 241, 243, 244, 245, 246
states, ix, x, 27, 30, 40, 47, 59, 72, 75, 77, 80, 91, 94, 96, 97, 106, 113, 114, 115, 117, 129, 146, 213, 214, 215, 216, 218, 219, 220, 221, 222, 225, 226, 227, 228, 229, 230, 231, 233, 234, 235, 236, 239, 240, 241, 242, 244, 245, 246
statistics, 187, 207, 209
stigma, 200
stimulus, 25, 45, 47, 48, 52, 56, 61, 79, 101, 102, 104, 105, 106, 116, 128
stomach, 64
storage, viii, 77, 78, 79, 81, 96, 98, 114, 117, 126, 128, 129, 130, 131, 132, 137
strain, 90, 104, 114
strategies, 53, 54, 55, 58, 59, 61, 68, 71, 98
strategy use, 176, 179
strength, 46, 56, 66, 106, 129, 130
stress, 39, 40, 41, 42, 44, 46, 51, 52, 55, 59, 60, 61, 62, 67, 68, 71, 72, 74, 75, 143, 145, 151, 152, 153, 177, 183, 187, 215
stress factors, 40, 52
stressful events, 61
stressful life events, 150, 178, 183, 186
stressors, 63, 73, 183
stretching, 90
striatum, 26
structural characteristics, 180
structure, vii, viii, 15, 26, 32, 68, 69, 77, 84, 85, 88, 95, 96, 98, 99, 100, 102, 104, 105, 106, 107, 108, 109, 110, 112, 113, 114, 115, 119, 120, 122, 123, 125, 128, 130, 132, 133, 134, 139, 206, 247
students, 74, 124
style, 23, 183, 185
subgroups, 156
substance abuse, 23, 24, 28, 32, 44, 215, 218, 219, 226, 227, 228, 229, 231, 233, 235, 239, 241, 245, 247
substance use, 32
substitution, 97, 121
substrate, 30, 53, 78, 116
suicidal behavior, 182
suicidal ideation, 184
suicide, viii, 196, 197, 198, 199, 200, 201, 202, 203, 204, 205, 206, 207, 208, 209, 210, 211
suicide rate, viii, 197, 198, 199, 200, 201, 202, 203, 204, 205, 206, 208, 209, 210, 211
superiority, 65
supervision, ix, 3, 27, 213, 218
supervisor, 50
supplier, 8
support staff, 11
suppression, 8, 127
surprise, 38
survival, vii, 30, 37, 55, 201, 202, 204
sustainability, 5
Sweden, ix, 199, 206, 207, 213, 235
Switzerland, 5, 12, 198, 200
symbols, 116, 119, 120, 122, 125, 127, 133
symmetry, 84, 86, 88, 90, 91, 99, 104, 115, 119, 120
symptom, 38, 50, 67
symptoms, 20, 22, 39, 40, 41, 42, 58, 63, 69, 70, 71, 73, 144, 148, 149, 156, 157, 158, 159, 160, 163, 164, 165, 166, 169, 170, 171, 177, 178, 179, 181, 183, 184, 187, 227, 228, 230, 244, 246
syndrome, 17, 18, 38, 42, 44, 227, 241, 247
synthesis, 23
Syria, 198

systems, 16, 28, 40, 85, 95, 98, 100, 123, 132, 133, 137

T

tactics, 235
target, 54, 106, 110, 125, 147, 217, 234, 239
targets, 55, 101
tariff, ix, 214, 218
task interference, 110
task performance, 53
tau, 85, 99, 100, 139
teacher support, 145
teachers, 143, 144, 153, 154, 155, 156, 165, 167, 169, 170, 171, 173, 174, 175, 177, 185, 187
teacher-student relationship, 147, 155, 163, 176, 179
teaching, 124
technical assistance, 8
techniques, 11, 54, 55, 57, 59, 63, 65, 66, 67, 68, 69, 73, 75, 125
technologies, vii, 1, 5, 11
technology, 3, 6, 9, 10, 11, 12
telecommunications, 11
telephone, 4, 10, 236
telephones, 8
telepsychiatry, vii, 1, 2, 3, 4, 5, 6, 7, 8, 9, 10, 11, 12
temperament, 34
temperature, 89
tempo, 116
temporal lobe, 27, 35, 98
temporal lobe epilepsy, 27, 35
tension, 41, 42, 45, 51, 56, 58, 60, 63, 64
territorial, 1
tertiary education, 227
test scores, 6
testing, 103, 120, 148, 160, 180, 222, 231
textbook, ix, 213, 217, 219, 238
textbooks, 237
texture, 83, 84, 85, 100
thalamus, 27
theft, 20
theory, viii, 25, 30, 74, 75, 77, 78, 80, 81, 82, 94, 101, 109, 113, 114, 115, 116, 119, 121, 123, 125, 127, 128, 130, 131, 132, 135, 137, 138, 139, 140
therapeutic approaches, 20
therapeutic change, 72
therapeutic interventions, 31, 40
therapeutic process, 47
therapeutic relationship, 3
therapeutics, 243
therapist, 44, 45, 47, 58, 59, 60, 62, 63, 68, 69, 71
therapists, 54, 58, 59, 64, 66, 68, 69
therapy, ix, x, 2, 6, 38, 49, 54, 55, 56, 57, 58, 59, 60, 61, 65, 66, 67, 68, 69, 70, 71, 72, 73, 74, 75, 213, 214, 215, 218, 221, 226, 233, 235, 236, 237, 238, 240, 246
thinking, 27, 48, 49, 57, 69, 125
third dimension, 82
Third World, ix, 214, 242
thoughts, 38, 41, 42, 43, 45, 49, 51, 53, 54, 55, 56, 59, 60, 61, 68, 69, 119
threat, 25, 39, 48
threats, 51
throws, 129
time, viii, 18, 23, 27, 39, 46, 48, 52, 56, 57, 58, 62, 63, 66, 67, 68, 77, 79, 81, 84, 85, 86, 87, 89, 90, 91, 92, 93, 94, 95, 96, 97, 98, 99, 100, 104, 105, 110, 112, 113, 115, 120, 123, 125, 126, 128, 129, 130, 131, 132, 134, 135, 136, 137, 138, 140
time commitment, 67
tin, 100
tobacco, 30, 187, 230, 232, 243
tobacco smoking, 187
tones, 24, 34
tracking, 87, 140
tradition, 101, 126
training, ix, 58, 61, 62, 63, 65, 66, 67, 68, 69, 71, 73, 142, 213, 216, 217, 222, 226, 236, 237, 238, 240, 241
traits, 17, 18, 19, 21, 23, 24, 25, 30, 31, 32, 33, 34, 47, 53, 184
trajectory, 92, 93, 94, 119, 125, 126
transference, 93
transformation, 83, 89, 90, 95, 100, 102, 103, 104, 114, 122, 124, 125, 158
transformations, 85, 90, 102, 104, 106, 107, 116, 119, 122, 123, 124, 158
transgression, 29
transition, 73
translation, 149
transmission, vii, 1, 9, 247
transportation, 194
trauma, 39, 42
traumatic events, 67
treatment, ix, x, 1, 3, 5, 6, 9, 11, 31, 38, 44, 47, 50, 54, 55, 56, 57, 58, 65, 66, 67, 68, 69, 70, 71, 72, 73, 74, 75, 93, 97, 177, 180, 201, 202, 203, 204, 205, 206, 214, 215, 221, 222, 223, 224, 225, 226, 227, 228, 230, 232, 233, 235, 236, 238, 240, 241, 242, 243, 244, 245, 246, 247
treatment methods, 68
trees, 103, 133
trend, 126
trial, 3, 5, 73, 75, 219, 220, 221, 222, 223, 224, 227, 229, 230, 232, 238, 241, 244, 245, 247

twins, 21

U

Ukraine, 198
uncertainty, 66, 87, 94, 96, 97
unconditioned, 29, 47, 48
uniform, 140, 192
united, 8, 189, 191, 197, 199, 205, 209
United Kingdom (UK), 8, 189, 197, 199, 200, 205, 206, 209, 247
United Nations (UN), 189, 191, 194
United Nations Development Programme, 191
United States, 199, 205
universe, 93, 94, 95, 133
universities, 240
urban, 181, 199, 205, 210
USA, x, 77, 209, 214
Uzbekistan, 198

V

valence, 25
Valencia, 12
validation, 160, 184, 187
validity, 70
valorization, 146, 155
valuation, 73, 74
values, 94, 100, 102, 103, 104, 111, 120, 121
valve, 98, 132
vandalism, 153
variability, 107
variable, 47, 95, 104
variables, vii, viii, 15, 47, 71, 74, 148, 150, 156, 157, 158, 159, 160, 164, 165, 169, 170, 171, 172, 173, 176, 178, 179, 180, 190, 192, 194, 202, 203, 204, 205, 207
variation, 23, 94, 104, 106, 110, 112, 131
variations, viii, 29, 174, 192, 197, 198, 200, 201
vascular dementia, 210
vector, 84, 88, 115, 129
velocity, 84, 85, 86, 87, 88, 90, 91, 94, 99, 103, 114, 131, 135
victimization, 144, 145, 147, 152, 155, 163, 165, 167, 169, 171, 173, 174, 177, 184, 191
victims, 17, 39, 71, 74, 155, 205, 210, 246
videoconferencing, vii, 1, 11
Viking, 138
violence, 17, 21, 30, 34, 35, 39, 43, 59, 147, 153, 155, 156, 163, 168, 170, 171, 172, 173, 175, 177, 180, 194, 195, 196
violent behavior, 34, 194
violent crime, 34, 190, 195, 196
violent offenders, 28
viruses, 61
vision, 41, 49, 79, 109, 133, 137, 139, 140
visions, 52
visual area, 85, 86, 99
visual stimuli, 25
visual system, 97
vitamin B1, 243
vitamin B12, 243
voice, 24, 116, 126
vulnerability, 21, 46, 50, 52, 53, 61, 72, 185
vulnerability to depression, 72

W

Wales, 199, 205, 206, 208, 209, 210
walking, 64, 97, 99, 114
Washington, 11, 35, 70, 71, 74, 138, 181, 185, 187
water, 8, 80, 82, 101, 105, 112, 117
weakness, 78
wealth, 86, 194
wear, 234
welfare, 206
well-being, 38, 51, 65, 147, 187
Western Cape Province, 227
Western Sahara, 2
white matter, 27
wildfire, 233
wind, 117
windows, 7
withdrawal, ix, x, 46, 213, 214, 215, 217, 218, 219, 220, 221, 222, 225, 226, 227, 228, 229, 230, 231, 232, 233, 234, 235, 236, 238, 239, 240, 241, 242, 243, 244, 245, 246, 247
word perception, 116
words, 16, 18, 28, 49, 52, 64, 69, 93, 101, 102, 104, 105, 110, 111, 112, 113, 116, 117, 119, 120, 126, 129, 130, 134, 137, 138, 140
work, vii, 16, 17, 27, 29, 37, 38, 39, 42, 49, 58, 59, 60, 62, 63, 69, 96, 122, 124, 131
work absenteeism, 38
workers, 11, 202, 203, 204, 205, 215, 216, 217, 226, 227, 235, 237, 238, 240, 241
working memory, 27, 91, 96, 135
World Health Organisation (WHO), 6, 13, 40, 44, 75, 182, 189, 191, 194, 195, 198, 199, 207, 208, 209, 210
worry, 42, 45, 62, 66, 115
writing, 94

X

xenon, 241

Y

yes/no, 151, 153
yield, 130, 179
young adults, 182, 186
young people, 182, 185, 186, 210